Rare and Uncommon Gynecological Cancers

Nicholas Reed • John Alan Green
David M. Gershenson • Nadeem Siddiqui
Rachel Connor
(Editors)

Rare and Uncommon Gynecological Cancers

A Clinical Guide

Springer

Editors
Nicholas Reed
Beatson Oncology Centre
Gartnavel General Hospital
1053 Great Western Road
Glasgow G12 0YN
UK
nick.reed@ggc.scot.nhs.uk

John Alan Green
School of Cancer Studies
University of Liverpool
Liverpool L69 3BX
UK
j.a.green@liverpool.ac.uk

David M. Gershenson
Department of Gynecologic Oncology
The University of Texas
M.D. Anderson Cancer Center
P.O. Box 301439
Houston, TX 77230-1439
USA
dgershen@mdanderson.org

Nadeem Siddiqui
Department of Gynaecological Oncology
Glasgow Royal Infirmary, 84 Castle Street
Glasgow G4 0SF
UK
nadeem.siddiqui@ggc.scot.nhs.uk

Rachel Connor
Department of Radiology
Victoria Infirmary, Langside Road
Glasgow G42 9TY
UK
rachel.connor@ggc.scot.nhs.uk

ISBN 978-3-642-13491-3 ISBN 978-3-642-13492-0 (eBook)
DOI 10.1007/978-3-642-13492-0
Springer Heidelberg Dordrecht London New York

Library of Congress Control Number: 2010933609

Cover design: eStudio Calamor, Figueres/Berlin

Printed on acid-free paper

Springer is part of Springer Science+Business Media (www.springer.com)

Contents

Part I

General Principles

Introduction

1

Nicholas Reed

1.1 Rationalef ort heT extbook

Do we need another textbook? Yes – this is an area that has been neglected and we believe we fill a void. It is not easy to find this kind of information in the standard textbooks. Rare conditions generally attract a disproportionate amount of interest compared to their rarity. Perhaps this is because unusual cases generate additional interest and also reflects the fact that for many of us, this presents a distraction from the humdrum of routine care where we are forced to think and seek out information. Rare editions of books, art or music attract collectors, perhaps for the same reasons. Nevertheless it is important when we are dealing with rare and uncommon disorders that we apply the highest standards. Many would argue that because of their rarity these conditions should be looked after by specialist teams. This allows a smaller number of expert teams to develop real expertise in this field. Furthermore, it would seem sensible to propose that there is a degree of centralisation of care for these conditions. Protocols for shared care may be developed in parallel and there are good examples available to follow such as in gestational trophoblastic tumours.

Why is there a need for such a book as this? The main rationale for the book is to provide the reader with some guidance on how best to manage these patients with rare and uncommon cancers. Access to information on these rare cancers can be difficult even in our modern age of rapid electronic communications and electronic repositories of information. Standard textbooks often contain little information apart from descriptive pathology. One can often find a wealth of information on the histopathology as pathologists usually cross-refer to each other and the main centres may develop an expertise in reviewing and reporting these cancers. However, for many of these conditions, modern and constructive management advice is hard to find. Surgeons and oncologists are not so good as pathologists in networking traditionally, although informal networks and "phone-a friend" may be carried out. Modern medical practice is breaking down these barriers. A book like this cannot be too proscriptive as there is often not the information available to allow such an approach, but our expert authors are recognised specialists in their field and have produced authoritative guidance on how to interpret the available literature. We cannot produce specific protocols for most situations but can guide the readers through the published literature and hopefully allow them to draw the right conclusions and apply them to their practice.

Of course the greatest weakness is that virtually from the moment the author completes the chapter, it is in danger of obsolescence as a new paper is published. However, with rare conditions this may be less of a risk and developments tend to occur more slowly as cases are so few, but occasional dramatic breakthroughs are seen such as the treatment of GIST with imatinib.

In this book we aim to review most of the relatively uncommon and rare gynaecological cancers. We cannot cover everything and if we are able to run to a second edition, maybe readers can provide suggestions to include what is missing! It is probably not realistic to include conditions where only a handful of anecdotes have been recorded in the literature. Ironically, it does seem that there are quite a number of these rare conditions in the gynaecological oncology area. Perhaps this reflects the fact that we are dealing with several

N.R eed
Beatson Oncology Centre, Gartnavel General Hospital,
1053G reatW esternR oad, Glasgow, G120Y N, Scotland, UK
e-mail:nic k.reed@ggc.scot.nhs.uk

N. Reed et al. (eds.), *Rare and Uncommon Gynecological Cancers*,
DOI: 10.1007/978-3-642-13492-0_1, © Springer-Verlag Berlin Heidelberg 2011

different organs and although many of them are thought to be of Mullerian tract origin they do develop in diverse ways. The major omission from the book is paediatric cancers as these are covered by other texts, but there will be an overlap with some cancers of adolescence which we have hopefully addressed. Maybe this is another chapter we can discuss with the publishers if we run to a second edition. Publishing is evolving very rapidly and electronic communication will predominate in the near future, so a series of e-appendices might be an option to consider.

1.2 Multidisciplinary Team Management

These conditions are best looked after by multidisciplinary teams so that there is the opportunity for surgeons and radiation and medical oncologists working with dedicated and specialist pathologists and radiologists to care for these patients. This will allow the best opportunity for the highest standards of care to be developed. In the United Kingdom we have further reinforced this by using Clinical Networks where agreed protocols and patterns of care are developed. Clinical Networks will bring together all the relevant disciplines in the field to work together and use agreed clinical protocols. In addition, data collection, registration and audit are key components to allow comparison with other networks as well as international comparisons of standards of care and outcome. Comprehensive cancer centres with multidisciplinary teams should be able to offer these same high standards.

1.3 Structure of the Book

We have attempted in this book to start with introductory chapters to cover broad topics. We had a dilemma in the subsequent chapters as to whether we would take each individual rare tumour in each individual organ or whether it would be better to group together the same histological types, and bring together the same pathological groups in one chapter. After much discussion and debate we have opted to use a pathologically oriented approach by putting together similar pathological types. This latter approach was chosen as it seemed to be more comprehensive. There are probably strong similarities between clear cell tumours of the ovary and uterus and it is better to consider them in this way. The chapters will highlight some of the differences that may be apparent.

We have tried not only to emphasise both the clinical and diagnostic issues but also to illustrate, where possible, some of the exciting new translational techniques and molecular pathways that are emerging. Exciting clues that are emerging from these molecular pathways may allow us to establish new treatments. A really exciting feature is the excellent review of imaging, which is as important as pathology. Working in centres which have developed expertise in pathology and imaging is essential to support the practising oncologists.

1.4 Databases, Registries and Tumour Banks

It is essential that we learn more about these tumours. One of the first apparent weaknesses in investigating the topic is the lack of real data. Thus, how rare is rare? Let us not get bogged down in a debate about actual numbers. Some diseases that are uncommon are given "orphan status" and this will apply to many of the tumours described here. Thus, one of the first priorities must be to set up reliable and accurate databases and registries. National cancer databases are often unreliable due to poor and incomplete recording and coding. Regional and national networks are ideally placed to capture and record this data. From this we may build a picture of the real size of the problem. Pathology registers are another valuable resource given that rare cancers do tend to get shown around, but we must be cautious about potential double counting!

Equally important is access to tissue and serum to allow clinical researchers and clinical scientists to expand our knowledge. Whilst tumour banks are immensely valuable resources, the creation of virtual tumour banks with modern IT has made this much easier. Thus, tracking of specimens and tissues can speed up new technological developments and registries should facilitate both of these functions. Our French colleagues have led the game with their "Observatoire National des Tumeurs Malignes Rares de l'Ovaire" (http://ovaire-rare.org/). These initiatives need to be replicated around the world and then linked up. The Gynaecological cancer InterGroup (GCIG) had tried to do this previously but failed mainly due to concerns over secure transfer of confidential data. By doing it nationally many of these issues should be overcome.

1.5 Clinical Trials

It is extremely challenging to run clinical trials in this setting and it is usually left to local champions to pursue this. The attitude of "why should I bother to go to all the trouble of putting through Ethics/IRB" is understandable when only one or two patients may be seen and their data entered. We need to rethink our approach to clinical trials in rare diseases; it is of course not just an oncology issue. In Europe, the misguided EU Clinical trials directive has backfired by stifling academic research and this particularly applies to rare cancers where pharmaceutical company-sponsored studies are uncommon and investigator-led studies predominate. We need to think creatively by looking at groups of rare tumour studies being submitted and approved together. Thankfully, there are still motivated and committed enthusiasts out there willing to make the effort to develop trials.

1.6 Tumour Sub-Types

It is becoming apparent that tumour sub-types maybe highly relevant. In the Western world clear cell and mucinous ovarian cancers make up around 5% of ovarian cancer cases; however their biology is different and their response to treatment, especially for mucinous tumours, is distinct. New trials are being developed specifically for these tumour types. It is possible that similar developments will occur with uterine cancers. Equally we are recognising that many sarcomas of ovary and uterus are not sarcomas; so, paradoxically, they may be included with epithelial cancers. Once again the role of the specialist pathologist becomes crucial to management.

1.7 Guidelines vs. Protocols

Given this sort of format we cannot produce protocols for clinical use, partly for medico-legal reasons but also because they would be outdated within a year or two. However, we can provide guidelines or simply guidance in the sense that they will help to direct the clinician to sources of references and the kind of approaches needed for management. However, the Cancer Networks and Comprehensive Cancer Centres should be developing their own or network-agreed protocols for care. If we cannot develop clinical trials, then we should try and coordinate care to try and treat rare diseases in a consistent manner and thus allow some useful data that can be used to develop new protocols.

We hope that this book will be useful as a handy reference for teachers, trainers and trainees. We run the risk that the book may become obsolescent fairly quickly but producing it in this format, we hope that it will be suitable to update it and maybe even produce an online edition that can be adapted for changes more readily. We have attempted to be as comprehensive as possible in our coverage; everybody will have their own definition of a rare and uncommon cancer and doubtless we will have omitted somebody's favourite rare tumour. Nevertheless, we hope that with the range of tumour types and histologies that we have covered, we have addressed most of the common issues that will arise. We hope readers will find this a valuable and useful resource, but the editors would also be receptive to feedback from readers so that we can adapt this if we come to a second or subsequent edition.

Epidemiologyand Dat abases

2

Nicholas Reed

There can often be confusion as to what we mean by rare or uncommon and whilst the dictionary may give a definition of what is meant by rare or uncommon, we have to take into account a number of modifying factors. These include the kind of practice that is run, the local geography, the part of the world where we work and local politics and arrangements. For example, clear cell cancers of the ovary are considered to be relatively uncommon in the Western world, accounting for only 3–5% of ovarian cancers, and yet in the Far East they may account for 15–20%. There are other examples where there are variations in the frequency of a condition on a global basis. From a different standpoint, an individual working in a small district cancer hospital seeing only 1,000 or 1,500 new cancers a year will see very few rare conditions, and yet those of us who work in major supra-regional or comprehensive cancer services will see a reasonable number of these so-called uncommon and rare cancers. Thus it is all relative to the kind of practice in which we work. In the introductory chapter we have already made reference to the fact that it may be argued that concentration of the care of these rare and uncommon cancers should be in the hands of a smaller number of regional or supra-regional centres, but of course there can be opportunities for shared care and networking between the smaller district hospital and the regional cancer centre. There is no "one size fits all" and it will be determined by local arrangements.

N.R eed
Beatson Oncology Centre, Gartnavel General Hospital,
1053G reatW esternR oad, Glasgow, G120Y N, UK
e-mail:nic k.reed@ggc.scot.nhs.uk

It is probably helpful at this point in time to list many of the types of tumours that we are discussing in this book. Firstly we are focusing on tumours of the ovary, uterine corpus, uterine cervix, vagina and vulva. We are concentrating mainly on tumours such as mucinous tumours, clear cell cancers, neuroendocrine tumours, sarcomas and sex cord and stromal tumours. Other less common cancers include serous uterine cancers, squamous cancers arising in ovarian dermoid tumours and melanomas of the vulva and vagina. We also cover uncommon situations like high grade borderline cancers which are worthy of merit not only because of their clinical infrequency but also because of their different biological behaviour. Fallopian tube cancers have not been specifically included as they are considered to be similar to ovarian cancers, and a recent provocative paper has suggested that Fallopian tube cancers may be the "mother of gynaecological epithelial tumours". Given the strong similarity between serous epithelial ovarian and tubal cancers, there is no attempt to distinguish them. The topic of gynaecological cancers arising in pregnancy is also a challenging one and we are fortunate to be able to include a chapter from the team based in Leuven who have been addressing this important topic. We also are pleased to be covering the controversial topic of pseudomyxoma peritonei (PMP). In the UK we have developed a National Service in Basingstoke and the chapter has been written by their team.

What has been omitted? We have not covered some important areas such as gestational trophoblastic tumours and germ cell cancers mainly because the management of these is usually relatively straightforward and there are already well established referral pathways and guidelines for centralisation of care.

N. Reed et al. (eds.), *Rare and Uncommon Gynecological Cancers*,
DOI: 10.1007/978-3-642-13492-0_2, © Springer-Verlag Berlin Heidelberg 2011

2.1 RareandU ncommon Gynaecological Cancers

We have already alluded to the difficulties in trying to define a rare or uncommon cancer and one of the challenges is trying to establish just how infrequent these tumours are. Cancer registers are very variable in their quality around the world but often reflect the quality of the data recorded at the time of initial diagnosis, and particularly for rare tumours the subsequent management and review of the case may indicate that we are dealing with a different final diagnosis. This revised diagnosis is unlikely to be routinely picked up by cancer registries. Internationally, there is huge variation in the way that this data is collected and one of the issues that we would like to address is the setting up of formal registries for these rare tumours. The Gynaecological Cancer Intergroup (GCIG) attempted an initiative a few years ago to try and set up a web-based register but unfortunately this faltered, mainly because of issues of how to deal with confidentiality and security. Transferring data globally presents major challenges and many felt that this was not securely achievable at present. However, other initiatives have shown that this can be done at least within a nation. The presentation at ESMO 2007 by Isabel Ray-Coquard on behalf of the French Rare Tumour Registry has shown how this can be done working within one nation and using a defined framework. The reader is referred to their website http://ovaire-rare.org/. Although this was set up partly to provide advice on the management of these rare cancers it has led the way forward in establishing how to collect data on these rare cancers.

The GCIG Rare Tumour Working Group has tried to lead the way in resolving how to overcome the challenges of setting up these databases internationally. One initiative would be to have a series of national registries and databases which could then be linked once the data had been suitably anonymised. However, to do this it would be necessary to have a common dataset. This could be in the format of a core dataset where the basic registration details with some form of unique identifier are kept. We would then have add-on modules in which we would collect specific details for the specific tumour types.

The benefits of this kind of registry are not simply that we would be able to collect data on the frequency of these tumours and establish whether they are truly rare or uncommon, but also that we could have a fantastic valuable resource for clinicians and scientists wanting to develop clinical research or translational studies in these areas. Using virtual tumour and serum banks we do not necessarily need to have tissues and serum flying round the world but can use identifiable tagging processes. We must use every opportunity to take advantage of modern technologies and these kinds of initiatives will hopefully lead the way in developing and progressing care.

We can also see whether, over the course of time, there are changes in patterns of disease. For example, uterine sarcomas were considered to be very uncommon tumours and yet, more recently, carcinosarcomas have become more frequently documented. Is this a genuinely increasing incidence or is this better recognition by pathologists using modern immunocytochemical techniques? For example, is the incidence changing due to exogenous oestrogens and use of tamoxifen for breast cancer? These kinds of issues can be addressed. We have to work together but the modern world is getting smaller and smaller due to the expanding use of electronic technologies. Many of the so-called Third World or low-income countries now have access to technology to match those of us in the Western world and no longer need to be excluded from these initiatives.

2.2 Definition: What is Rare?

There can often be confusion as to what we mean by rare or uncommon and whilst the dictionary may give a definition of what is meant by rare or uncommon we have to take into account a number of factors.

How do we define rare? Is there a simple definition? One definition is "few in number and widely separated from each other (in space or time)" and another is "of a kind, class or description seldom found, met with or occurring: unusual, uncommon, exceptional". This does not help as no numbers are given and it has already been commented that what is rare in a small centre may be seen more often in a big centre. Recently the National Institute of Health and Clinical Excellence (NICE) in the UK suggested that a cancer with less than 7,000 cases per annum would be proposed as uncommon. This would be considered generous by most standards and many intermediate incidence cancers like renal and oesophagus would be included. A reasonable proposal might to be to suggest fewer than 50 cases per million population but the author has never seen such a figure proposed and we have to start somewhere! This will include virtually all of the cancers listed below.

What kinds of examples can we consider? Listed below are some of the other rarer cancers.

2.3 Exampleso fR are and Uncommon Cancers

- Ophthalmicc ancers
- Thyroidc ancers
- Neuroendocrinec ancers
- Soft Tissue and Bone sarcomas
- Braina ndC NSc ancers

However, we are looking often at subsets of the more common gynaecological cancers as well as the rarer types; these have been listed below.

- Sub-sets of commoner gynaecological cancers
  - Smallc ella ndne uroendocrinec ancers
  - Clear cellc ancers
  - Mucinousc ancers
  - Serouse ndometrialc ancers
  - Sarcomas/carcinosarcomas
  - Sexc ordtumours

Having thus set the scene, it is now time for the reader to review the contents and it is to be hoped that we have done our best to address most of the issues likely to be raised. In the next section of the book we have brought together all the rarer types into sections as listed, but we recognise that there are differences between some of the tumour types. In each section we have attempted to have a template format of epidemiology, diagnosis, imaging and treatment with particular emphasis on the multi-modality and multi-disciplinary treatments. It will be noticed that the chapters and sections vary in their detail, but this reflects the amount of information that is known about a condition and the degree of controversy about their management and care. We have attempted to include not just the clinical aspects but the molecular pathology and the associated biomarkers as appropriate.

Whilst we accept that there are differences between mucinous or clear cell cancers within the ovary, uterus and cervix, it is felt that this commonality of approach is justifiable because there are similarities in their aetiology and in their clinical behaviour. The increasing use of molecular markers to diagnose tumours has indicated that the pathways to cancer development may be similar. This is increasingly being reflected in the use of cell signalling pathway inhibitors as part of the therapeutic armamentarium. It is very likely that by the time the book is published, our knowledge will have leapt further forward, but nevertheless, we hope that this is an accurate reflection of the state of the art atthe time ofw riting.

Rare and Uncommon Gynaecological Cancers: A Clinical Guide

3

W. Glenn McCluggage and David Millan

3.1 Pathology

The female genital tract, comprising the vulva, vagina, uterine cervix and corpus, fallopian tubes and ovaries, as well as the pelvic peritoneum as part of the secondary Mullerian system, is characterised by the occurrence of a greater range of tumour types than any other organ system in the body. This is especially so in the ovary where numerous diverse tumours, benign and malignant, occur. There are three main groups of primary ovarian neoplasm comprising tumours in the surface epithelial-stromal, germ cell and sex cord-stromal categories (Table 3.1) [1]. Within each of these categories, several rare and uncommon tumour types exist. Metastatic tumours are also quite common in the ovary. Clinical correlation is of great importance in the recognition of rare tumour types; for example, the occurrence of hypercalcaemia in a young woman with a small, round blue cell ovarian tumour assists in establishing the diagnosis of a small cell carcinoma of hypercalcaemic type.

It is beyond the scope of this chapter to describe in detail the pathological features of the many individual tumours, but a few general points are made. The first is that generous sampling by the pathologist with the examination of multiple tissue blocks may assist in histologically problematic cases by revealing more diagnostic areas. For example, primary neuroendocrine carcinomas within the ovary may be associated with a component of usual surface epithelial-stromal tumour and generous sampling may reveal such areas, providing strong evidence that the neuroendocrine carcinoma represents a primary ovarian neoplasm rather than a metastasis from elsewhere. Careful sampling may also assist in cases in which a particular tumour is closely mimicked by another neoplasm. For example, some ovarian endometrioid adenocarcinomas may closely mimic a sex cord-stromal tumour, such as a granulosa cell tumour or a Sertoli cell tumour. Generous sampling may reveal areas of more typical endometrioid adenocarcinoma or foci of squamous differentiation or endometriosis, all of these features in this diagnostic dilemma being characteristic of an endometrioid neoplasm. Sampling may also help to identify mixed neoplasms; for example, in the uterus, mixed endometrioid and serous carcinomas are not rare and extensive sampling may reveal a minor component of a particular tumour type. If the minor component constitutes a more aggressive neoplastic type, this may be therapeutically and prognostically important. Sampling is also particularly important in primary ovarian mucinous neoplasms. These are typically extremely large neoplasms with a heterogeneous admixture of benign, borderline and malignant elements. If not adequately sampled, a small area of invasive carcinoma may be potentially missed which may have an adverse effect on the outcome. Additional sampling can be carried out subsequently after the first set of slides have been examined, if these reveal a borderline mucinous tumour at the upper end of the spectrum with intraepithelial carcinoma.

Given the wide range of potential tumours in the female genital tract, some of which are extremely rare such that an individual pathologist may not see a particular neoplasm in his or her lifetime, it may be useful to seek a specialist opinion. This has the added advantage of resulting in accrual of case series of unusual

W.G. McCluggage (✉)
Department of Pathology, Royal Group of Hospitals Trust, Grosvenor Road, Belfast BT12 6BA, UK
e-mail: glenn.mccluggage@belfasttrust.hscni.net

D. Millan
Department of Pathology, Glasgow Royal Infirmary, 84 Castle Street, Glasgow G4 0SF, UK

N. Reed et al. (eds.), *Rare and Uncommon Gynecological Cancers*,
DOI: 10.1007/978-3-642-13492-0_3,

Table3.1 Threema ingr oupsof pr imaryo varianne oplasm

Surface epithelial-stromal
Germc ell
Sexc ord-stromal

neoplasms where clinical information and pathological features can be documented. It is in this way that new entities are described and significant new information emerges regarding uncommon neoplasms.

Immunohistochemistry has contributed significantly in recent years as an aid to diagnosis in the field of gynaecological neoplasia and several reviews are available on this subject [2–6]. There are many scenarios in which immunohistochemistry may be extremely useful, including in the diagnosis of rare and uncommon ovarian neoplasms. For example, new markers of ovarian sex cord-stromal tumours have been described, including inhibin, calretinin and CD56 [7–9]. These markers may be of value in confirmation of a sex cord-stromal neoplasm and in excluding other neoplasms. It has been already pointed out that it may be difficult to distinguish a sex cord-stromal tumour from an endometrioid adenocarcinoma and the aforementioned sex cord markers may be useful in conjunction with epithelial markers, such as epithelial membrane antigen (EMA) and cytokeratin 7, which are positive in endometrioid neoplasms and negative in sex cord-stromal tumours. Immunohistochemistry has also been of value in helping to confirm that in pseudomyxoma peritonei, the appendix is usually the site of the primary tumour and the coexistent ovarian mucinous neoplasm is due to spread from the appendix; differential cytokeratin staining has shown that the mucinous epithelium in the appendiceal, peritoneal and ovarian neoplasms is CK20 positive and CK7 negative, in keeping with a large intestinal phenotype [10]. These markers, in conjunction with others, such as CA125, CA19.9, CEA, CDX2, TTF1 and hormone receptors, may also be of value in diagnosing metastatic adenocarcinomas within the ovary and in determining the primary site in an adenocarcinoma of unknown origin. They may also be used in cytology specimens, for example, peritoneal and pleural fluids. Neuroendocrine markers (chromogranin, synaptophysin, PGP9.5, CD56) are of value in confirmation of a neuroendocrine neoplasm and melanocytic markers (S100, melan A, HMB45) in the diagnosis of malignant melanoma. Other markers useful in a diagnostic setting in gynaecological pathology include WT1, which is positive in most ovarian, tubal and peritoneal serous carcinomas [11, 12]. Interestingly, this marker is usually, although not always, negative in uterine serous carcinomas and this may be helpful in ascertaining the site of origin of a disseminated serous carcinoma [13]. p16 is a useful surrogate marker in the cervix of the presence of high-risk human papillomavirus (HPV) [14]. HPV-related cervical neoplasms, including squamous carcinomas, adenocarcinomas and neuroendocrine carcinomas, are usually diffusely positive. However, some non-HPV-related tumours, such as serous carcinomas of the ovary and uterus and uterine leiomyosarcomas, may be p16 positive [15–17].

A few general points are made regarding the use of immunohistochemical markers in a diagnostic setting. The first is that immunohistochemistry is used as an adjunct to pathological examination and that the results should always be interpreted in the light of the gross pathological and morphological features; consideration of the clinical scenario and imaging findings may also be of value. A panel of markers should always be chosen and this should be focused depending on the differential diagnosis under consideration. In general, markers should be chosen which are expected to be positive and negative in the various neoplasms considered in the differential diagnosis. It is stressed that no marker is specific for any given tumour, and as experience with many markers increases, they are often found to be less specific than was originally thought. One example of this is the recent demonstration that thyroid transcription factor 1 (TTF1), which was considered to be a relatively specific marker of pulmonary and thyroid neoplasms, has now been shown to be positive in some gynaecological adenocarcinomas [18, 19]. Thus, there is always the possibility of unexpected positive and negative staining reactions and the pathologist needs to be aware of this.

In general, immunohistochemistry is most valuable and used most often in a diagnostic setting and, as yet, in the field of gynaecological pathology there are few markers which are of value in a prognostic or predictive sense. However, it is anticipated that this will change in the future and that large studies will identify markers of prognostic or predictive value in a particular tumour type. It is also anticipated that targeted therapies will be developed against specific proteins, the presence of which will be demonstrated on tissue sections of neoplasms using immunohistochemistry. Immunohistochemistry is already used in certain scenarios in a therapeutic sense. For example, the demonstration of hormone receptor (oestrogen receptor and progesterone receptor) positivity in a recurrent or metastatic gynaecological neoplasm may be used to predict a response to hormonal agents, such as gonadotropin releasing hormone agonists.

Currently, molecular pathology has a relatively minor role in the broad field of diagnostic gynaecological pathology. Identification of HPV types by polymerase chain reaction (PCR) can now be done with relative ease. This can be used to confirm an HPV-related neoplasm. For example, in a metastatic adenocarcinoma, the identification of HPV is helpful in pointing to the cervix as the site of origin. HPV studies may also be useful in the sometimes problematic distinction between an endometrial and an endocervical adenocarcinoma. HPV studies have also assisted in establishing that two distinct types of vulval squamous carcinoma exist, a non-HPV-related squamous carcinoma, usually of keratinising type, and an HPV-related type, usually with basaloid morphology [20]. Molecular studies have also demonstrated characteristic genetic abnormalities in different tumour types and this has been paramount in establishing the histogenesis of various neoplasms. As an example, high-grade serous carcinomas in the uterus and ovary have been demonstrated to consistently harbour p53 mutations, while endometrioid adenocarcinomas arising in the same organs not uncommonly exhibit microsatellite instability and mutations in beta catenin, k-RAS, PIK3CA and PTEN genes [21]. Molecular studies have also been instrumental in demonstrating that there are two distinct types of ovarian serous carcinoma, termed low-grade and high-grade serous carcinoma [22, 23]; these are two different neoplastic types rather than high-grade and low-grade variants of the same neoplasm. The much more common high-grade ovarian serous carcinomas are characterised by p53 mutations and BRCA1 and BRCA2 abnormalities, while low-grade serous carcinomas are characterised by k-RAS and BRAF mutations. The demonstration of identical p53 mutations in the epithelial and mesenchymal components of carcinosarcomas has helped to confirm that these are monoclonal neoplasms and, in effect, carcinomas with sarcomatous metaplasia rather than collision tumours [24, 25]. Some gynaecological tumours have relatively specific chromosomal translocations. For example, many endometrial stromal sarcomas (low-grade endometrial stromal sarcomas) harbour a characteristic chromosomal translocation t (7; 17) (p15; q21), which results in the JAZF1-JJAZ1 gene fusion product [26]. This may be useful in the diagnosis of problematic cases and in the exclusion of other neoplasms.

The establishment of carefully regulated and funded tissue banks is vitally important both in common tumour types and in unusual gynaecological neoplasms. Such tissue banks will enable the procurement of significant numbers of uncommon neoplasms by combining samples from different banks. This will facilitate future research into biomarkers and molecular markers of use in a diagnostic setting as well as in apre dictiveorprognos tics ense.

References

1. Tavassoli FA, Devilee P, editors. World Health Organization Classification of Tumours. Pathology and genetics. Tumours of the breast and female genital organs. Lyon: IARC; 2003.
2. McCluggage WG. A critical appraisal of the value of immunohistochemistry in diagnosis of uterine neoplasms. A critical appraisal of the value of immunohistochemistry in diagnosis of uterine neoplasms. Adv Anat Pathol. 2004;11: 162–71.
3. McCluggage WG. Immunohistochemical and functional biomarkers of value in female genital tract lesions. Int J Gynecol Pathol. 2006;25:101–20.
4. McCluggage WG, Young RH. Immunohistochemistry as a diagnostic aid in the evaluation of ovarian tumors. Semin Diagn Pathol. 2005;22:3–32.
5. McCluggage WG. Recent advances in immunohistochemistry in gynaecological pathology. Histopathology. 2002;40: 309–26.
6. Mittal K, Soslow R, McCluggage WG. Application of immunohistochemistry to gynecologic pathology. Arch Pathol Lab Med. 2008;132:402–23.
7. McCluggage WG, Maxwell P, Sloan JM. Immunohistochemical staining of ovarian granulosa cell tumors with monoclonal antibody against inhibin. Hum Pathol. 1997;28: 1034–8.
8. McCluggage WG, Maxwell P. Immunohistochemical staining for calretinin is useful in the diagnosis of ovarian sex cord-stromal tumours. Histopathology. 2001;38:403–8.
9. McCluggage WG, McKenna M, McBride HA. CD56 is a sensitive and diagnostically useful immunohistochemical marker of ovarian sex cord-stromal tumors. Int J Gynecol Pathol.2007; 26:322–7.
10. Ronnett BM, Shmookler BM, Diener-West M, et al. Immunohistochemical evidence supporting the appendiceal origin of pseudomyxoma peritonei in women. Int J Gynecol Pathol.1997; 16:1–9.
11. McCluggage WG. WT1 is of value in ascertaining the site of origin of serous carcinomas within the female genital tract. Int J Gynecol Pathol. 2004;23:97–9.

12. Al-Hussaini M, Stockman A, Foster H, McCluggage WG. WT-1 assists in distinguishing ovarian from uterine serous carcinoma and in distinguishing between serous and endometrioid ovarian carcinoma. Histopathology. 2004;44:109–15.
13. Hirschowitz L, Ganesan R, McCluggage WG. WT1, p53 and hormone receptor expression in uterine serous carcinoma. Histopathology. 2009;55:478–82.
14. O'Neill CJ, McCluggage WG. p16 expression in the female genital tract and its value in diagnosis. Adv Anat Pathol. 2006;13:8–15.
15. Phillips V, Kelly P, McCluggage WG. Increased p16 expression in high grade serous and undifferentiated carcinoma compared with other morphologic types of ovarian carcinoma. Int J Gynecol Pathol. 2009;28:179–86.
16. O'Neill CJ, McBride HA, Connolly LE, Deavers MT, Malpica A, McCluggage WG. High grade ovarian serous carcinoma exhibits significantly higher p16 expression than low grade serous carcinoma and serous borderline tumour. Histopathology.2007; 50:773–9.
17. O'Neill CJ, McBride HA, Connolly LE, McCluggage WG. Uterine leiomyosarcomas are characterized by high p16, p53 and MIB1 expression in comparison with usual leiomyomas, leiomyoma variants and smooth muscle tumours of uncertain malignant potential. Histopathology. 2007;50: 851–8.
18. Kubba LA, McCluggage WG, Liu J, et al. Thyroid transcription factor-1 expression in ovarian epithelial neoplasms. Mod Pathol. 2008;21:485–90.
19. Siami K, McCluggage WG, Ordonez NG, et al. Thyroid transcription factor-1 expression in endometrial and endocervical adenocarcinomas. Am J Surg Pathol. 2007;31:1759–63.
20. McCluggage WG. Recent developments in vulvovaginal pathology. Histopathology. 2009;54:156–73.
21. Matias-Guiu X, Catasus L, Bussaglia E, et al. Molecular pathology of endometrial hyperplasia and carcinoma. Hum Pathol.2001; 32:569–77.
22. McCluggage WG. My approach to and thoughts on the typing of ovarian carcinomas. J Clin Pathol. 2008;61:152–63.
23. Shih IM, Kurman RJ. Ovarian tumorigenesis. A proposed model based on morphological and molecular genetic analysis. Am J Pathol. 2004;164:1511–8.
24. McCluggage WG. Malignant biphasic uterine tumours: carcinosarcomas or metaplastic carcinomas? J Clin Pathol. 2002;55:321–5.
25. McCluggage WG. Uterine carcinosarcomas (malignant mixed mullerian tumors) are metaplastic carcinomas. Int J Gynecol Cancer. 2002;12:687–90.
26. Koontz JI, Soreng AL, Nucci M, et al. Frequent fusion of the JAZF1 and JJAZ1 genes in endometrial stromal tumors. Proc Natl Acad Sci USA. 2001;98:6348–53.

The Contribution of Diagnostic Imaging inR areG ynaecologicalMal ignancies

4

Rachel Connor

4.1 Introduction

The goal of imaging at initial patient presentation is to pre-operatively predict gynaecological malignancy, potentially identify a tumour type and to provide appropriate staging information which will influence management and likely inform patient prognosis. Following treatment, imaging allows assessment of response and differentiation of potential relapse from treatment related complications. The identification of localised relapse, before it is clinically apparent, has the potential to offer selected patients a chance of curative salvage therapy.

Unfortunately, many gynaecological tumours are too rare to provide an evidence base for reliable, specific predictive imaging information. Some tumours will be characterised by particularly aggressive or unusual behaviour and for these tumours, modifying either initial investigation or a follow-up imaging strategy can be helpful.

Radiology has embraced major advances in technology with developments within the modalities of ultrasound, CT, MRI, CT/PET and nuclear medicine and there are exciting future prospects for targeted molecular imaging. This anatomic and functional imaging is changing survival data not only by more accurate initial staging, but by assessing response to therapy early on in a treatment cycle, allowing individual, tailored changes in management. All these modalities have their place in the optimal management of these patients with rare tumours.

R.C onnor
Department of Radiology, Victoria Infirmary,
LangsideR oad, GlasgowG 429TY , UK
e-mail:ra chel.connor@ggc.scot.nhs.uk

Many of the rare tumours will only be seen once in a career by many general radiologists and the importance of referral to a dedicated Gynaecological Oncology multi-disciplinary team, before surgery, cannot be underestimated to provide the best treatment plan, tailored to improve the chance of patient survival.

4.2 ImagingT echniquesf orEval uating the Primary Gynaecological Malignancy

4.2.1 Ultrasound

Ultrasound is inexpensive, readily available and is often the initial imaging modality used to assess patients with symptoms and signs suspected to be of gynaecological origin. More than other modalities, ultrasound is limited by patient obesity and excessive bowel gas. It is also limited by operator experience and initial hard copy images have a more limited value in external review. Nevertheless, transvaginal imaging is the modality of choice to evaluate patients with post-menopausal bleeding [1], providing an accurate measurement of assessing endometrial thickness, overall uterine morphology and the presence or absence of adnexal masses and ascites. Although ultrasound will detect adnexal masses and effectively triage patients with unscheduled bleeding into those who will then require endometrial biopsy and hysteroscopy, it is not accurate in staging endometrial or uterine neoplasms. Ultrasound morphology is useful to characterise benign vs. malignant adnexal masses, particularly when this is combined with Doppler assessment and this forms the basis of a risk of a malignancy index (RMI) when combined with CA 125 levels and the patient's menopausal status [2, 3].

N. Reed et al. (eds.), *Rare and Uncommon Gynecological Cancers*,
DOI: 10.1007/978-3-642-13492-0_4,

Adoption of an RMI will triage patients into groups which require either intervention or follow-up. When trying to determine whether an adnexal mass is benign or malignant, MRI is more accurate than either ultrasound or CT, by providing exquisite soft tissue detail and additional tissue characterization not possible with other modalities [5]. Both CT and MR will stage the abdomen more comprehensively than ultrasound, but MR is more accurate than CT for nodal staging in the abdomen and pelvis [6].

4.2.2 CT

CT is an imaging modality that is now widely available in developed countries and newer multi-slice machines are rapid, with scan times of a just a few minutes to cover the entire chest, abdomen and pelvis, which removes some of the problems associated with movement artifact, particularly in unwell or poorly cooperative patients. CT is preferable to MR in assessing the lungs and thorax and this is particularly important in tumours with a propensity for haematogenous metastases or in advanced or relapsed disease. In gynaecological malignancy, it is important that scan coverage for the whole chest, abdomen and pelvis includes the supraclavicular fossa, (where there may be unexpected involvement of supraclavicular nodes), without contiguous mediastinal involvement, extending to inguinal node regions. However, until there is confirmation of a malignant pelvic mass, there is no evidence base to support scanning the entire thorax, although imaging of lung bases is essential to detect possible pleural effusions or enlargement of paracardiac nodes [7]. Multi-slice CT allows volume acquisition of data and isotropic multi-planar reconstructions for example in coronal or sagittal planes. CT scans should be performed with intravenous and either positive or negative intraluminal bowel contrast. Despite advances, CT still does not have the soft tissue discrimination of MRI and it has the major drawback of ionising radiation.

Cumulative diagnostic radiation dose is now recognised as an increasingly important issue. Females and young patients in particular are at increased risk for stochastic, or long-term effects of ionising radiation. Although exact risks are difficult to establish, the likelihood of inducing a solid cancer or leukaemia from a single CT scan of the abdomen or chest (dose 10 mSv) in a female, is estimated at approximately 1:1,000 depending on patient age [8].

Most CT scans of chest abdomen and pelvis will result in a dose in the 15–20 mSv range. For young patients requiring long term follow-up, e.g. those patients with ovarian granulosa cell tumours or leiomyosarcoma (LMS), the cumulative radiation burden of repeated CT imaging should be considered and ultrasound or MRI imaging substituted [9].

4.2.3 CT/PET

CT/PET is now increasingly utilised in the staging and follow-up of some categories of gynaecological malignancy. CT/PET is more accurate than either CT or PET alone in the detection of metastatic disease. This technique involves fusion of images from a PET scanner, after the patient is injected with a suitable isotope (most commonly 18 – fluorodeoxyglucose – 18 FDG PET) with images from an in-line CT scanner, which provides the anatomic resolution lacking in pure PET images. FDG-PET essentially relies on the higher metabolic activity of most neoplasms having increased affinity for the injected glucose isomer. It is therefore not specific to tumour cells and uptake is also seen in other metabolically active normal tissue, such as heart and bowel as well as inflammatory tissues. False negative uptake is also seen in neoplastic tissue with low metabolic activity or very small tumour foci. This results in the sensitivity of PET diminishing rapidly in lymph nodes less than 5 mm in size. The use of SUV (standard uptake values) provides quantitative measurement of PET activity which can help to differentiate benign from malignant processes. The exam preparation requires patients to fast and diabetic patients need to control blood sugars within normal ranges. PET scans can be limited in grossly obese patients in whom MR and CT can still provide morphological nodal assessment (Fig. 4.1).

The role of CT/PET has increased in many centres to encompass the role of assessing response to chemoradiotherapy after completion of treatment and determining which patients will be most likely to relapse and which will benefit from salvage therapy, before significant disease progression has occurred. These selected patients then appear to have improved prospects for long term survival [18].

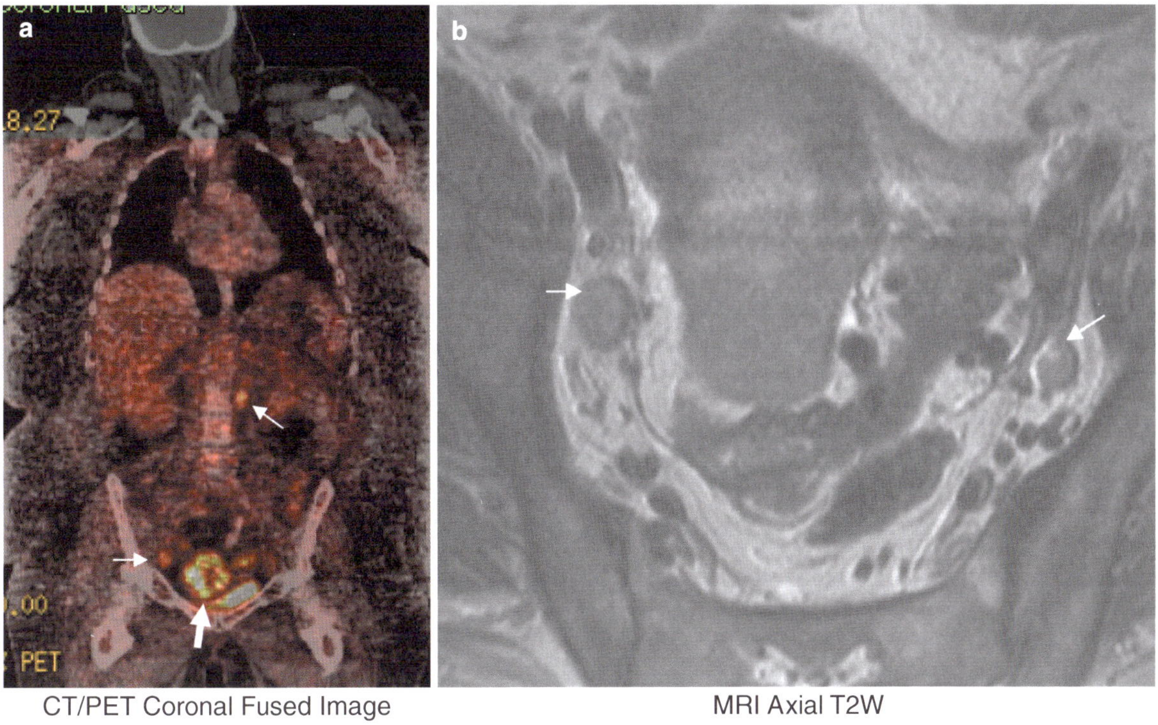

Fig. 4.1 (**a**) CT/PET coronal fused image. Note poor image quality due to gross obesity. (**b**) Corresponding MRI T2W axial. Grossly obese patient. High para-aortic node and right obturator node confirmed in patient with Stage 2B cervical carcinoma (*broad arrow*) with bowel uptake and obesity obscuring left pelvic adenopathy. MR scan detects bilateral obturator nodes only, with small focus of necrosis on left (*arrows*)

CT/PET results in higher levels of diagnostic Ionising radiation (approximately 25 mSv) and the same considerations of accumulated dose apply for the routine use of this modality in long term follow-up as for CT.

Future developments in PET imaging include fusing FDG-PET images with MR. Preliminary reports suggest this will improve accuracies for detection of involved lymph nodes by combining the better soft tissue discrimination and spatial resolution of MRI, with the functional/metabolic discrimination of PET imaging. Reported sensitivity and specificity of CT/PET and fused MR/PET, 44.1, 93.9 and 54.2 and 92.7% respectively [21, 36].

New horizons in functional PET tumour imaging include mapping uptake of radiopharmaceuticals isotopes of copper (Cu^{60} and Cu^{64} – copper(II)-diacetyl-bis(N4-methylthiosemicarbazone)(copper-ATSM). This assesses of the degree of tumour hypoxia which has been found to correlate with prognosis in cervical and other cancers, as hypoxic tumours respond less favourablytoc hemoradiotherapy [22].

4.2.4 MRI

MRI is particularly useful for evaluating gynaecological masses and when compared to ultrasound and CT, it is the most accurate modality for characterising adnexal masses with accuracy of 60–95% in discriminating benign from malignant masses [4]. In elderly, unfit and obese patients, with vaginal or cervical stenosis, the attendant risks of anaesthesia can make endometrial sampling impossible and MRI in particular, is useful for assessing a pelvic mass in the presence of post-menopausalble eding(Fig. 4.2).

MR can also characterise soft tissue, accurately identifying fluid, fat and blood products Blood less than 3–4 weeks old (methaemoglobin) will characteristically show increased signal on T1 weighted sequences and decreased signal on T2 sequences (Fig. 4.3). Chronic blood products (haemosiderin) will be of low signal on all MR sequences. This helps to characterise endometriomas and haemorrhagic cysts, vs. other solid or cystic adnexal masses as well as identifying haemorrhagic uterine tumours. Macroscopic fat within tumours

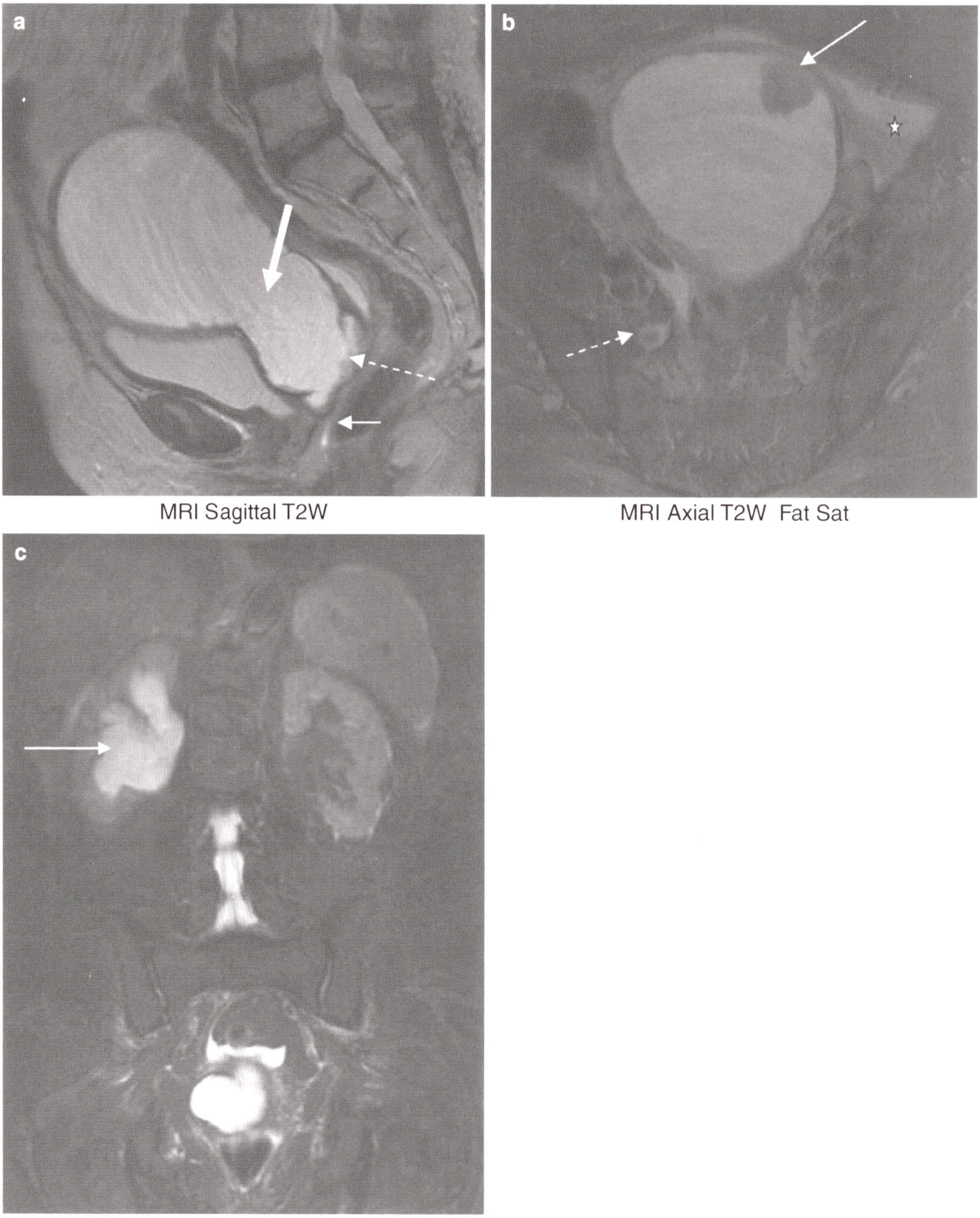

Fig. 4.2 Serous Endometrial cancer Elderly patient with scant vaginal bleeding, vaginal stenosis and a pelvic mass. Treated 20 years previously with radiotherapy for cervical cancer. (**a**) Distended endometrial cavity and endocervical canal (*arrow*); endocervical tumour seeding (*broken arrow*); vaginal stenosis (*thin arrow*); (**b**) polypoid endometrial serous neoplasm (*arrow*); ascites (*star*); obstructed right ureter due to serosal and parametrial involvement (*broken arrow*). (**c**) Unexpected right hydronephrosis (*arrow*)

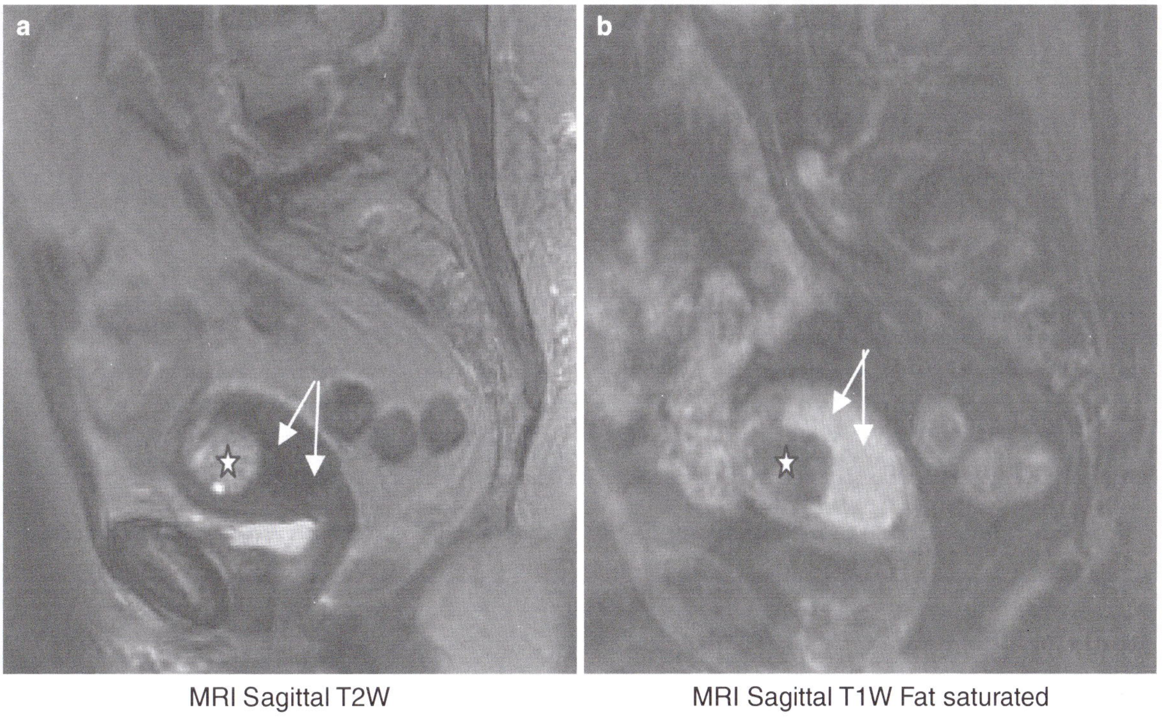

Fig. 4.3 (**a**) MRI sagittal T2W. (**b**) MRI sagittal T1W fat saturated. Post-menopausal patient with vaginal bleeding and cervical stenosis. Endometrial cavity is distended with blood (*arrows*) bright on T2 weighted sequences and dark on T1 weighted sequences. A typical hyperplastic benign high signal fundal polyp is present (*star*). Note change of subcutaneous fat from bright on T2 weighted image, to dark on fat saturated image increasing conspicuity of high signal blood products (and proteinaceous fluidi nbo wel)

e.g. Teratomas, will follow the signal of subcutaneous fat, appearing dark on fat saturated sequences and bright on T1, and most T2 weighted images. Unfortunately, MRI has significant limitations in identifying calcification, seen clearly on CT exams, which contributes important imaging characteristics to both epithelial and non-epithelial ovarian malignancy.

With MRI, it is therefore important to routinely include a range of sequences to characterise an unknown, complex adnexal mass and these should include, T1 and T2 weighted as well as pre and post-contrast fat saturated T1W sequences.

In gynaecologic imaging generally, an anti-peristaltic bowel agent, such as hyoscine butylbromide, is also routinely recommended, to reduce artefact from bowel movement and allow better discrimination of tissue margins.

MR examinations are contraindicated in patients with some metallic implants e.g. pacemakers and may not be suitable for claustrophobic or acutely unwell patients. Most current MR scanners have a magnetic field strength of 1.5 Tesla (T), necessitating long scan times with sequences usually taking 4–5 min each, and an examination of pelvis and abdomen requiring between half to 1 hour. This may be reduced with increasing availability of 3 T scanners. MRI does not use ionising radiation and is therefore more suitable for repeated imaging and scans in pregnant patients. Routine use of MR is not recommended in the first trimester of pregnancy, but is a preferable alternative to CT. The use of gadolinium contrast in MR provides additional information in characterising adnexal and uterine masses and in staging, particularly of endometrial neoplasms, but as gadolinium crosses the placenta, its use is not recommended in pregnancy.

Recent developments in dynamic contrast imaging sequences, allow quantitative measurements of tissue enhancement with contrast over time. This can help to distinguish for example, the rapid uptake of contrast by tumour tissue from radiation induced fibrosis in a potential recurrent cervical cancer.

Diffusion weighted MR imaging is an established technique in neurological imaging, but more recently utilised in body imaging. This non-invasive technique utilises the difference in movement of free water molecules in normal and abnormal tissues, to distinguish benign from malignant tissue characteristics and has been successfully used for imaging cervical and endometrial tumours and assessing response to therapy [13]. Whole body diffusion imaging also shows a promise as a method of surveying for metastatic disease.

4.3 LymphN odeI maging in Gynaecological Malignancy

The correct, pre-operative identification of metastatic nodal disease, particularly when this extends beyond conventional pelvic radiotherapy fields, still remains a great diagnostic challenge. The identification of affected lymph nodes changes the prognosis and FIGO staging for most categories of gynaecological malignancy.

Ultrasound has limited value in identifying metastatic adenopathy, largely due to the deep retroperitoneal location of lymph nodes. The exception is in the assessment of enlarged, superficial inguinal nodes, most often secondary to vulval or vaginal cancers, but occasionally involved in aggressive ovarian or uterine malignancy through retrograde spread along round ligament lymphatics. High resolution and Doppler ultrasound can accurately identify these abnormal nodes by morphology and vascularity and provide image guided fine needle node aspiration if necessary [14].

Both MRI and CT will identify macroscopic involvement of pelvic and para-aortic lymph nodes, primarily by virtue of size criteria, with round (instead of oval) and large nodes more likely to reflect metastatic disease. The shortest diameter measurement of a lymph node is more reproducible and is regarded as standard for a single axis measurement. Pelvic and para-aortic nodes greater than 10 mm short axis diameter, have a high likelihood of neoplastic involvement, but this size cut-off results in a low sensitivity for metastatic disease. An upper limit of 8 mm in the pelvis is preferable and will increase sensitivity without significant loss of specificity [16]. MRI can also identify macroscopic extra-capsular nodal spread which appears as a slightly speculate outline (Fig. 4.4) [17] and when combined with nodal tissue characterisation, is more sensitive in detecting nodal neoplasia than CT.

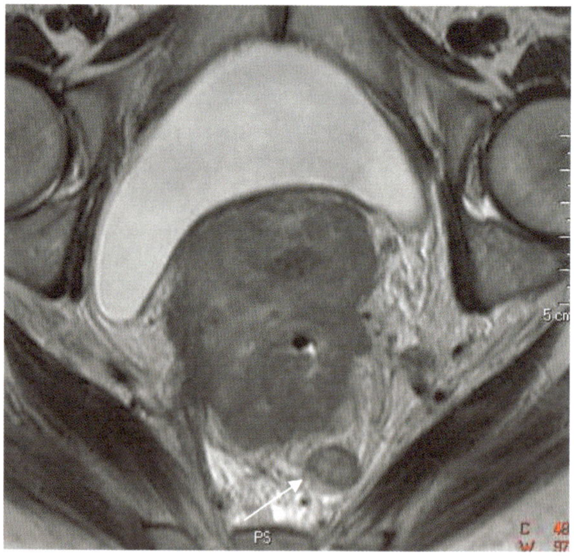

MRI Axial T2W

Fig. 4.4 Stage 4 cervical carcinoma extending posteriorly to involve the rectum. Enlarged pre-sacral nodes (11 mm short axis) show slightly irregular spiculated margin (*arrow*)

Nodal necrosis, seen as fluid attenuation within the node on both CT (density less than 20 HU) and high signal on T2 weighted MRI, (Fig. 4.1) has a reported positive predictive value of 100% for neoplastic involvement [32]. Unfortunately, both CT and MRI still have limited overall sensitivities and specificities for detection of neoplastic lymph node involvement; in the pelvis sensitivity 40–60%, specificity 80–90% and para-aortic region sensitivity 43% and specificity 91%. This is a consequence of metastases occurring in nodes smaller than 8 or 10 mm and large, reactive nodes enlarging greater than 10 mm.

With the advent of conformal and intensity modulated radiotherapy fields, MR or CT identification of nodal chains provides a necessary treatment-related road map for accurate planning of radiotherapy fields and the reporting of involved lymph nodes outside normal radiotherapy fields (Fig. 4.4) is therefore essential [16, 34].

More recently, non-invasive MR diffusion weighted imaging has been used to identify involved lymph nodes but early results do not appear to be as accurate as CT/PET.

Newer imaging techniques using specific nanoparticle iron oxide lymphographic contrast agents (ultra small particles of iron oxide – USPIO) in magnetic resonance lymphangiography (MRL) has shown great promise. This MR contrast agent is taken up by the reticuloendothelial system from an intravenous injection and on specific MR (T2* weighted) sequences, neoplastic deposits appear as non-functioning, contrast negative areas within affected lymph nodes. Although, prostate cancer has been most extensively assessed to date [33, 35], smaller studies in patients with endometrial and cervical cancer have identified metastases in nodes less than 5 mm short axis [16] at a size when PET sensitivity becomes limited. Studies indicate that the negative predictive value of this technique results in a false negative rate of less than 4%. At present, this lymphographic agent; Ferumoxtran-10, is not yet licensed for routine radiological use.

CT/PET is rapidly becoming the modality of choice for more accurate whole body nodal and metastatic staging, but it is a scarce resource and there are some pitfalls associated with its use. In cervical and uterine cancers, overall patient sensitivities of 50–73% and overall accuracy of 80–89% for detection of involved lymph nodes have been reported, although results are significantly better with cervical cancer and nodes greatertha n1c m [19, 20, 30].

CT/PET has limitations in detecting disease in nodes less than 1 cm for endometrial cancer [27] with recently published sensitivity of 67% and specificity of 94%. This may in part be due to the lower metabolic activity of low grade endometrial cancers, so that for nodal staging, the role of CT/PET in most endometrial cancers has not produced the same benefits as for cervical and ovarian cancer.

CT/PET is particularly useful in characterising enlarged pelvic and para-aortic nodes that have been detected as a result of other imaging. This can justify targeted surgical lymph node sampling, either laparoscopically or at routine laparotomy with frozen section to confirm potentially malignant nodes and reduce the need for full para-aortic and pelvic lymphadenectomy. Occasional false positive FDG PET uptake in reactive or inflammatory lymph nodes still necessitates caution and tissue confirmation of malignancy, where an unexpected finding of potential metastasis is likely to fundamentally change patient management. False positive nodal uptake can occur with pelvic inflammatory disease, such as tuberculosis or endometriosis, but also occurs in the presence of large, necrotic, either cervical or occasionally uterine tumours (Fig. 4.5).

Sentinel node mapping for cervical tumours, when both radiocolloid isotope and blue dye injections into the cervix are combined, has shown an excellent detection rate for selective lymph node sampling, identifying primary draining nodes with micrometastases [23, 24]. In a recent meta-analysis [30], sentinel nodes have been identified in over 90% of patients when these techniques are combined, allowing selective pre-operative sampling to detect patients with involved nodes unsuitable for radical hysterectomy. Unfortunately, there remains a small, but significant false negative rate of 3.2% which at present cannot accurately determine surgical candidates requiring selective vs. complete lymphadenectomy but it is particularly of benefit to patients requesting fertility sparing surgery or where pelvic lymphadenectomy is technically challenging.

4.4 StagingC onsiderations

4.4.1 Uterus

Clinical examination has been shown to be an unreliable predictor of stage, understaging by up to 22% in endometrial cancer [51]. As a consequence, FIGO has recommended surgical staging since 1988. Referral for imaging with cervical or uterine malignancy is usually preceded by preliminary results from uterine or cervical biopsy. In endometrial sampling, it is recognised that there is a pre to post-operative histopathological sampling error rate of approximately 20%, with usually a higher grade reassignment occurring when complete post-operative specimens are available for analysis. Various grades of adenocarcinoma often coexist with rare tumour types such as serous or clear cell differentiation and this may not always be identified in pre-operative sampling.

MRI, with pre and post-contrast sequences is the recommended imaging modality for pre-operatively staging endometrial cancer, with overall staging accuracy of between 85 and 93% [1, 51]. Administration of intravenous contrast, preferably as a dynamic run, with imaging in arterial, portal venous and equilibrium phases, will not only allow better determination of the degree of myoinvasion, but may demonstrate a hypervascular mass, unusual for most endometrial adenocarcinomas, thus raising the possibility of an unusual tumour, such as a sarcoma. Cervical invasion is also best determined with MRI.

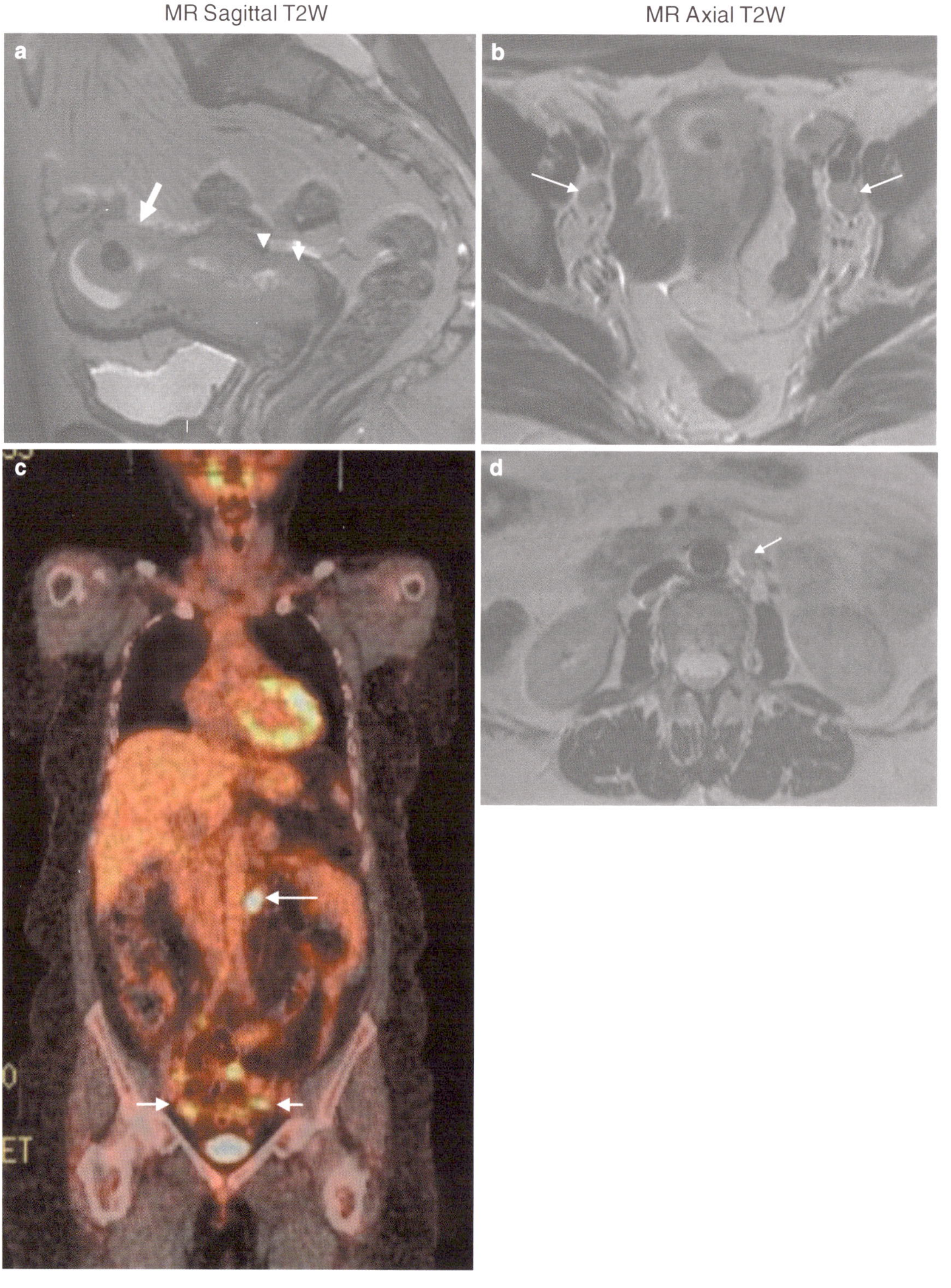

Fig. 4.5 Extensive clear cell endometrial tumour, but clinically confined to the uterus. (**a**) MR imaging demonstrates extension to involve the cervical stroma (*arrowheads*) and serosal surface of the uterus (*arrow*). (**b**) Pathologically enlarged external iliac lymph nodes (*arrows*). (**c**) CT/PET confirms significant uptake in suspect node (*arrow*), as well as pelvic lymph nodes. (*small arrows*). (**d**) Corresponding axial MRI with 8 mm para-aortic adenopathy (*arrow*). Post-operative pathology revealed metastatic para-aortic node, but pelvic lymph node dissection revealed onlyr eactive,e nlargedpe lvicnode s

Although cervical stromal invasion is a key determinant in upstaging endometrial cancers, this does not constitute a change in stage for uterine sarcomas [12, 25].

With rare uterine tumours there is a paucity of evidence, but it seems likely that MRI for local tumour assessment, combined with CT or CT/PET to determine metastatic status, is ideal to optimally stage most of these patients. A few prospective studies using CT/PET in endometrial sarcoma and carcinosarcomas have shown avid uptake of FDG PET within both the primary tumour and within metastases, correlating well with high metabolic tumour activity in the few patients studied to date. This ability to accurately detect the extent of metastatic disease was shown to have a direct effect on patient management [21, 37, 50].

The rationale for local tumour staging with MRI is usually to determine resectability and plan the extent of surgery, for example the requirement for pelvic lymph node excision vs. sampling, or for identifying bowel or bladder involvement requiring extensive resection. In high grade adenocarcinoma, as well as more unusual but aggressive tumour types such as clear cell, serous, carcinosarcoma or adenosquamous histology, metastases or unexpected local invasion occurs early, when the primary tumour is confined to the inner myometrium and these cancers are often significantly underestimated on clinical examination alone (Figs. 4.5 and 4.6). Unexpected serosal disease, with ascites and peritoneal dissemination will favour chemotherapy and a less aggressive initial surgical approach. But it is usually the detection of more distant extra pelvic metastases which will change a proposed management plan from extensive lymph node dissection, or a change in planned radiotherapy fields, or consideration of neoadjuvant chemotherapy, or a change to a palliative approach. These tumours therefore, require additional imaging of the abdomen and chest, with either CT or CT/PET.

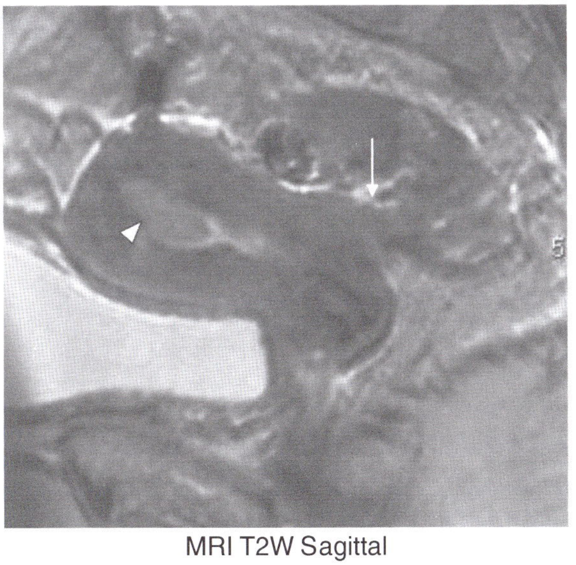

MRI T2W Sagittal

Fig. 4.6 Clear cell carcinoma. Normal sized uterus. Endometrial "plug" of tumour, (*arrowhead*) with serosal extension through lower segment of myometrium to involve adjacent recto sigmoid colon (*arrow*)

4.4.2 Cervix

Most cervical malignancy will have been diagnosed on biopsy, prior to a request for imaging and MR is pivotal in providing a rational management plan. Clinical examination, even under anaesthesia is associated with a significant understaging error, which increases from almost a third of patients with stage 1B, to over half of stage 4 patients. MRI is the most accurate method for assessing primary tumour volume and extent and for identifying suspicious adenopathy in the pelvis and lower abdomen. It will also determine whether fertility sparing surgery is an option.

Although punch biopsy does not usually affect staging, cone or loop excision (LLETZ) of the cervix produces difficulty in accurately determining original tumour size and cervical oedema can cause problems in determining the correct depth of stromal invasion. MRI of pelvis and lower abdomen should therefore be obtained prior to cone or loop excision of the cervix.

The large component of dense connective tissue in the cervical stroma results in low signal on T2 weighted MR. Most tumours are bright against this background and with this natural contrast, there is usually no need for intravenous contrast, although this has been used to detect early 1A2 and 1B tumours against the background of higher signal cervical mucosa (Fig. 4.7).

In pregnancy, from the second trimester onwards, into the immediate post-partum period, cervical stroma loses its low signal on MR and together with increase in the parametrial vascularity, the accurate staging of tumour size, stromal infiltration and parametrial extension can become very difficult(Fig. 4.8).

MR sequences to stage cervical tumours should include thin section T2 axial and sagittal images of the pelvis, as well as thin 3–4 mm axial images perpendicular to the axis of the cervix. Abdominal sequences,

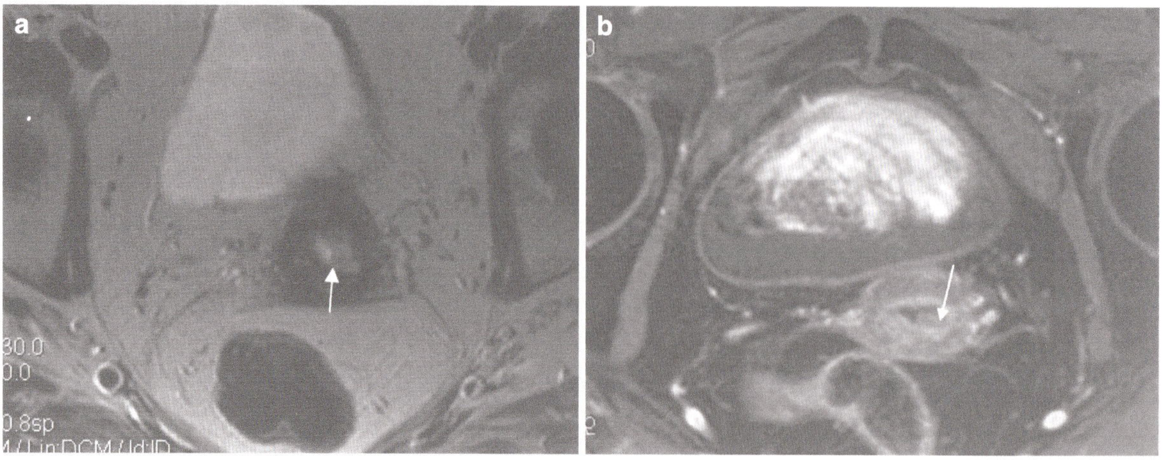

MRI Axial T2W MRI Axial T1 Fat Sat Post Contrast

Fig. 4.7 Squamous cervical cancer: Very small 1B tumour is seen clearly against natural contrast of dark cervical stroma (*arrows*). Post-contrast, the tumour enhances relative to the stroma, but there is loss of natural contrast. (**b**) Enhancement of cervical mucosa deep to the tumour is indicative of minimal or no significant stromal invasion

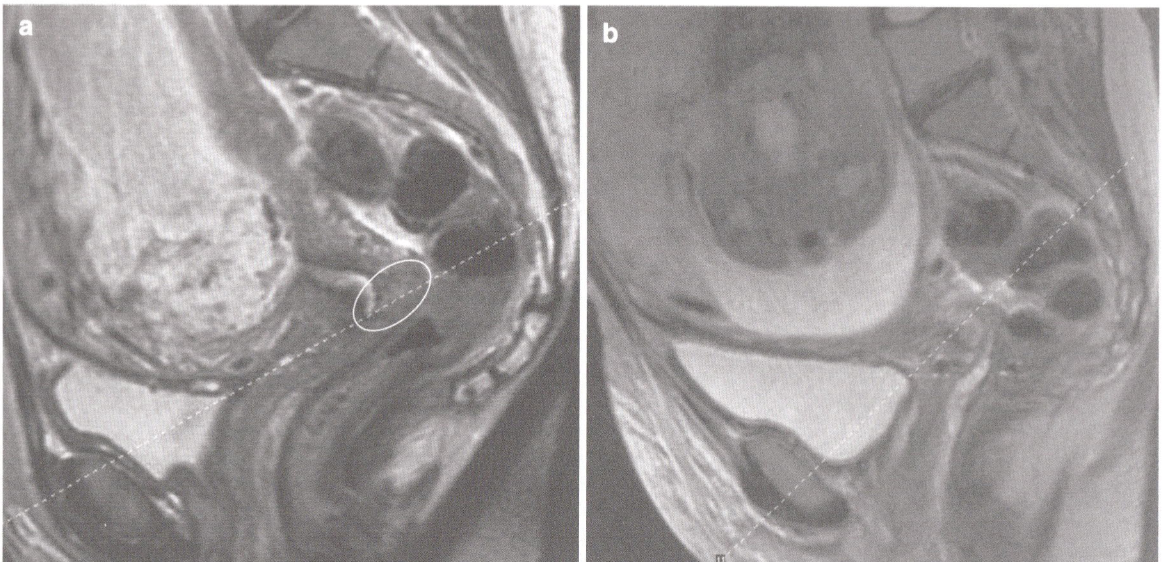

T2W Sagittal Detailed Section MRI Sagittal T2W

Fig. 4.8 Squamous cervical Cancer: Twelve and twenty six week pregnancy. (**a**) There is loss of Later in pregnancy the tumour becomes invisible against the increased stromal signal normal dark cervical stromal signal. The small 1B tumour on the posterior lip of the cervix becomes difficult to identify (*ellipse*) (**b**) In early third trimester, the tumour becomes invisible against thei ncreaseds ignalf romc ervicals troma

which will allow adequate assessment of retroperitoneal nodes and potential dilatation of renal tracts should also be included. CT, or CT/PET is an alternative to staging the abdomen and pelvis in patients who are not suitable for MRI.

Most cervical cancers will metastasise to lymph nodes in an orderly fashion, involving preferentially external iliac or obturator nodes before involving common iliac or para-aortic chains. However, direct drainage to para-aortic nodes from cervical cancer has occasionally been identified with sentinel node imaging. A normal pattern of spread can be altered if there has been previous pelvic surgery or pelvic inflammatory disease and primary spread to para-aortic or groin

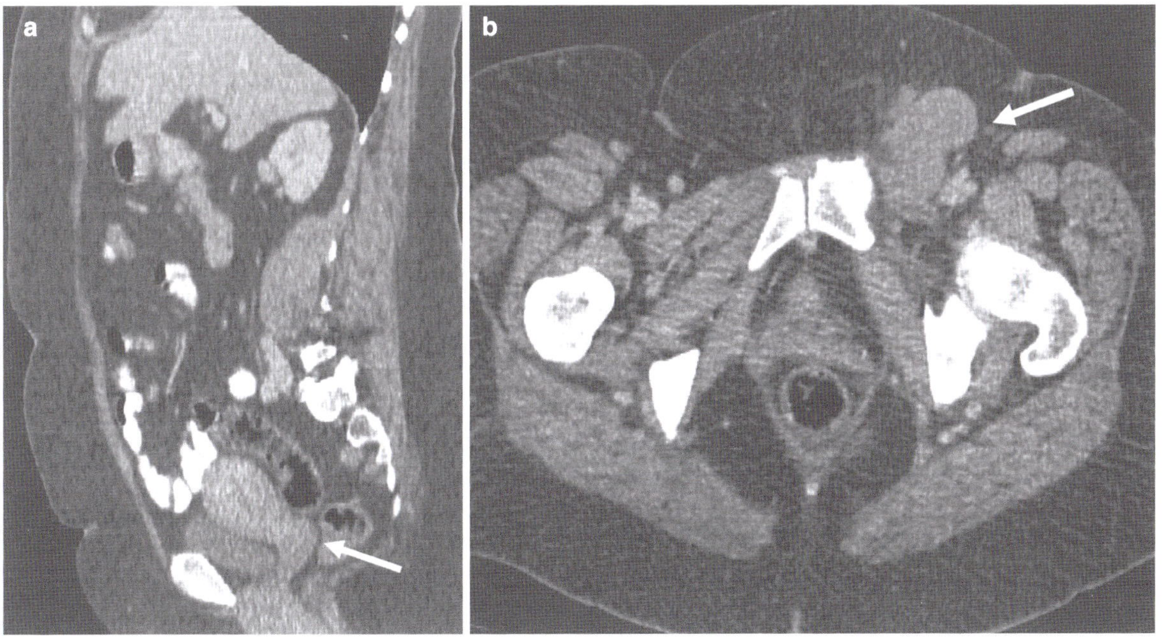

Fig. 4.9 (**a**) CT small cell cervical cancer with small primary tumour bulk (*arrow*) and minimal parametrial extension but, (**b**) bulky inguinal adenopathy (*arrow*)

nodes may then occur which is also seen with aggressive tumours such as small cell carcinomas (Fig. 4.9).

Gross involvement of pelvic lymph nodes by tumour will also increase the likelihood of retrograde involvement of groin nodes.

4.4.3 Vagina

Local staging of vaginal tumours is best assessed with a combination of clinical assessment and MRI. Soft tissue detail from thin section (3–4 mm) axial and sagittal images provides good local tumour staging and macroscopic evidence of depth of tumour invasion to determine resectability. With detailed soft tissue discrimination, MR can readily identify penetration of tumour through the vaginal wall, paravaginal tissue and identify involvement of adjacent pelvic floor muscles and urethra (Fig. 4.10). As the lower third of the vagina drains predominantly to inguinal nodes, MR imaging should include the groins as well as the remainder of the pelvis to determine likely nodal involvement. As inguinal nodes are the primary nodal drainage station from the legs, they are often prominent, with a short axis diameter up to 15 mm and a normal fatty hilum. These reactive nodes can be easily seen on MR and CT in these reactive nodes.

CT/PET is indicated if exenterative surgery is considered, to exclude nodal involvement and more distant disease, but it cannot accurately assess potential surgical resection margins or primary tumour stage as well as MRI.

4.4.4 Vulva

Lymph node staging in vulval carcinoma is the key to prognosis and FIGO has held surgical staging as the gold standard since 1988. New FIGO staging in 2009 [12] gives weight to the prognostic importance of numbers of lymph nodes involved, as well as local invasion of perineal structures such as urethra and vagina. Thorough inguinofemoral lymph node dissection, particularly if bilateral, is a particularly morbid procedure, often performed in an elderly patient which in retrospect post-operatively, may be unnecessary, as the size of the primary tumour does not always correlate with nodal metastases. Up to 75% of early stage vulval cancer will have negative nodes after groin dissection. Sentinel node imaging, using a combination of blue dye and radiocolloid isotope has been successfully utilised to identify and

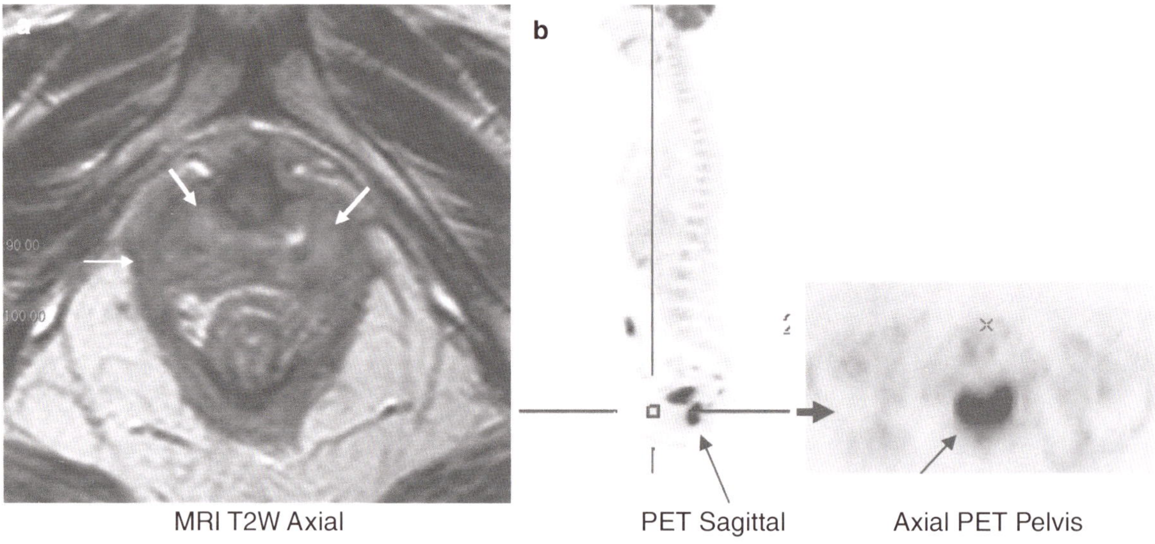

Fig. 4.10 Vaginal carcinoma (*broad arrows*) with concentric involvement of vaginal mucosa and muscularis. Penetration through adventitial tissue (*arrow*) is evident to adjacent levator ani muscle. Which shows high signal on MR. (**b**) PET confirms tumour localised to central pelvis (*arrow*), but it cannot accurately show invasion of pelvic floor

allow excision of the primary draining nodal stations this avoids inguinofemoral node dissection in node negative patients, with a resulting 97% 3-year survival. A 0–2% false negative rate has been reported for sentinel nodes when followed by formal lymphadenectomy [28].

A further advantage of this procedure is the pre or intraoperative identification of patients with positive sentinel nodes, allowing appropriate selection for radiotherapy instead of surgery, with reduced morbidity compared to patients subjected to extensive surgery followed by radiotherapy.

Due to the superficial position of inguinal nodes, high resolution ultrasound, as in head and neck cancer imaging, is not only able to measure nodal size, but is able to characterise morphology and likelihood of neoplastic change by virtue of Doppler assessment and fine needle aspiration if necessary, producing combined ultrasound and cytological sensitivity of 93% and specificityof10 0% [14].

Cross sectional imaging is not usually necessary in assessing vulval carcinoma unless it is clinically advanced. However, the exquisite soft tissue detail afforded by small field of view MR can non-invasively assess important perineal structures, as well as assist in staging lymph nodes in groins and in the pelvis, although sensitivity is limited and normal sized nodes would not preclude nodal dissection (Fig. 4.11).

4.4.5 Ovary

While Ultrasound is important in discriminating benign from malignant adnexal masses, it has less value in staging either routine epithelial or unusual ovarian malignancy. On abdominal ultrasound, abdominal ascites, omental cake and obstructed kidneys may be apparent and although specificity is high, the sensitivity of ultrasound to diagnose peritoneal disease, retroperitoneal adenopathy and unresectable bulk disease is poor. Distant thoracic metastatic disease is unlikely to be seen on ultrasound with the exception of pleural based deposits, when they are surrounded by pleural fluid.

While MRI is the preferred modality for characterising a complex adnexal mass and has a 60–95% accuracy in differentiating benign from malignant masses, [5, 6, 26] CT scan of abdomen and pelvis, following intravenous and oral contrast, is generally recommended as the preferred imaging modality for comprehensive staging. This determines suitability for either primary, or delayed debulking surgery. Multi-slice CT facilitates multi-planar reconstruction with coronal and sagittal images which is particularly useful to determine whether there is likely to be irresectible disease. Pre-operative imaging with a CT scan, rather than relying solely on findings from ultrasound imaging, also has the advantage of depicting an unexpected primary neoplasm arising from elsewhere,

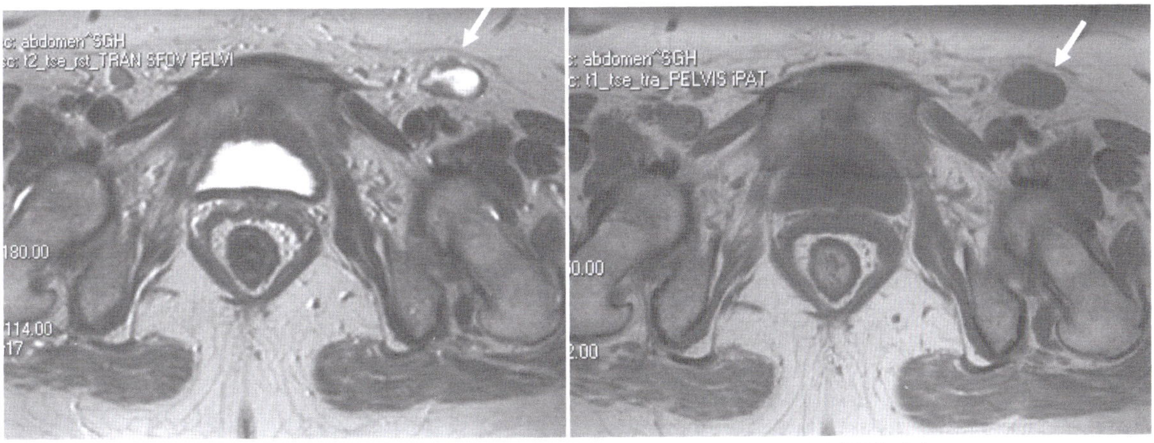

Fig. 4.11 Advanced vulval carcinoma. Enlarged necrotic left inguinal lymph nodes, typical for squamous cancer, showing high, fluid signalonT2w eighteds equences

originating, for example, in the gastrointestinal tract or pancreas, with metastases to the ovaries and peritoneum as the presenting complaint (Krukenberg tumour).

In rare tumours, CT can guide the extent of primary surgery required, which may allow conservation of fertility. Once there is tissue confirmation of ovarian malignancy, particularly if this is either of advanced stage, or of unusual histopathology, then CT of the chest is more sensitive than a chest radiograph in the detection of lung and pleural metastases.

CT/PET is being used increasingly in patients to detect relapse of epithelial ovarian cancer, particularly when prompted by a rise in CA125 levels. It has a reported sensitivity of 80–90%, which is greater than that afforded by CT or MRI and recent studies suggest it may be more sensitive than increasing CA125 levels inde tectingre currence [15].

However, there are false negatives in detecting microscopic disease in lesions less than 5 mm [15, 39] and its greatest value may be in its positive predictive value for assessing potentially localised disease and suitability for repeat limited surgical resection. The value of CT/PET in staging and following up non-epithelial ovarian cancer has not been established.

In the follow-up of recurrent disease, a recent study have shown no survival advantage in the treatment of asymptomatic women with rising CA 125 levels, [41] as opposed to waiting to treat symptomatic women. As a consequence, it may be that detecting disseminated recurrence any earlier with imaging adds to costs, produces anxiety and confers no survival advantage.

4.5 ImagingC haracteristics of Specific Tumours

4.5.1 *Uterus*

4.5.1.1 ClearC ellandSer ous Endometrial Tumours

Serous endometrial tumours are the most aggressive epithelial tumours, with a poor prognosis. Although serous and clear cell tumours account for only 10% of endometrial neoplasms, they contribute to 50% of deaths with a 42% 5-year survival for stage1B tumours. These high grade, type 2 endometrial cancers are 2–6 times more likely to occur in patients with previous breast cancer [29].

They are frequently advanced at presentation with deep myometrial invasion, lymphovascular invasion and often involvement of the serosal surface of the uterus. Involvement of the serosal surface rapidly produces a pattern of tumour dissemination comparable to epithelial ovarian cancers with peritoneal and omental disease. Trans tubal dissemination will also produce peritoneal disease and positive washings, even when the tumour appears confined to the endometrium.

Serous tumours in particular, have a propensity for early nodal dissemination and haematogenous metastases. These nodal metastases may be massive, mimicking the imaging appearances of lymphoma, with bulky, confluent para-aortic and pelvic lymphadenopathy(Fig. 4.12).

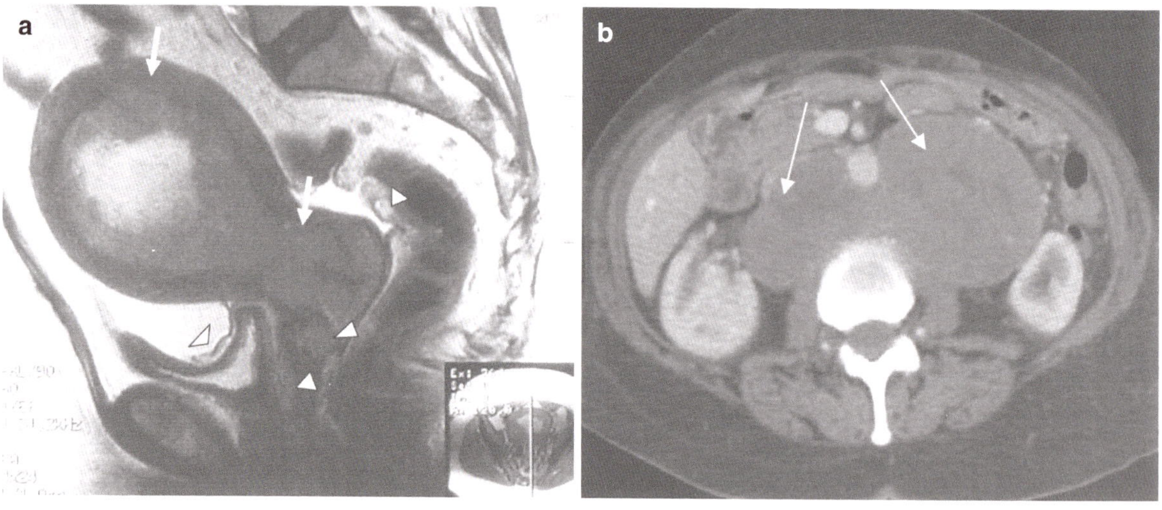

Fig. 4.12 (**a**) Serous endometrial tumour just extending to outer half of myometrium, but with extensive cervical stromal involvement (*arrows*) and deposits in vaginal fornix, vesico-vaginal septum and serosal peritoneal surface with ascites (*arrowheads*). (**b**) Massive retroperitoneal para-aortic adenopathy (*arrows*)

Nodal spread in cancers of the uterine corpus tends to be more disorderly than in cervical cancer, due to differences in normal uterine lymphatic drainage, so that involvement of para-aortic nodes, or rarely inguinal nodes, can occur in the absence of pelvic adenopathy. When cervical stroma is involved, aggressive endometrial tumours will behave more like cervical cancers, spreading to the parametrium, obstructing ureters and involving adjacent bowel and bladder.

This propensity for peritoneal dissemination and distant metastases should prompt careful imaging evaluation of the chest, abdomen and pelvis with MRI for local staging to determine resectibilty, in addition to a CT or CT/PET scan (Figs. 4.1 and 4.5).

In common with serous tumours, clear cell tumours have a poor prognosis, frequently presenting with disease extending beyond the uterine corpus, even in the presence of clinically small volume disease (Fig. 4.6). Nodal metastases are often unsuspected (Fig. 4.5). This supports the need for pre-operative MRI in this group of patients with endometrial cancer.

Uterine clear cell carcinomas may have an association with endometriosis [42] and adenomyosis, although clear cell and other adenocarcinomas are more frequently associated with ovarian or extragonadal endometriosis, rather than the uterus.

Adenomyosis is identified accurately on MRI, with widening and heterogeneity of the junctional zone of the myometrium (Fig. 4.13). Evidence of the complications of endometriosis, such as endometriomas, obliteration of the Pouch of Douglas, with characteristic endometriotic plaques in the pouch of Douglas and bowel adhesions may be present on pre-operative MR scans. Complications and increased morbidity for both surgical resection and radiotherapy, more often indicated in high grade endometrial cancer, can be highlighted if these sequelae of endometriosis can be identified preoperatively (Fig. 4.14).

4.5.1.2 Carcinosarcoma

On imaging, uterine carcinosarcomas (previously called mixed mesodermal mullerian tumours), initially appear to behave in the same way as high grade endometrial adenocarcinomas. That is, they are tumours centred on and producing widening of the endometrium, rather than masses centred initially in the myometrium [44, 56]. They also have the same age and risk distribution characteristics as endometrial adenocarcinomas [43]. There is an increased incidence following long term Tamoxifen for previous breast cancer. Previous pelvic irradiation is also a predisposing cause, which in addition, can make clinical assessment difficult (Fig. 4.2).

Carcinosarcoma tends to present as a bulky, advanced tumour, (Figs. 4.15 and 4.16) often extending outside the uterus. In common with other sarcomas, it not infrequently presents as a large irregular heterogenous pelvic

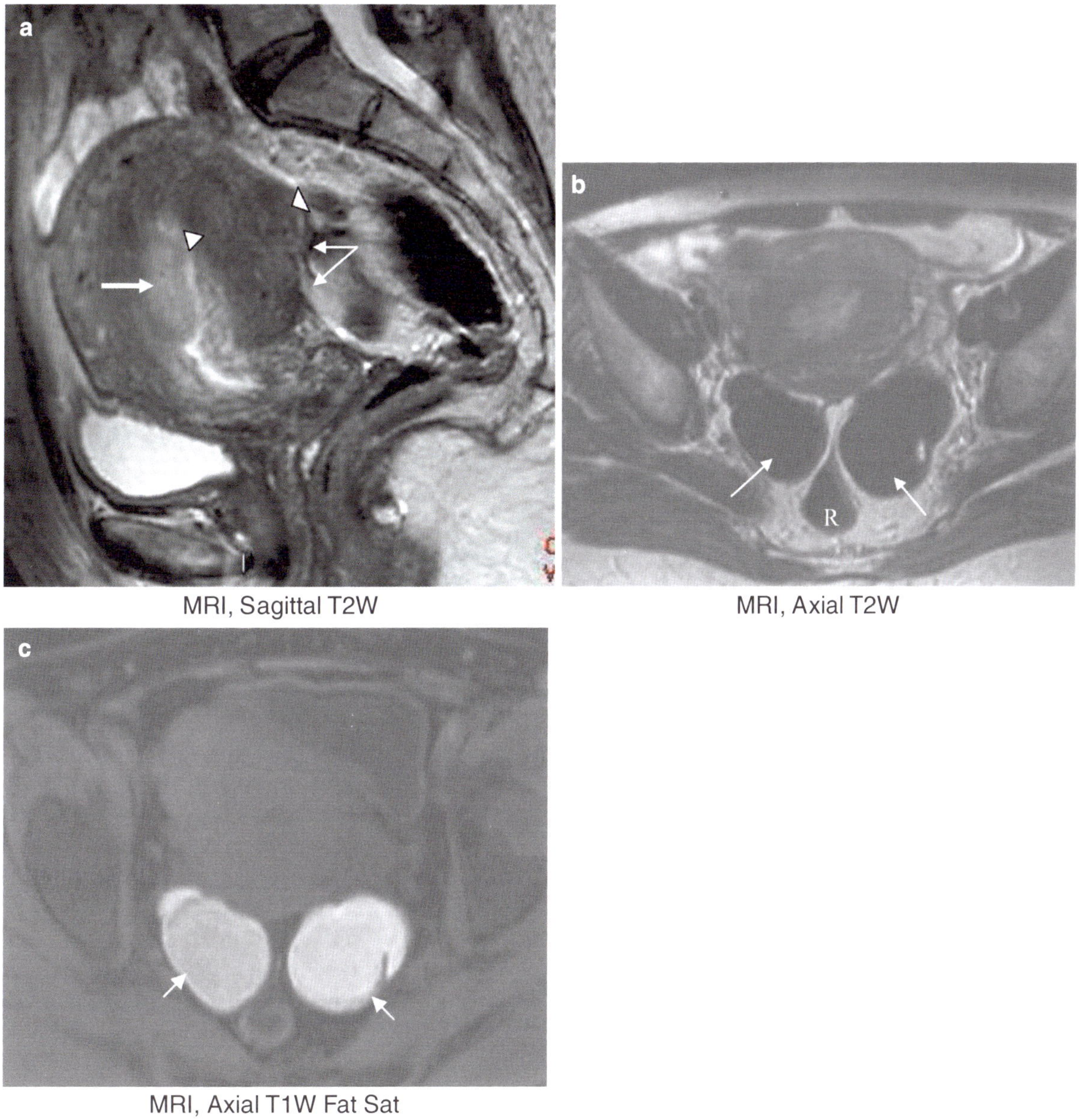

Fig. 4.13 MRI: (**a**) 1A clear cell endometrial carcinoma confined to inner myometrium (*bold arrow*), with adenomyosis reflected in widened junctional zone of uterus (*arrowheads*). Note obliteration of the uterovesical pouch, and pouch of Douglas secondary to chronic endometriosis (*thin arrows*). (**b**) Low signal (T2W) endometriotic cysts either side of rectum (R) produce a compressive effect (*arrows*). (**c**) Fat saturated T1W sequence confirm endometriomas, with blood (methaemaglobin) within the cysts (*arrows*) with high signal on T1 and low signal on T2W

mass with serosal and extrauterine invasion to adjacent bowel loops or other pelvic structures, when it can be difficult to determine the organ of origin. Over twenty percent of patients are likely to be upstaged at surgery and twenty percent of these to stage 4 [43]. Spread to adjacent pelvic organs and lymph node metastases occurs 3 times more frequently than for adenocarcinoma, with omental involvement a particularly common site of distant metastasis and nodal disease occurring in 16–18% of patients.

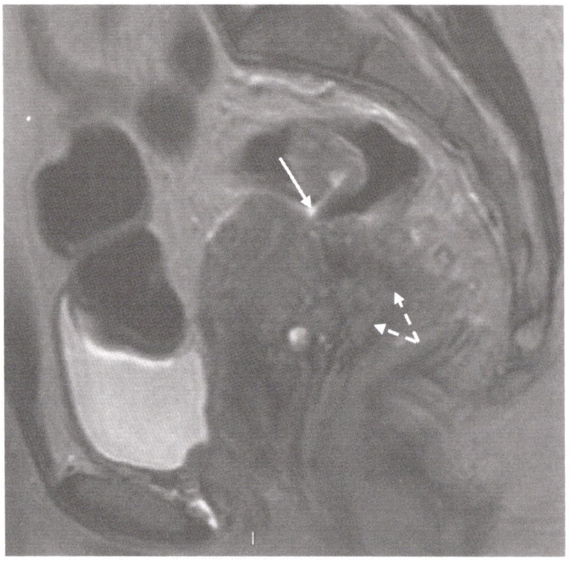

Fig. 4.14 MRI T2W. Adhesions of bowel to endometriotic plaque (*arrow*) at cervico-uterine junction in Pouch of Douglas with obliteration of the peritoneal recess. Note large endometriotic deposit (*broken arrows*) invading rectum, clinically potentiallymis takenf or tumour

If there is no pre-operative imaging to identify the extent of metastatic disease, primary surgical resection is more likely to be incomplete. As gross residual tumour following surgery appears to have the most important adverse prognostic effect on survival [43, 54], pre-operative identification of tumour spread is particularly important. Unfortunately, pathological identification of carcinosarcoma from pre-operative endometrial biopsies is limited in up to 25% of patients [43] so that the need for pre-operative imaging may not be realised.

Pre-operative imaging assessment should follow the format for other aggressive uterine tumours with MRI for local staging and complete distant staging with CT or CT/PET, in order to plan the extent of surgery, lymphadenectomy or determine non-surgical options.

Carcinosarcomas are mostly hyper-intense with respect to myometrium on T2W sequences, often presenting as a polypoid mass expanding the endometrial cavity. As size increases, tumours become more heterogenous, with striations and areas of increased or decreased signal (Fig. 4.15) usually due to foci of haemorrhage or necrosis. Pre and post-contrast sequences are critical for accurately identifying the extent of invasion. Following contrast, the tumour is mostly hypovascular with respect to normal myometrial enhancement, but areas of increased vascularity, persisting into delayed, portal-venous phases, appear toc orrelatew ithmore s arcomatouse lements [45].

Both high grade, type 2 endometrial carcinomas, and carcinosarcomas tend not to invade pre-existing myometrial leiomyomata, (Fig. 4.16) which may help to differentiate from the appearances of endometrial sarcoma.

There are no specific imaging features that clearly distinguish this tumour from other high grade endometrial neoplasms, apart from the propensity for early aggressive behaviour and some post contrast features. However, there appear to be some imaging features which may be helpful in differentiating carcinosarcoma from endometrial stromal sarcoma and LMS.

4.5.1.3 LeiomyosarcomaandEndo metrial Stromal Sarcoma

Leiomyosarcoma (LMS) and endometrial stromal sarcomas (ESS) are rare mesenchymal tumours of the uterus, comprising 1–3% of all uterine malignancies, occurring more commonly in black races and occurring in younger, often pre or peri menopausal patients, rather than in older post-menopausal patients who have a higher incidence of carcinosarcoma and high grade endometrial adenocarcinoma.

ESS closely resembles normal endometrial proliferative stromal cells and usually arises from the endometrium or from foci of myometrial adenomyosis. Although, low grade tumours have a 5-year survival of approximately 80%, in high grade tumours this is reduced to approximately 50%.

Macroscopically these are often fleshy, polypoid tumours distending the endometrial cavity. Stromal sarcomas almost invariably involve the myometrium, although this may not always be apparent on imaging. When there is direct communication of tumour with the endometrial cavity, diagnosis is possible from an endometrial biopsy and pre-operative imaging will be precipitated. But in some patients, there may be minimal involvement of the endometrium, with a predominantly myometrial mass and appearances may be interpreted as a leiomyoma, particularly at ultrasound. The diagnosis may then only be made post-operatively after an inappropriate simple hysterectomy, polypectomy or myomectomy to treat abnormal vaginal bleeding.

The MR imaging appearances are governed not only by the tumour grade, but by the location of the bulk of the tumour. Thus the tumour may protrude as

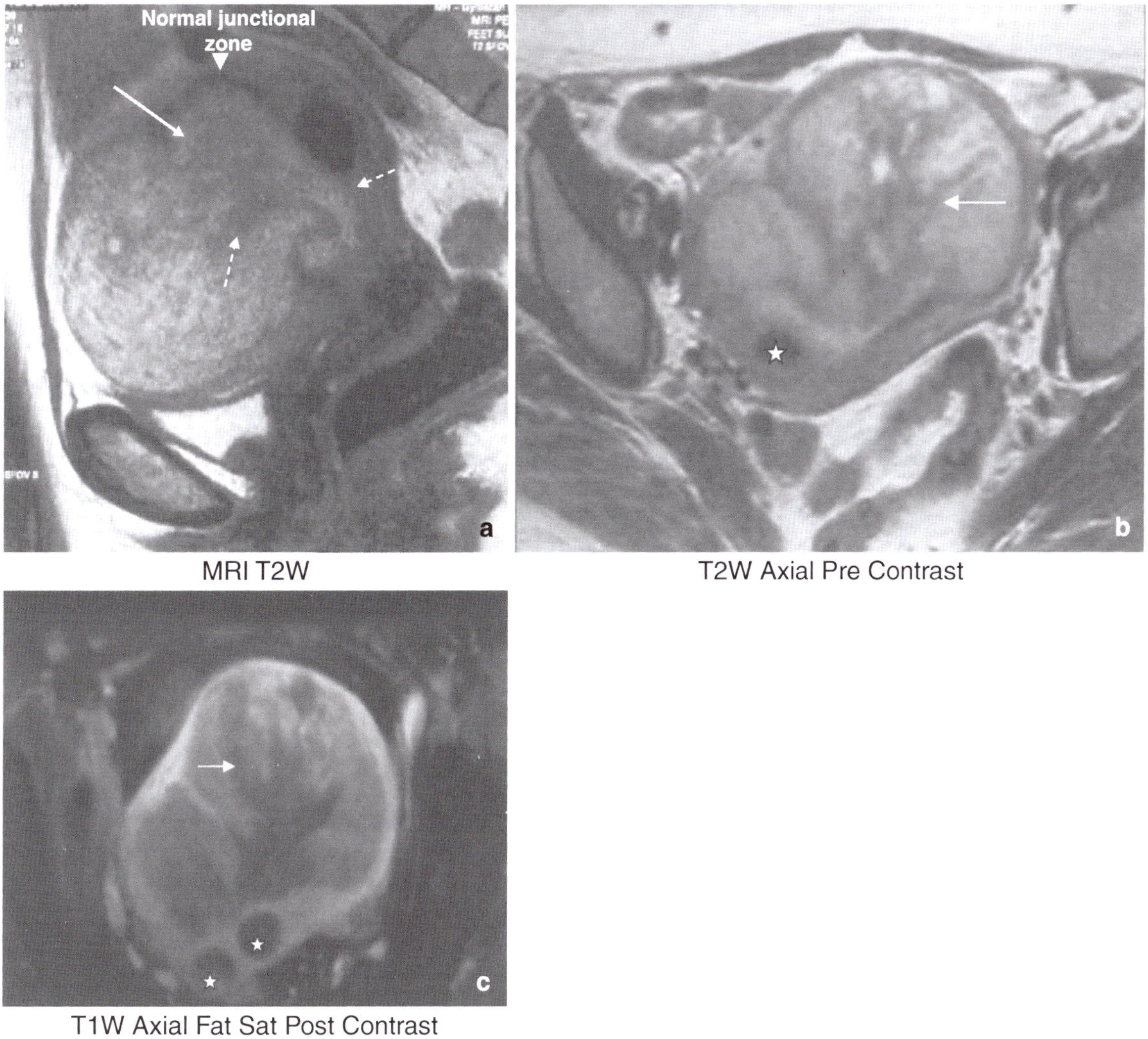

Fig. 4.15 (**a**) Carcinosarcoma. Extensive, hyperintense tumour centred on endometrium, (*arrow*) with foci of necrosis, but with disruption of junctional zone (*broken arrow*) and extensive myometrial involvement to cervix and serosal surface of uterus (**b** and **c**). Low signal avascular "straie" of necrosis within the central tumour with no enhancement (*arrow*) on delayed post-contrast images. Pre-existing, non-enhancing mature fibroids (*)

an intermediate signal T2W polypoid mass into the endometrial cavity, (Figs. 4.3 and 4.17) where on imaging alone it can be mistaken for a hyperplastic polyp, or it may predominantly infiltrate the myometrium and junctional zone of the uterus sometimes with associated endometrial thickening.

Although the tumour may be confused on MR with cystic or hyaline degeneration of a fibroid, in contrast to simple leiomyomata, these are often larger, hypervascular masses, particularly notable in a post-menopausal patient. The myometrial margin of the mass is usually poorly defined, but the endometrial tumour margin is frequently well defined and lobulated and may be outlined by endometrial fluid. In younger patients, lower grade tumours are more common and when these infiltrate the myometrium, there are characteristic low signal bands on T2W sequences which correspond pathologically to bands of normal myometrial fibres interspersed with infiltrating tumour spindle cells. Higher grade tumours, more common in older patients, tend to lack these low signal bands and more frequently have areas of haemorrhage and necrosis, which can

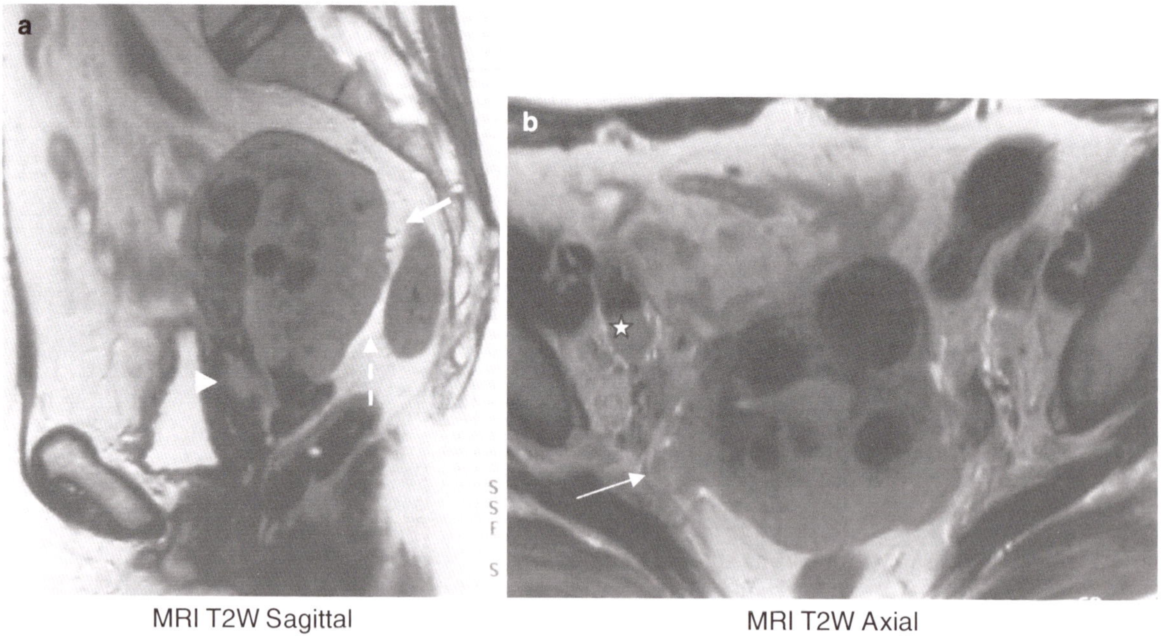

Fig. 4.16 Uterine carcinosarcoma, infiltrating myometrium with sparing of pre-existing fibroids. (**a**) Spiculated extension to serosa (*arrow*) and cervix (*arrowhead*), with small amount of ascitic fluid (*broken arrow*). (**b**) Unexpected extension through serosa to pelvic side wall and piriformis muscle (*arrow*) enlarged external iliac nodes (*)

also be identified on MRI [45] (Fig. 4.17). The tumour bulk generally enhances less than normal myometrium, but there are areas of increased vascularity within the tumour and areas of myometrial invasion identified by contrast enhancement greater than, or equal to, normal myometrium [46] (Fig. 4.17). In contrast, infiltrating endometrial carcinoma is usually hypovascular with respect to normal myometrium. Although, post-contrast enhancement is also often seen in benign leiomyomata, in sarcomatous tumours vascularity tends to be more prominent and disordered [55, 56].

ESS tumours are also characterised by lympho-vascular invasion and nodular serpiginous extension of tumour into blood vessels, surrounding structures and tissue planes, even when pathology is reported as a low grade with little cytological atypia. At initial presentation, this can produce a similar appearance to benign intravenous leiomyomatosis where plugs of benign tissue are seen within large pelvic veins or the inferior vena cava. Slow growth of venous deposits can result in a strikingly delayed recurrence, more than 10 years later, with tumoural venous thrombosis and metastaticdis ease(Fig. 4.18).

The current FIGO staging (2009) [25] for ESS takes into consideration involvement of pelvic and/or para-aortic lymph nodes and so pre-operative imaging should include assessment of chest, abdomen and pelvis in view of the propensity for haematogenous metastases, even when the primary tumour is small. MRI is most appropriate for local tumour staging and assessment of resectability, but CT scan of chest and abdomen (or CT/PET) should also be performed for complete staging.

Fig. 4.17 (**a**-**e**) (**a**) MRI: post-menopausal patient with high grade endometrial stromal sarcoma. High signal heterogenous tumour (*arrow*) distends the endometrial cavity, thinning the myometrium. (**b**) Low signal junctional zone (*broken arrow*) is maintained apart from site of myometrial invasion (*broad arrow*). (**c**) Foci of high signal haemorrhage on T1W sequences (*arrow*). (**d**) Dynamic contrast enhanced MRI: arterial phase shows intense irregular enhancement of tumour equal to myometrium. Low signal junctional zone is maintained, except at site of invasion (*broken arrow*) Non-enhancing central avascular clefts or necrosis (*). (**e**) Delayed equilibrium phase (4 min) continued tumour enhancement with overall enhancement less than adjacent myometrium

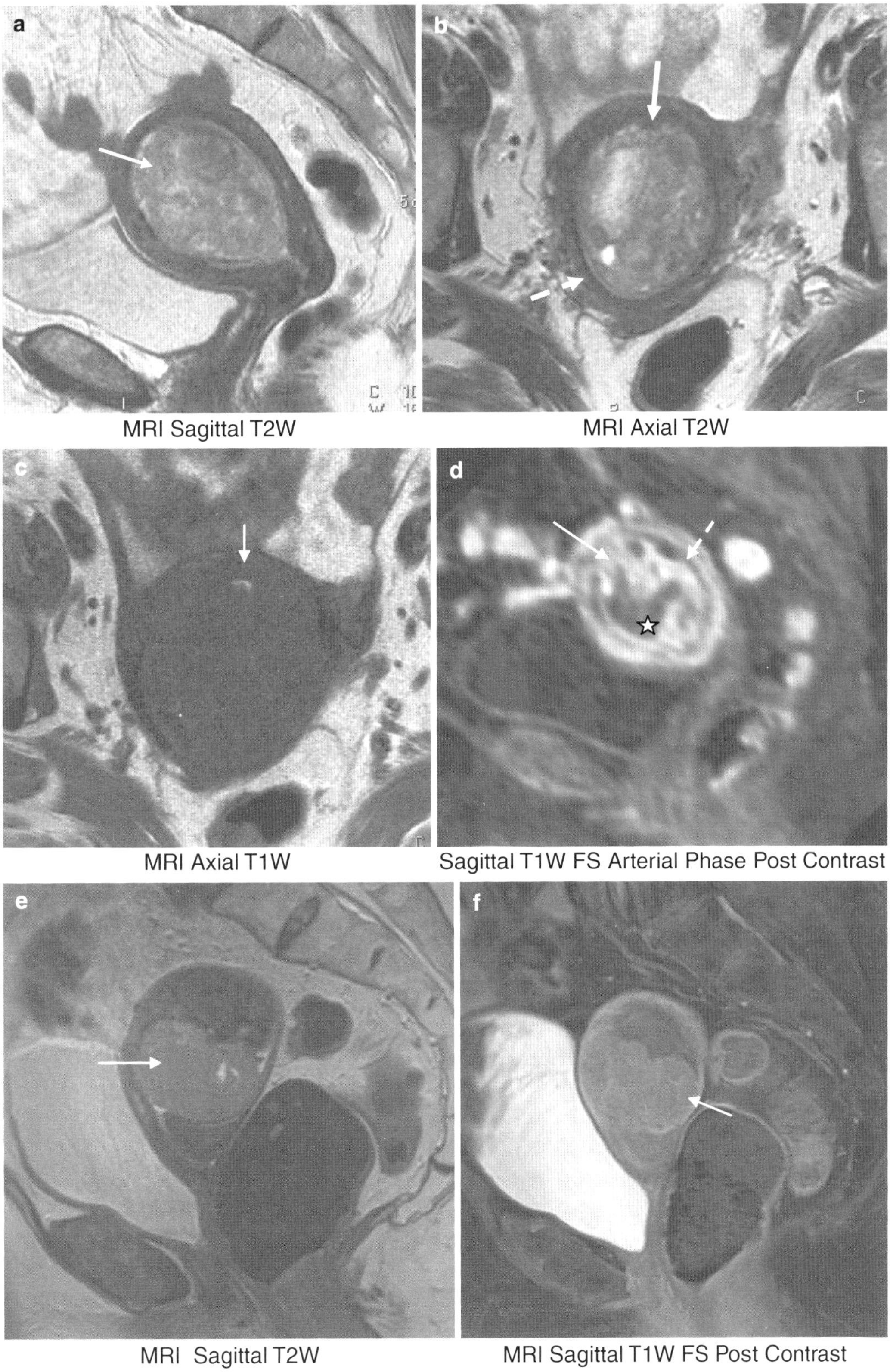
a
b
MRI Sagittal T2W
MRI Axial T2W
c
d
MRI Axial T1W
Sagittal T1W FS Arterial Phase Post Contrast
e
f
MRI Sagittal T2W
MRI Sagittal T1W FS Post Contrast

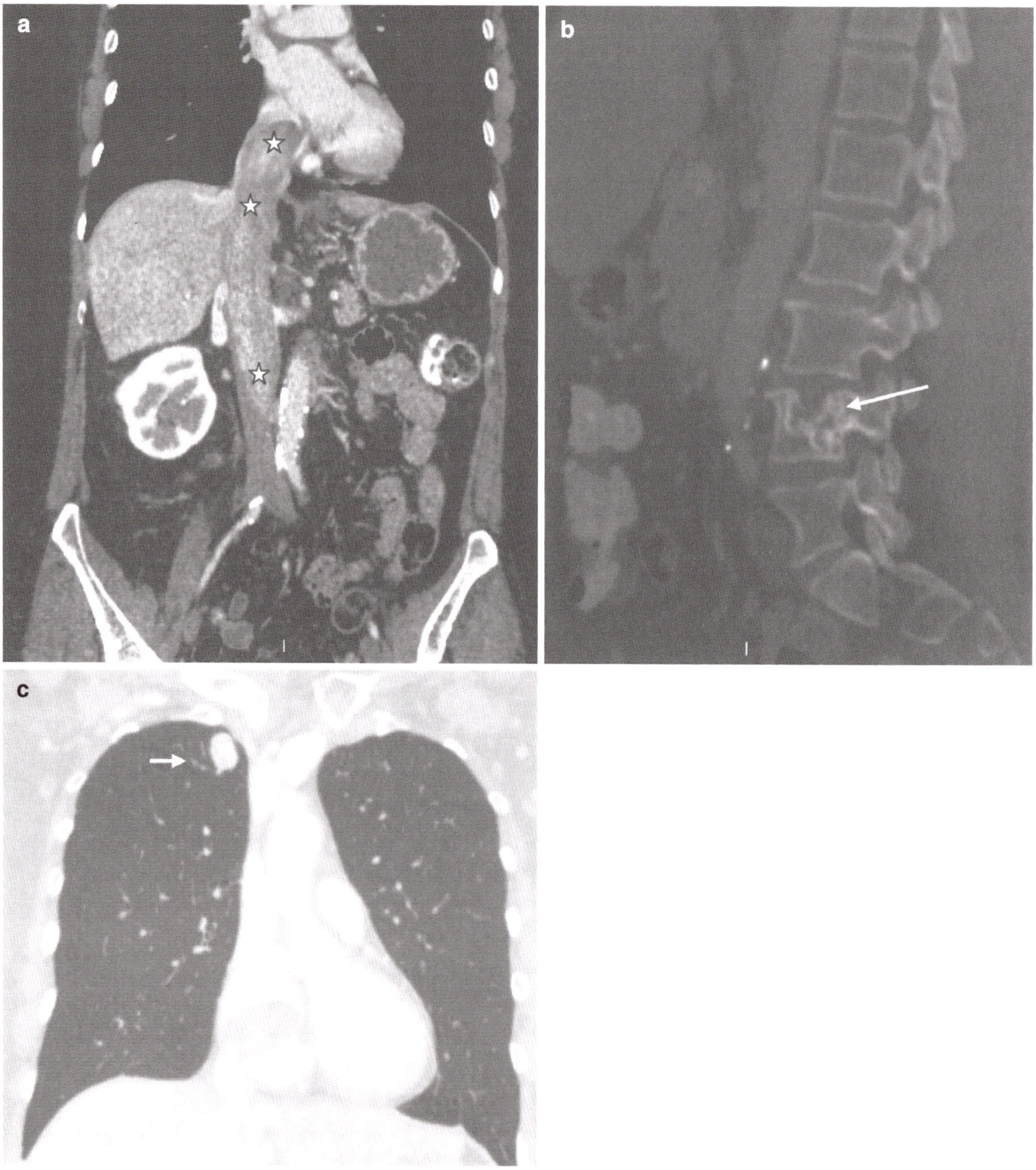

Fig. 4.18 Low grade endometrial stromal sarcoma resected with TAH and BSO 29 years previously. (**a**) CT scan post contrast: recurrence of extensive venous tumour thrombus in pelvic veins, IVC, and extending to right atrium (*stars*) (note vascular enhancement of tumour thrombus). (**b**) Well-defined lytic/sclerotic bone metastasis to L4 vertebral body (*arrow*). (**c**) Lung metastasis (*arrow*)

4.5.1.4 Leiomyosarcoma

LMS usually arise de novo within the myometrium, and only rarely arise in a pre-existing fibroid. Rapid growth of a fibroid or uterine enlargement is not a reliable indicator of malignancy. In a retrospective review of 1,332 patients having surgery for leiomyoma, only 0.23% had uterine sarcoma (including carcinosarcoma). Even for patients having surgery for rapidly enlarging leiomyoma, the incidence of sarcoma is reported as 0.27% [57].

In high grade tumours, there is usually rapid progression to involve the endometrium which then presents with abnormal vaginal bleeding, prompting earlier investigation and intervention. However, with low grade tumours in particular, diagnosis may be an unexpected finding at hysterectomy for other indications. Thus pre-operatively, the diagnosis of leiomyosarcoma is not only difficult clinically, but is often not diagnosed from uterine biopsy or hysteroscopy. If pre-operative imaging is performed, MR appearances may be able to suggest a leiomyosarcoma.

Unlike endometrial carcinomas and carcinosarcomas, LMS tend to arise within the myometrium and compress, rather than enlarge the endometrial cavity, which can therefore be difficult to identify (Figs. 4.19–4.21). Initial appearances may be very similar to a benign leiomyoma and indeed, sarcomatous elements may rarely be found within an otherwise benign leiomyoma (Fig. 4.19). As the tumours enlarge, cystic necrosis and haemorrhage often occurs (Fig. 4.20). High grade LMS are more likely

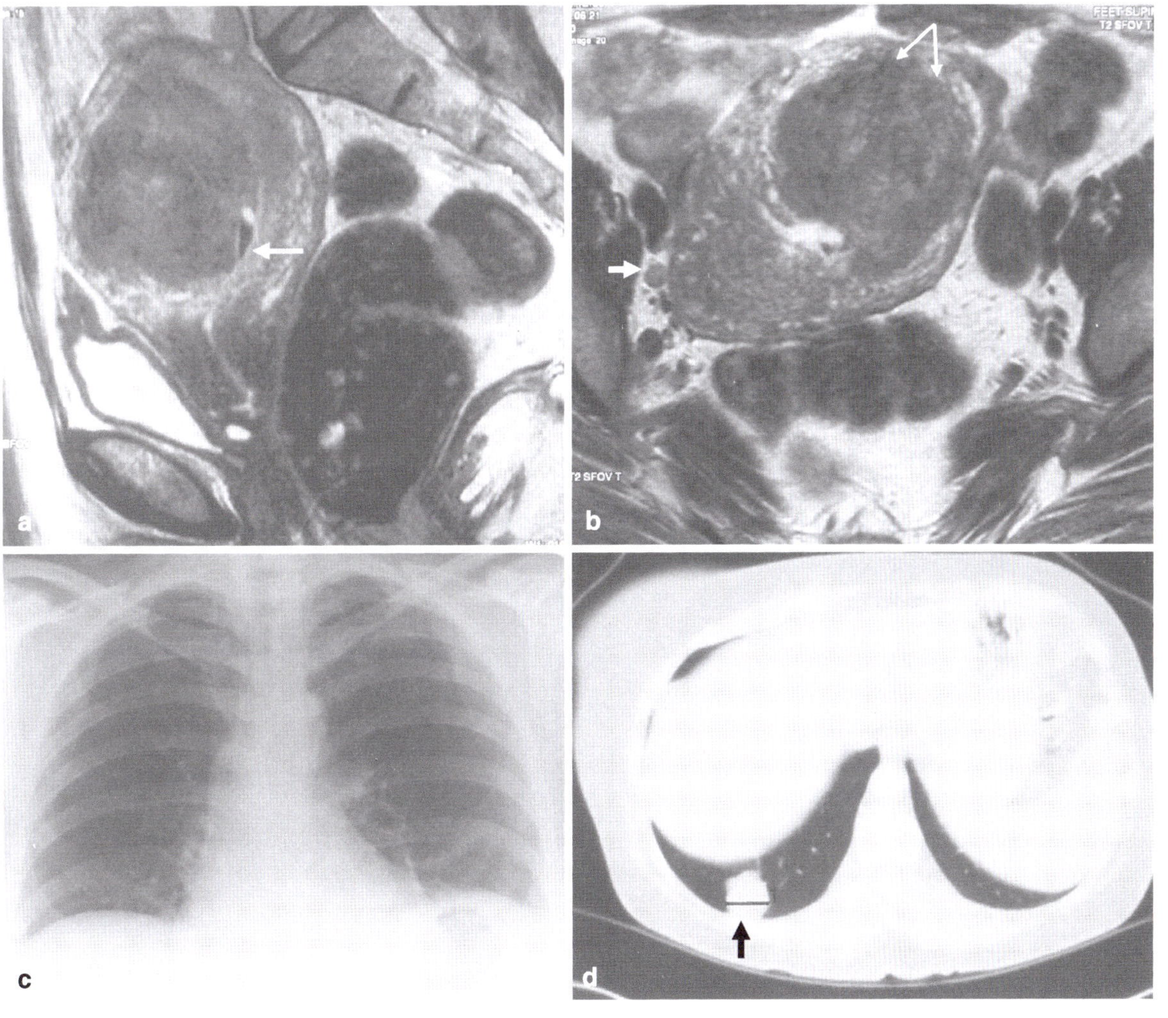

Fig. 4.19 Unexpected leiomyosarcoma post-hysterectomy for presumed benign fibroid disease. Post-menopausal bleeding. (**a**) Endometrial cavity containing a small amount of blood (*arrow*), is compressed by large leiomyoma eroding endometrium and containing sarcomatous elements. (**b**) Image shows heterogeneous myometrial mass, poorly marginated in places, (*double arrows*) and small right pelvic external iliac node (*broad arrow*). (**c**) Post-operative normal chest X-ray, (**d**) CT shows a prominent metastasis (*arrow*) within posterior costophrenic recess, not seenonc hestr adiograph

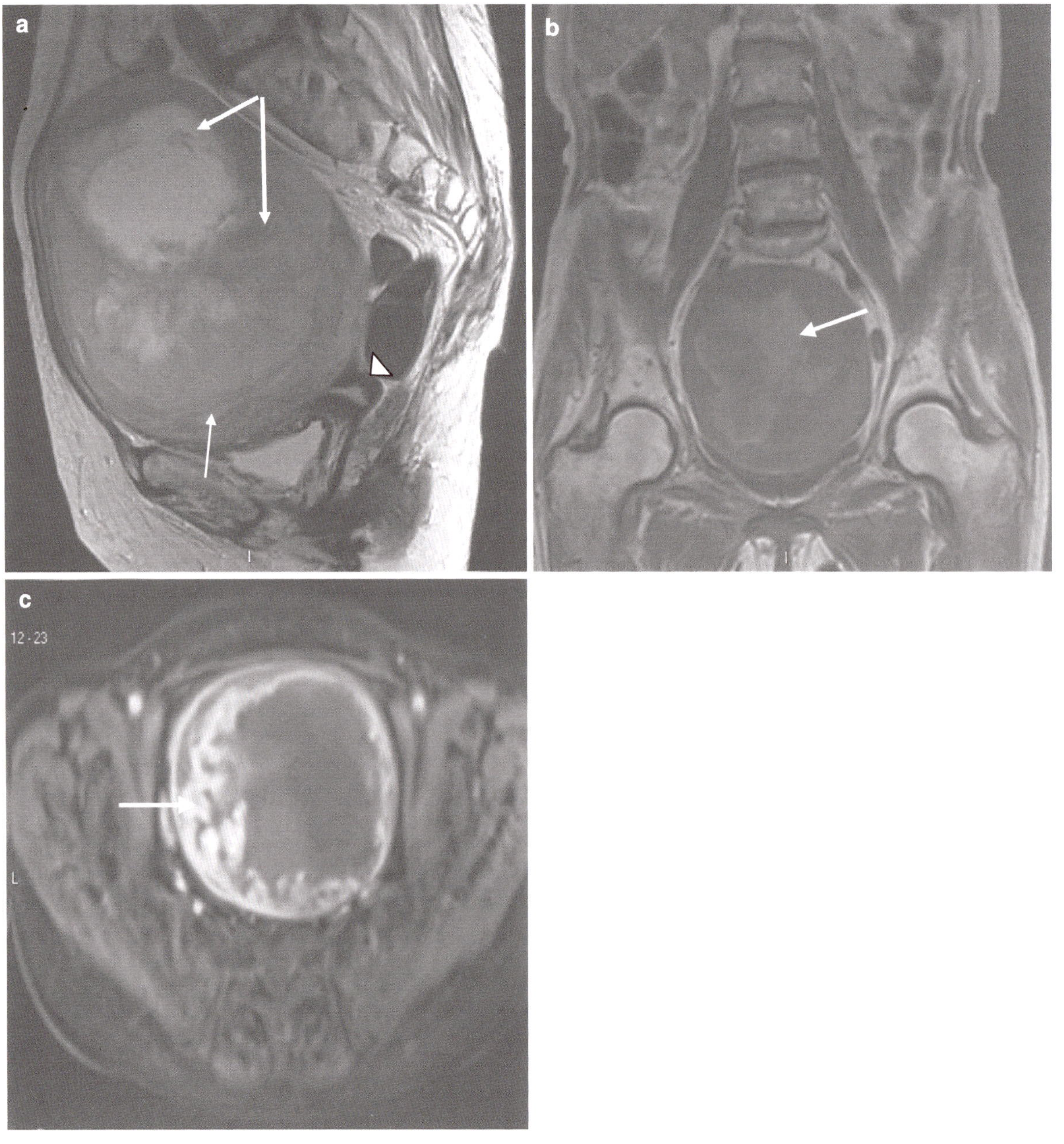

Fig. 4.20 LMS in post-menopausal patient: (**a**) MR Sagittal T2W large necrotic tumour (*double arrows*) shows invasion and compression of endometrial cavity (*single arrow*) normal cervix (*arrowhead*). (**b**) Coronal T1W: increased signal indicating haemorrhagic necrosis (*arrow*). (**c**) Axial post contrast: Marked bizarre tortuous vascular enhancement of solid area, (*arrow*) withnon- enhancingc entralne crosis

to show invasion of endometrium, uterine serosa, cervix and extend into parametrium or adjacent soft tissue (Fig. 4.21) [57, 58].

On imaging appearances, haemorrhage may be difficult to differentiate from "red" haemorrhagic degeneration in a benign fibroid. In elderly patients, most mature leiomyomas return a consistent low signal on all MR sequences due to their high fibrous content, and acute cystic and red degeneration of benign fibroids is uncommon, so that these appearances will then raise the pre-operative possibility of a sarcoma. Following injection of intravenous contrast, a dynamic study with a late

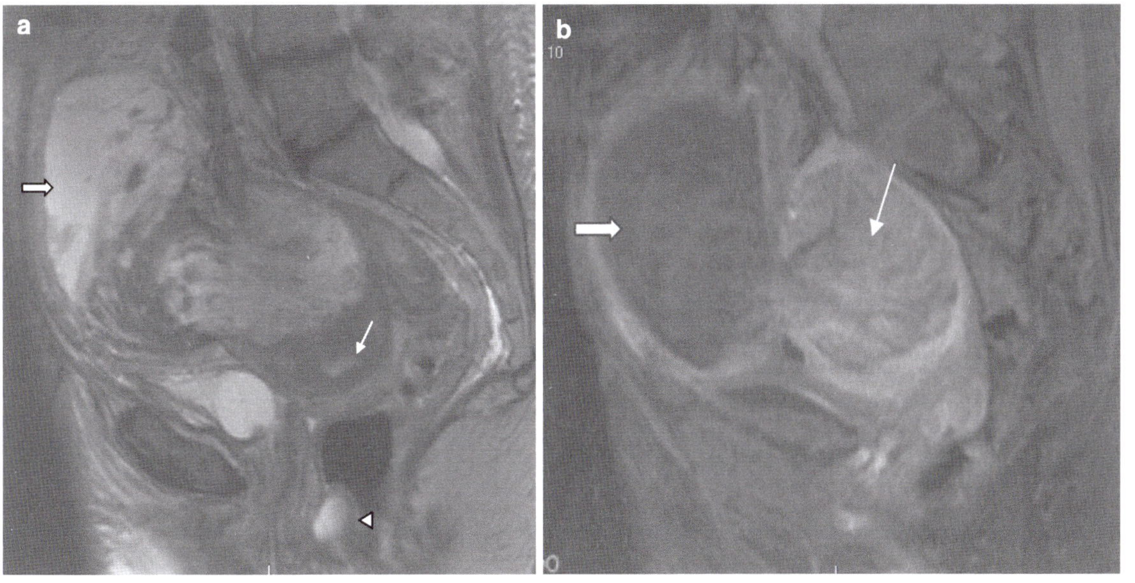

Fig. 4.21 (**a**) LMS with areas of necrosis, (*broad arrow*) compression of endometrial cavity (*arrow*) and metastasis to rectovaginal septum (*arrowhead*). Urinary catheter is in situ. (**b**) Marked early vascular enhancement of solid tumour with linear hypovascular striations (*arrow*) non-enhancing necrosis (*broad arrow*)

arterial phase, (Fig. 4.20c) may demonstrate tortuous vessels and later, a bizarre enhancement pattern not seen with benign fibroids. Areas of non-enhancement, probably correspond to haemorrhagic necrosis, and have been reported to be a differentiating feature of LMS and smooth muscle tumours of uncertain malignant potential [58]. However, these distinctive changes may not be appreciated with small tumours, or in small areas of sarcomatous change within an existing leiomyoma.

Diffusion weighted MRI may have a place in helping to differentiate benign leiomyomas from sarcomas [59]. This would have value particularly in patients being assessed for non-invasive treatment of leiomyomas, for example by ultrasound ablation or interventional vascular embolisation, where histopathological assessment of the uterus will not be available. Unfortunately, at present, there remains some overlap between benign and malignant tissue diffusion values and this technique cannot yet be used solely for definitive diagnosis of malignancy.

Revised FIGO staging (2009) for uterine LMS reflects the wide variation in survival between small, low grade tumours and the abysmal survival in high grade LMS where survival is measured in months, depending on mitotic index, size and lymphovascular invasion of the primary tumour. If pre-operative CT imaging has not been performed, or MRI was confined to the pelvis, a post-operative CT of chest, abdomen and pelvis is recommended at about 6–8 weeks to provide a baseline and exclude distant metastases, 80% of which are likely to be extrapelvic. A chest X-ray is insufficient to exclude lung metastases; the commonest site for distant disease (Fig. 4.19). In line with some other soft tissue or bone sarcomas, solitary lung parenchymal metastases may be considered for resection with curative intent.

CT/PET is sensitive and highly specific in the detection of high grade sarcomas; both of the primary tumour and its' metastases, and its use has been shown to change patient management [37]. However, low grade tumours have a low 18-FDG uptake and SUV, which is likely to make detection insensitive, until there is a significant mass or volume of tumour recurrence which is then likely to be evident on CT or MR imaging.

Even if the primary tumour is small, (Fig. 4.19) there may be unexpected haematogenous dissemination as well as a propensity for local, peritoneal, or retro peritoneal recurrence (Fig. 4.22). However, there is a spectrum of behaviour and low grade sarcomas can demonstrate an indolent behaviour, with metastases to lungs, peritoneum or other solid organs, or venous invasion occurring more than 20 years after initial resection. The pattern of recurrence of low grade sarcoma is unusual to the point that if the patient presents with an solid peritoneal or retro peritoneal tumour even two decades after initial treatment, recurrent sarcoma should be considered.

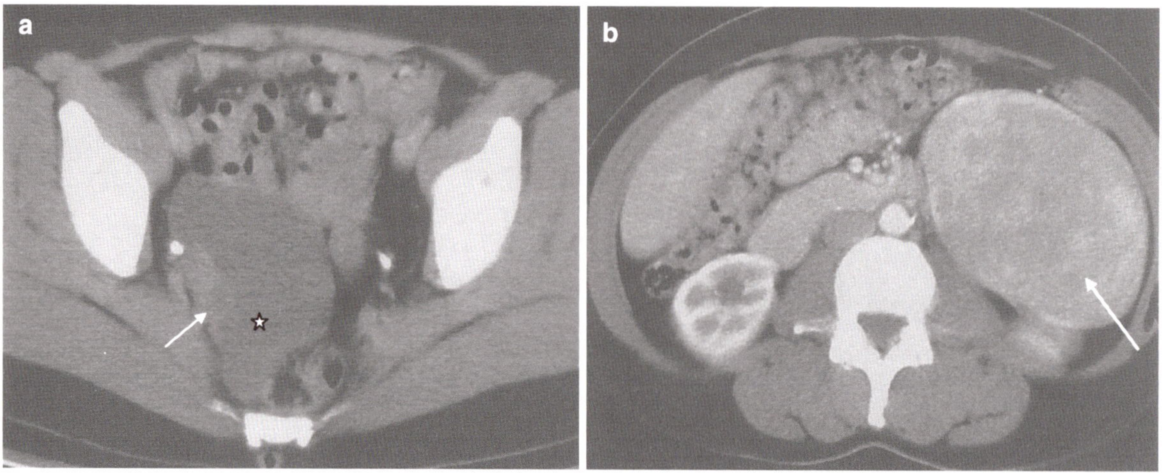

Fig. 4.22 CT recurrent leiomyosarcoma post-hysterectomy and bilateral oophorectomy. (**a**) Ascitic fluid (*star*) within Pouch of Douglas with peritoneal deposit (*arrow*) adherent to right pelvic side wall. (**b**) Solid, well-defined and large vascular metastasis (*arrow*)i nferiort ol eftki dney

There is an unusual propensity for lower grade sarcomatous tumours to invade venous structures and metastasise as an extending plug of vascular tumour into pelvic veins and inferior vena cava even extending into the right atrium and ventricle (Fig. 4.18), in the same way as occurs with tumour thrombus from renal cell carcinoma. This may present with venous obstruction and cardiovascular related signs many years after the primary tumour resection. Tumour thrombus can be differentiated from normal venous thrombus by vascular enhancement. Contrast studies will also differentiate a tumour "plug", which can be removed fairly easily by thrombectomy, or whether there is actual vascular invasion of the vessel wall. It is not possible on imaging, to differentiate this venous "plug" from benign intravascular leiomyomatosis, and a previous history of even a low grade sarcoma is the key to correct diagnosis.

These patients need long term follow up, for ten years or more, but tumour markers are not helpful and there is little published guidance on the frequency of imaging. Further imaging should be guided by factors governing prognosis: patient age, tumour grade and mitotic index and stage at presentation. For younger patients, with low grade tumours, follow-up annual chest films with MR scans of abdomen and pelvis would be worthwhile for 5 years. Following this, a 2-yearly MR scan might be more appropriate, depending on resource. Frequent screening with whole body CT scans should be avoided due to the cumulative radiationdos e.

4.5.1.5 Adenosarcoma

This uncommon mesenchymal tumour comprises approximately 8% of uterine sarcomas and presents in the same way as most uterine cancers – with unscheduled vaginal bleeding in a post-menopausal patient. These are usually large polypoid endometrial tumours that at histology contain homologous uterine elements such as smooth muscle and stromal cells or heterologous, non-uterine tissues such as striated muscle, cartilage and fat. On MR imaging this tumour is usually apparent as a partly cystic/solid, septated mass distending the endometrial cavity. There is usually early macroscopic evidence of myometrial invasion. The solid areas are of intermediate to low signal on T2 weighted sequences, but in common with other sarcomas, show prominent post-contrast enhancement, in addition to areas of haemorrhage and necrosis. This tumour has a poor 5-year survival, in the order of 10–25% and staging and follow-up should be as for other aggressive endometrial cancers such as carcinosarcomas [38].

4.5.2 Cervical Cancers

Squamous and adenocarcinomas are the commonest sub types of epithelial cancer, constituting over 95% of all cervical neoplasms. Non-epithelial cancers; Lymphomas, rhabdomyosarcomas and other sarcomatous tumours are extremely rare and may occur as a direct extension from the uterus. Unfortunately, with few exceptions, imaging appearances cannot usually differentiate specific histological tumour types in the cervix, but occasionally, appearances can suggest, or correlate with a more unusual or aggressive tumour type, particularly if a large cervical neoplasm presents as an interval screen detected cancer.

Although squamous carcinoma is the commonest epithelial cancer, adenocarcinoma is now occurring with increased frequency, comprising 10–20% of cases, often in older women and with a worse prognosis, stage for stage, than squamous cancer.

Most cervical malignancy originates at the squamocolumnar or transformation zone in the cervix. As this migrates cephalad with increasing age, becoming endocervical, adenocarcinomas in elderly patients can be almost completely endocervical [66]. This may result in a "barrel shaped" enlarged cervix with clinically a grossly normal appearance to the ectocervix and preservation of the endocervical canal [47]. If biopsy results indicate an adenocarcinoma, differentiation from an advanced or aggressive endometrial cancer involving the cervix can be difficult. MR can help to determine the origin of tumour in these patients by identifying the greatest bulk and site of tumour and by weighting the imaging behaviour of cervical vs. endometrial tumour extension, for example by suggesting a uterine origin when there is little or no parametrial tumour extension in the setting of a large mass involving the lower uterine segment and endocervical canal (Fig. 4.23).

Adenoma Malignum (also known as minimal deviation adenocarcinoma) is a sub type of mucinous adenocarcinoma, with a prevalence of 1.3–3% of all cervical adenocarcinomas (Fig. 4.24). It has a worse prognosis than adenocarcinoma, being less responsive to chemoradiation. There is an association with Peutz-Jeghers syndrome, which also has an increased incidence of ovarian mucinous tumours and sex cord tumours with annular tubules (SCTAT) of the ovary [61]. The usual presentation is with watery discharge and unscheduled bleeding. MRI appearances are of prominent endocervical glandular proliferation extending into the cervical stroma, sometimes with solid areas, which are almost indistinguishable from prominent Nabothian cysts, or endocervical mucosal hyperplasia [62, 66]. However, if contrast sequences are obtained then solid elements within the tumour will enhance distinguishing tumour from adjacent cervical stroma and simple benign cystic disease [40].

The deep penetration into the stromal tissue by endocervical glands requires a deep mucosal biopsy for diagnosis, rather than a PAP smear.

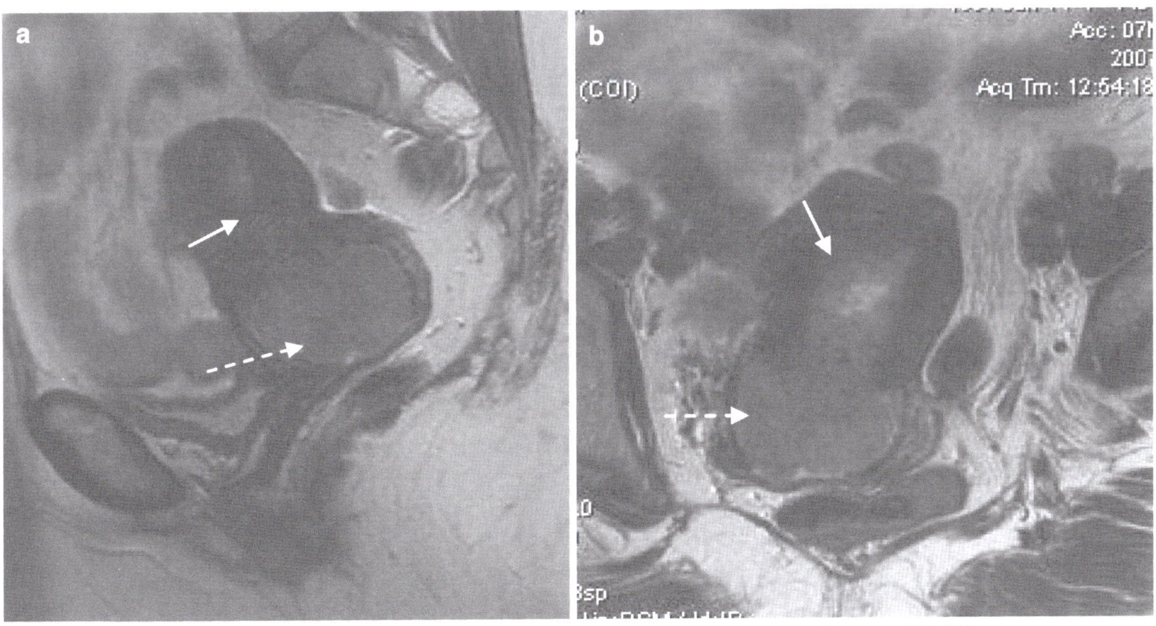

MRI Sagittal T2W

MRI Coronal T2W

Fig. 4.23 Endometrial neoplasm clinically presenting as a large cervical adenocarcinoma. Extensive tumour is seen in the endometrial cavity (*arrows*) extruding through internal os, involving cervical stroma and distending cervix (*broken arrow*), but withoutpa rametriale xtension

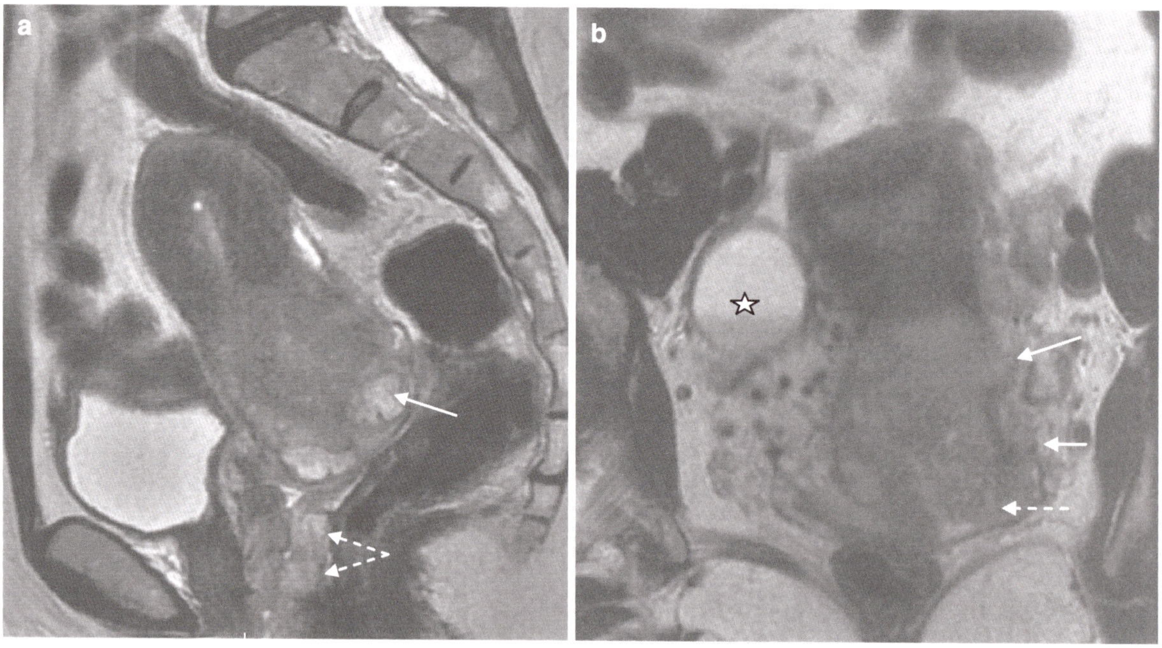

Fig. 4.24 Adenoma malignum. (**a**) Sagittal and (**b**) coronal T2W MR – large, high signal tumour, replacing cervix and containing multiple large and small foci of mucinous fluid (*arrow*) mimicking nabothian cysts. Vaginal metastases (*broken arrows*). (**b**) There is complete cervical stromal invasion by tumour, with foci of high signal mucin (*broken arrows*) with extension into the parametria (*arrows*). Incidental right ovarian cyst (*star*)

The detection of lymph node metastases on MRI may be more difficult with mucin secreting tumours (as occurs with mucin secreting rectal tumours), as this can result in high signal on T2 weighted sequences similar to background fat appearances.

Glassy cell, Adenosquamous cervical carcinoma is a poorly differentiated neoplasm, more common in younger women with an incidence of 1.5–7.5%. On MRI it is usually a solid tumour, hyperintense to cervical stroma. It has a poor prognosis and is often advanced at the time of presentation, with reported 5-year survivalof13–30% [63].

4.5.2.1 SmallC ellC arcinoma

There is a spectrum of rare neuroendocrine tumours which may arise in the cervix. These rare tumours account for 0.5–6% of cervical tumours. Small cell cervical tumours are renowned for their highly aggressive behaviour and advanced stage at presentation. Prognosis is poor with a 35–60% 3-year survival and almost 0% 5-year survival for tumours greater than stage 1B1 [48, 64]. Tumours enlarge rapidly and patients often present with large, lobulated inoperable tumours with widespread lymphtic and haematogenous dissemination (Figs. 4.25 and 4.26). The diagnosis may be suspected when there is grossly disseminated disease, particularly in the presence of biochemical abnormality such as hypercalcaemia, or when extensive disease occurs in an interval screen detected cancer. If small cell carcinoma is evident from cervical biopsy, then although MRI is helpful for optimal local staging to determine whether surgery is an option, complete assessment of metastatic disease is recommended with CT, or CT/PET, of chest, abdomen and pelvis. Even when tumours appear confined to the cervix, without obvious nodal involvement, there is increased likelihood of distant metastatic disease. Although comprehensive imaging is important, it is important that imaging does not delay initiation of treatment, particularly with chemotherapy. Small cell cervical tumours should be regarded in the same way as small cell lung cancers i.e. as a systemic disease and treatment should be initiated as soon as possible.

On MRI there is often a bulky lobulated tumour with extensive parametrial extension, with increased signal on T2 weighted sequences and avid post-contrast enhancement with foci of necrosis and haemorrhage (Fig. 4.26). Most squamous and adenocarcinomas

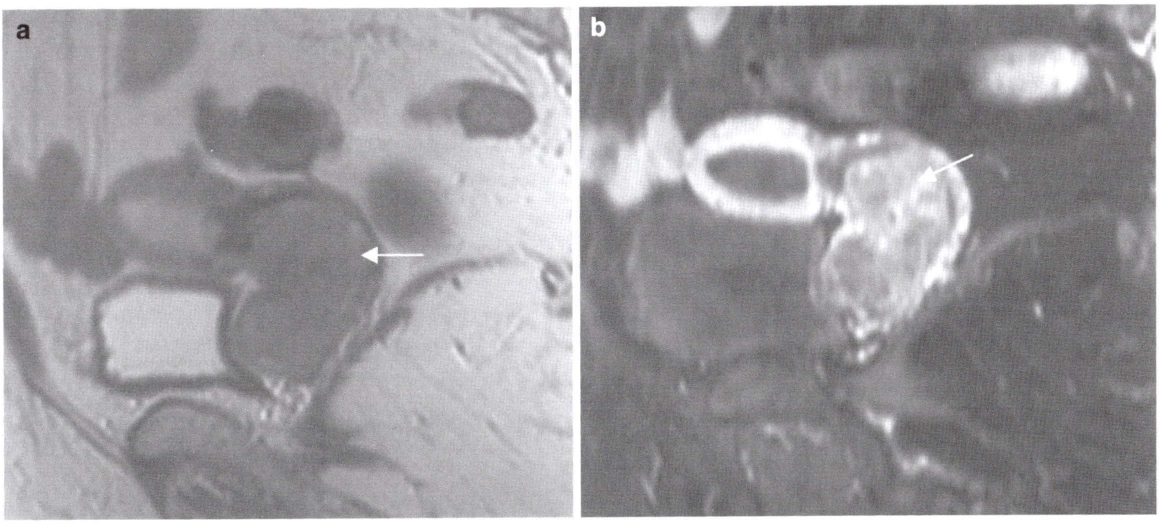

Fig. 4.25 Small cell cervical cancer, Clinical stage IB in post menopausal patient: Liver metastases were present (not shown). (**a**) A small uterus with hydrometra is seen, secondary to cervical occlusion by high signal tumour with marked exophytic "mushroom" appearance (*arrow*). (**b**) Post contrast, there is rapid heterogenous enhancement, but with areas of non-enhancement correspondingt one crosis

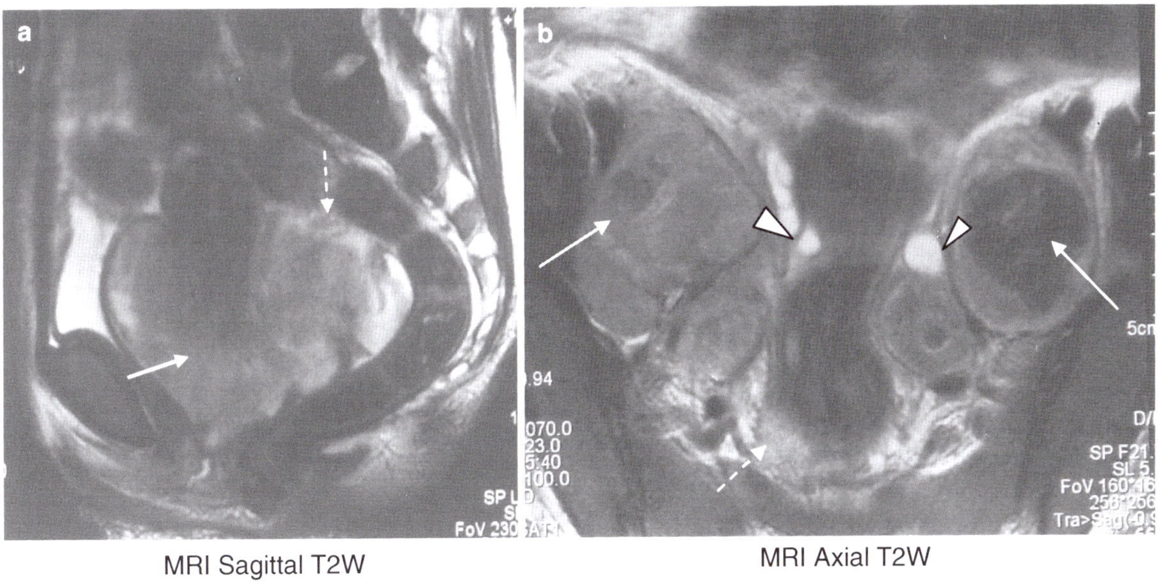

Fig. 4.26 Small cell cervical cancer, pre menopausal patient: (**a**) Extensive 'mushroom' of ectocervical tumour (*arrow*) extending to parametria, involving rectum (*broken arrow*). (**b**) Gross pelvic lymphadenopathy with necrosis (*arrows*), obstructed ureters (*arrowheads*), rectal involvement is present (*broken arrow*)

of the cervix are of increased signal on T2W sequences compared to cervical stroma, but generally only show intermediate post-contrast enhancement. Bulky, widespread nodal metastases, often showing central necrosis on CT or MRI is usually present, even when the primary tumour is less than 4 cm in diameter. There is also a propensity to involve unusual nodal groups e.g.inguina lnode s(Figs . 4.9a nd 4.26).

4.5.3 Uterine and Cervical lymphoma

Primary lymphoma affects the cervix more often than the uterine corpus, although the uterus is more often involved than the cervix as a secondary site for lymphoma(Fig. 4.27).

It is a rare tumour comprising less than 1% of primary cervical neoplasms [65]. On MR imaging, the tumours are bulky, poorly defined and usually hyperintense on T2 and hypointense on T1 weighted sequences with respect to myometrium, with a diffuse infiltration. Distinguishing features are that the endocervical epithelium may be preserved in the presence of extensive stromal tumour and that unlike other large neoplasms, necrosis is rarely evident. Nodal metastases are also unusual until the tumour becomes advanced. Lymphoma involving the uterine corpus may also show extensive bulky tumour but with preservation of the endometrium [43].

Post contrast, there is fairly homogenous tumour enhancement which is almost as prominent as normal myometrium, in contrast to poorly enhancing endometrial adenocarcinomas or hypervascular sarcomas.

In common with other lymphomas, CT of chest abdomen and pelvis is recommended for initial complete staging and to exclude secondary involvement of the uterus from primary lymphoma elsewhere.

4.5.4 Cervical Sarcomas

Cervical sarcomas, comprising mostly LMS and rhabdomyosarcomas, are extremely rare and with a few exceptions for more differentiated sub-types, are associated with a poor prognosis. Most have early haematogenous metastases and initial staging should include CT of chest, abdomen and pelvis.

Rhabdomyosarcomas may be suspected by the presence of a bulky, vascular tumour replacing the cervix in an adolescent, although gynaecological rhabdomyosarcomas occur more commonly in the vagina or vulva.

LMS occur in the 4th to 6th decades, involving the cervix are usually bulky, lobulated, heterogenous hypervascular masses with extension into adjacent tissue planes at presentation [40, 41]. They have similar features to uterine LMS.

4.5.5 Vaginal Tumours

Primary vaginal malignancies, comprise 1–2% of gynaecological malignancies, although vaginal metastases, especially from other gynaecological tumours, are not uncommon, accounting for more than 80% of vaginal neoplasia. Involvement of the vaginal vault following resection of previous gynaecological malignancy is a particularly a common manifestation of recurrence. The majority of primary tumours (over 85%) are squamous cancers, usually with the same epidemiological risk

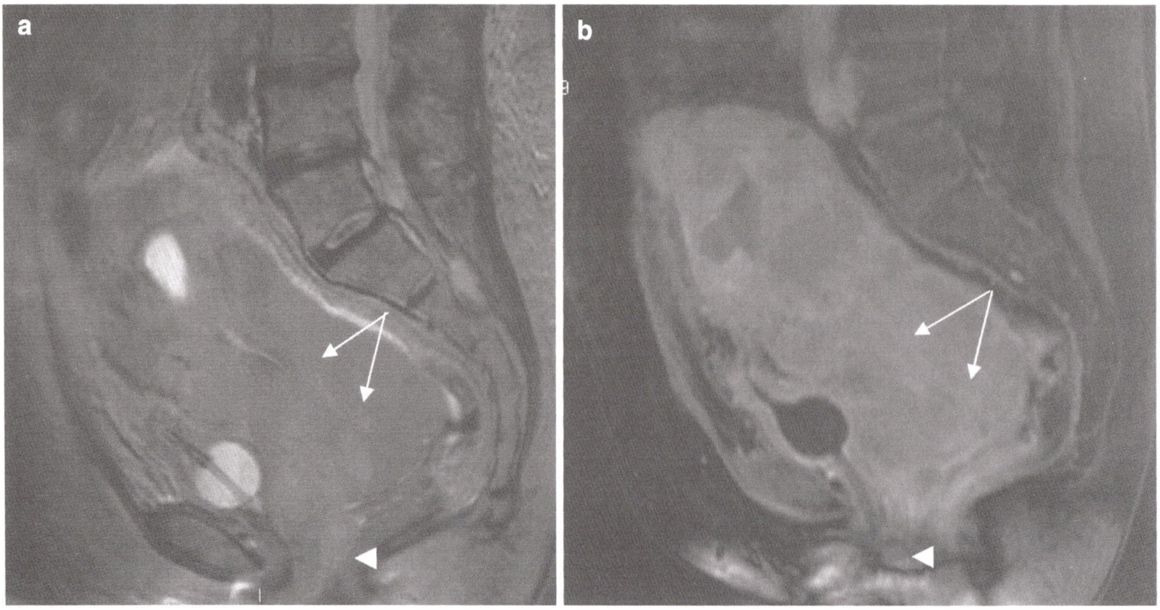

Fig. 4.27 (**a**) Primary lymphoma of uterus and cervix (*arrows*) expanding and destroying normal zonal architecture and hypodense cervical stroma. Overall organ shape is maintained. Further extension to vaginal wall (*arrowhead*). (**b**) Post contrast, tumour enhances almost as well as myometrium (cf. endometrial cancers). Note abnormal enhancement and expansion of cervix but with normal configurationof e ndocervicalc anal

factors as for cervical cancers. Although it can be difficult to decide the site of origin if the cervix is involved, 75% of squamous vaginal tumours arise in the cervix and this is then considered to be the site of origin. The FIGO classification regards any tumour involving the external os as a cervical primary tumour, regardless of the size of the vaginal component.

Most primary vaginal squamous tumours arise in the posterior, upper third, which may be related to repeated coital trauma and this may be preceded by vaginal intraepithelial malignancy (VAIN).

Adenocarcinomas, melanoma, sarcoma and metastases account for the remaining tumours, often occurringina younge ra gegroup [67, 69].

Adenocarcinomas are associated with in utero exposure to diethylstilbestrol (DES), predominantly used in the USA up until the 1970s.

There is an increased incidence of squamous carcinomas occurring more than 10 years after successful radiotherapy for cervical carcinoma (Fig. 4.28) [67]. Although it is difficult to exclude primary vaginal neoplasms occurring as a result of persistent risk factors, in our experience, some of these tumours have occurred at slightly atypical locations, often at the penumbra of the previous radiotherapy field. An increased incidence of vaginal LMS has also been reported more than 5 years following radiotherapy.

Clinical presentation is usually with irregular vaginal bleeding or discharge, pain, urinary symptoms and

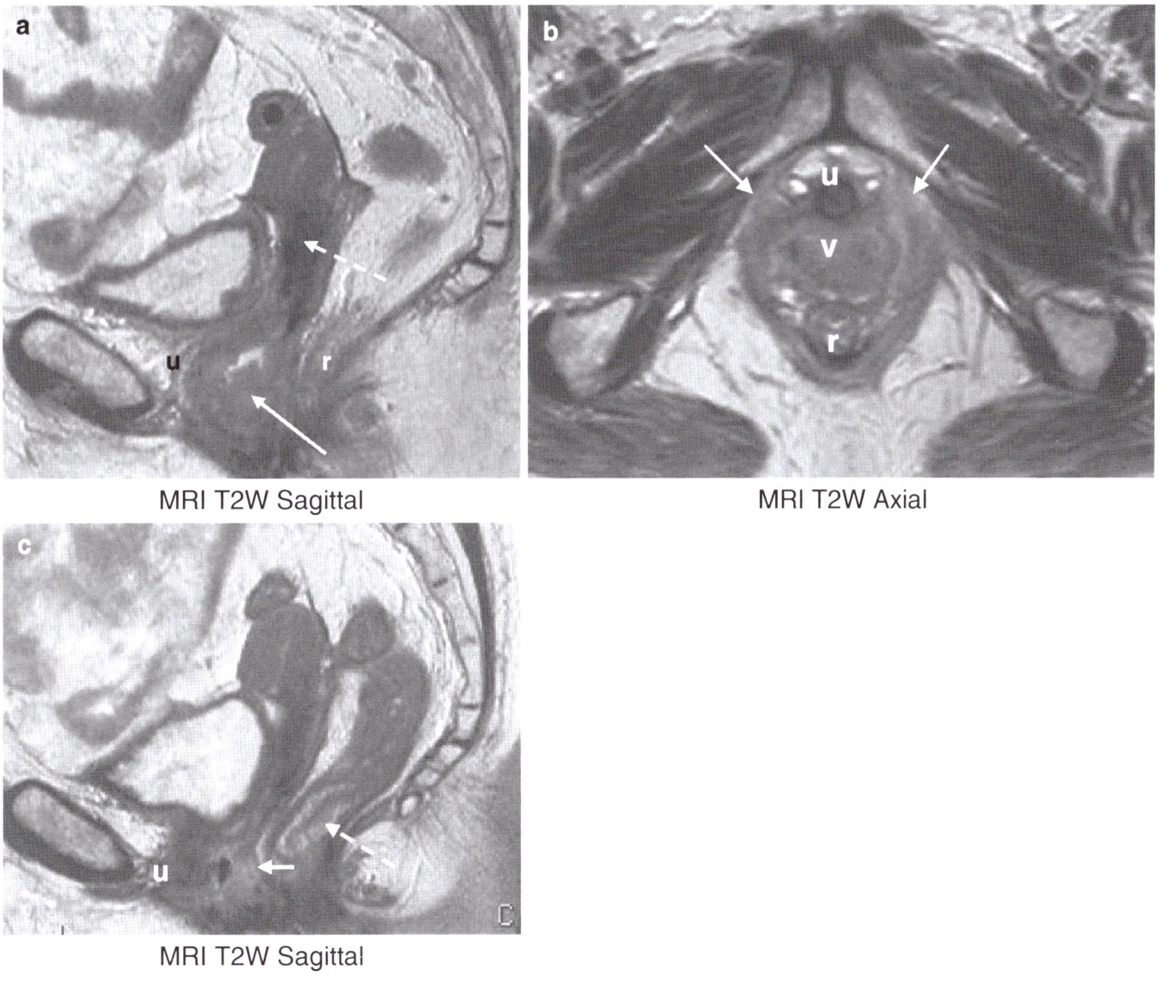

Fig. 4.28 Squamous Vaginal Carcinoma arising in lower vagina 20 years after radiotherapy for cervical carcinoma. MRI Sagittal T2W (**a**) Tumour (*arrow*) encircling lower vagina and invading urethra (not shown) chronic post-radiotherapy changes to cervix and uterus (*broken arrow*). (**b**) T2W Axial section lower vagina (v): extensive infiltrating tumour (*arrow*) involving puborectalis muscle bilaterally (*arrows*). Normal appearance of urethra (u) and anorectal (r) junction at this level. (**c**) Four months post-radiotherapy shows good response of vaginal tumour (*arrow*). Acute radiotherapy related change in rectum (*broken arrow*)

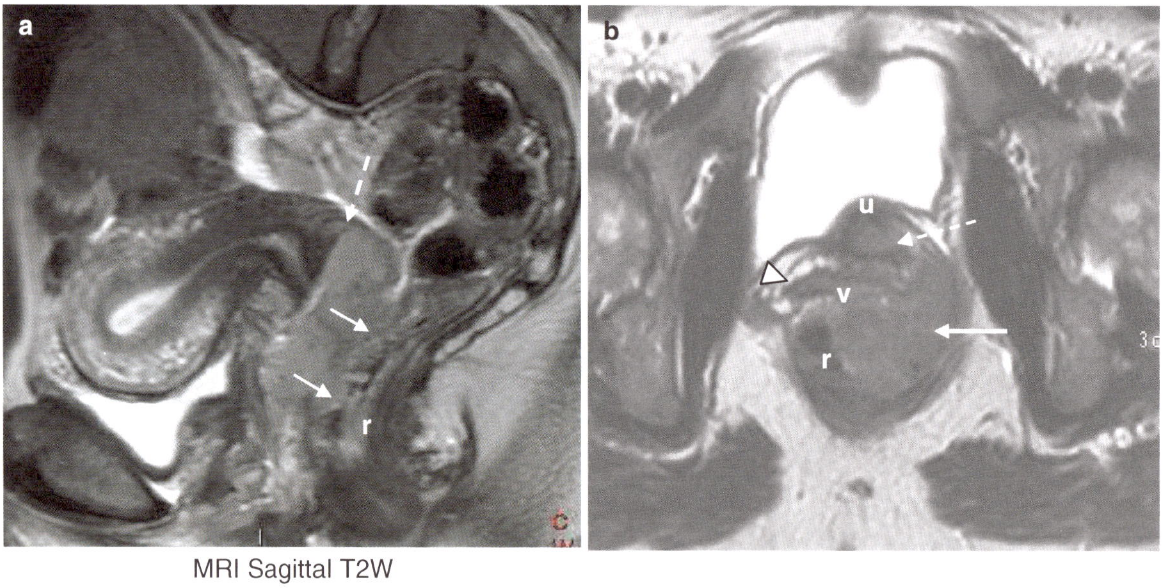

Fig. 4.29 Squamous Carcinoma developing in mature teratoma: Squamous Vaginal carcinoma stage 4 a) primarily involving (**a**) posterior upper two thirds (*arrow*). Involvement of mucosal surface of cervix (*broken arrow*) extension to rectum (r) through rectovaginal septum (*small arrows*). (**b**) Axial section through upper vagina. Tumour (*arrow*) extending to left levator and urethral muscle (*broken arrow*) (u-urethra, v-vagina, r-rectum) Note normal low signal of uninvolved right vaginal wall muscle (*arrowhead*)

a feeling of a mass. Clinically, tumours are usually visible as an ulcerating or fungating mass and less often as a constricting or annular lesion. Imaging is important to determine stage and potential resectability. Tumours are usually advanced at presentation, with infiltrative margins which spread easily to urethra, bladder base and rectum due to lack of adjacent peritoneal or anatomic fascial planes. Nodal metastases occur early and these may include inguinal as well as intrapelvic nodes [68]. Extension to pelvic muscles (Figs. 4.28 and 4.29), precludes successful surgical resection.

Most tumours are of intermediate to high signal on MRI T2 weighted sequences. The high signal intensity of the tumour allows accurate determination of tumour penetration through the normal low signal muscular wall of the vagina (Fig. 4.29b) providing staging information and suitability for surgery. Tumours with very high signal, approximating to fluid, suggest either areas of necrosis in an aggressive squamous carcinoma or mucin secretion tumour in an adenocarcinoma. The latter occur more commonly on the upper anterior wall and without previous DES exposure are thought to arise in foci of adenosis or endometriosis. These tend to be bulky tumours, correlating with clinical findings.

Vaginal Melanomas are less common than vulval melanomas. There are only a few reports of imaging appearances with MRI. Melanin has a paramagnetic effect giving increased signal on MR, so depending on the amount of melanin in the tumour, they can present with a solid tumour that may show increased signal on both T1 and T2W sequences, although this can be confused with intratumoural haemorrhage. Amelanotic tumours will have a low signal on T1W sequences; thus an absence of increased signal does not exclude melanoma [69].

LMS are extremely rare aggressive tumours, with a reported increased incidence following previous radiotherapy. Imaging appearances have been reported as being similar to uterine and cervical LMS; with bulky, heterogenous and vascular enhancing tumours. Areas of haemorrhage and necrosis may be apparent. The latter appearances may help to differentiate this from benign vaginal leiomyomas, which usually have the same imaging characteristics as mature uterine leiomyomas; typically low signal on T1 and T2 weighted sequences due to the mature fibroustis sue(Fig. 4.30).

4.5.6 Rare Ovarian Tumours

Most patients with rare ovarian cancers will present with the same symptoms and signs as common epithelial tumours. But those rare tumours associated with abnormal biochemistry, or hormone secretion will often be present with clinical signs or symptoms related to that functional activity.

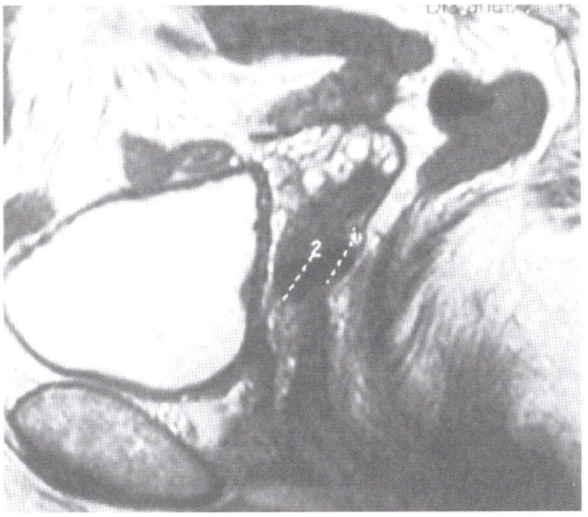

Fig. 4.30 Vaginal Leiomyomas: Seventy-two year old woman with vaginal discharge. Previous hysterectomy for benign disease. Low signal masses T2W (and T1W not shown), consistent withl eiomyomas

Age at presentation is a particularly important discriminatory factor so that in the first three decades a germ cell or sex cord stromal tumour is the commonest ovarian malignancy. Hormonally functioning tumours, such as granulosa tumours (GCT), with increased oestrogen levels, may present with effects secondary to endometrial hyperplasia Conversely, virilisation may prompt diagnosis of a Sertoli Leydig tumour. Small cell ovarian carcinomas often have accompanying metabolic disturbances such as hypercalcaemia or struma ovarii tumours that of associated hyperthyroidism [88]. This additional clinical information will influence the radiological interpretation of an adnexal mass and add clues to allow a specific diagnosis based on imaging interpretaion.

4.5.7 Germ Cell Tumours

These can be broadly divided into teratomatous and non-teratomatous. Teratomatous tumours are further divided into benign and malignant categories, with further subdivision of malignant types into monophasic, such as carcinoid tumours and polyphasic which includes malignancy developing in benign mature teratomas, and immature teratomas with several malignant elements.

Non-teratomatous germ cell tumours comprise dysgerminoma, yolk sac tumour, non-gestational choriocarcinoma and gonadoblastoma.

4.5.8 Teratoma

Mature teratomas are most frequent in children and premenopausal women, with up to 10% bilateral. These tumours contain mature adult tissue from at least two of three germ cell layers: ectoderm, endoderm and mesoderm and radiologically are usually easily identified on CT, MRI, and often on ultrasound, by the characteristic appearance of fat, calcification or bone, and hair or sebaceous elements. The latter is often seen as an oily layer, perhaps containing a hair ball, floating on the fluid component of a cyst (Fig. 4.31). Hair, bone and teeth commonly arise from a solid "Rokitansky" nodule, an avascular solid nodule projecting intraluminally from the cyst wall [90]. Post-contrast enhancement of a Rokitansky nodule is suspicious, but not specific for malignant transformation [90]. When the combination of fatty and calcified elements are missing, the imaging diagnosis of a benign dermoid cyst is more difficult.

Monodermal teratomas, arising from one germ cell line, can give rise to struma ovarii, primary carcinoid or neural tumours and some of these tumours have a more specificima ginga ppearance [71, 72].

Malignant transformation of elements of a mature teratoma has a reported incidence of less than 1%, and can occur in any one of the three germ cell layers, although squamous carcinoma, arising from epithelial elements occurs most commonly, accounting for 80% of cases [73, 90]. Malignant transformation of a mature teratoma generally has a poor prognosis, occurring typically in a patient beyond the fourth decade of life, with a large, greater than 10 cm cyst, which is rapidly increasing in size. On imaging, there is often a prominent, irregular and vascular/enhancing solid component (Figs. 4.31 and 4.32) which can be seen to extend beyond the cyst margin and infiltrate adjacent tissue planes. Peritoneal involvement may produce ascites (Fig. 4.32). Metastases may be either lymphatic, haematogenous or intraperitoneal. Local tissue invasion of the pelvic side wall often results in incomplete surgical excision and recurrence, particularly if this is not identified pre-operatively with referral to a specialist unit.

These malignant teratomas may be associated with elevated Squamous Carcinoma Antigen, CA125 and CEA levels, which may be helpful in surveillance monitoring, with rising levels triggering further imaging [71].

Struma Ovarii is a mature monodermal cystic teratomas composed entirely or predominantly of thyroid tissue, containing variable sized follicles with colloid material. Thyroid tissue is not infrequently part of a mature teratoma. Thyrotoxicosis can occur in about

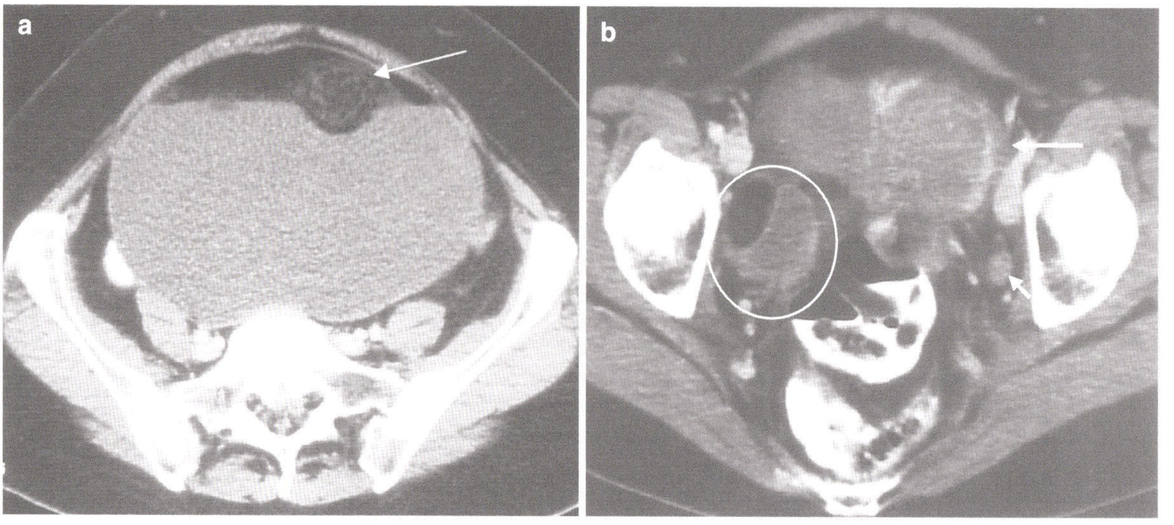

Fig. 4.31 Squamous Carcinoma developing in mature teratoma: Squamous Cancer arising in mature teratoma: 50-year-old patient with increasing abdominal girth and pain. Bilateral, mature teratomas with development of cancer in left teratoma. (**a**) Typical fat fluid level and floating hair ball (*arrow*) within upper margin of large cyst. (**b**) Inferiorly, large vascular component to the solid element which, extends through the cyst wall (*arrow*). Enlarged, malignant left obturator node (*small arrow*). Coexisting small right mature teratoma (*ellipse*)

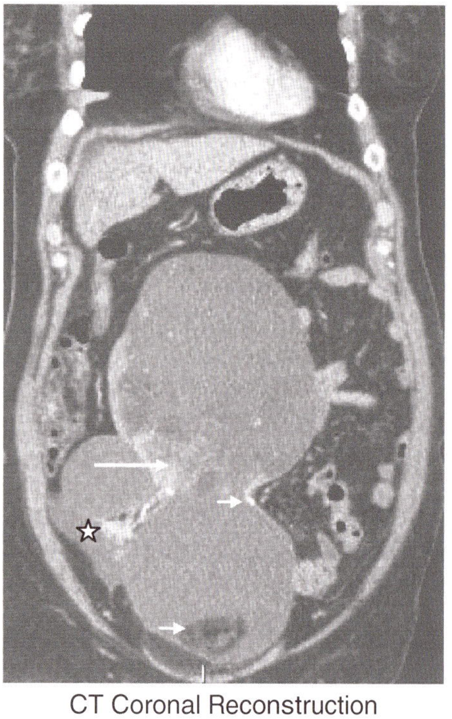

CT Coronal Reconstruction

Fig. 4.32 Sebaceous gland tumour arising in a mature teratoma: Note large size of cyst with irregular enhancing solid area (*arrow*) in addition to foci of fat and calcification (*short arrows*). On other sections, areas of capsular invasion are seen with a pocket of abdominal ascites (*)

5% of cases and thyroid carcinoma can occur rarely, behaving in a similar manner to primary thyroid malignancy. This will require specific imaging with radioactive iodine and possibly CT/PET, with management similar to that of a primary thyroid malignancy, but likely to involve total thyroidectomy to allow follow-up surveillance with serum thyroglobulin levels.

The imaging appearances of struma ovarii are complex, often with multiple cystic and solid areas. On MRI, these cystic locules show variable signal intensities secondary to the thick, gelatinous colloid material which varies in proteinaceous or haemorrhagic content, causing changes in MR signal within each of the locules (Fig. 4.33). Despite this, when hyperthyroidism is not present, it can be difficult to differentiate appearances from other causes of complex cystic adnexal masses, both benign and malignant, such as endometriosis, tuboovarian abscesses and cystadenocarcinoma [71].

4.5.9 Carcinoid Tumours

These are the second commonest monodermal ovarian teratomas after struma ovarii and these are regarded as malignant.

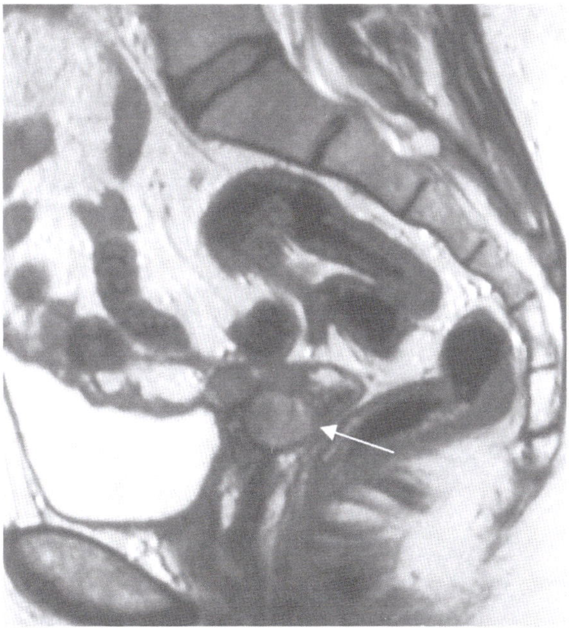

Fig. 4.33 Recurrent malignant struma ovarii (thyroid carcinoma) to vaginal vault (*arrow*) post total hysterectomy and oophorectomy. Similar appearance to primary tumour, with multipleloc ulesw ithdi fferent" shading"onM RI

Primary ovarian carcinoids tumours are usually slow growing, medium sized (8 cm) unilateral, solid hypervascular, tumours occurring in post-menopausal patients [72].

Functioning tumours are generally greater than 10 cm in size and arise from the progenitor neuroendocrine cells of respiratory or gastrointestinal epithelium in teratomas. Approximately, one quarter to one third of primary ovarian carcinoid tumours (almost always of insular type) will result in the carcinoid syndrome. Unlike gastrointestinal carcinoid tumours, secretion of serotonin analogues into the systemic ovarian veins directly will bypass the breakdown by hepatic enzymes and result in the carcinoid syndrome, without the presence of hepatic metastases; thus the development of the syndrome and resultant cardiovascular effects is likely to be proportionally higher than for GI carcinoids. Patients may initially present with the valvular effects of right heart failure, in the absence of a symptomatic pelvic mass.

Most patients will present with stage one disease, localised to the ovary, although image interpretation may be confused by the cardiac effects of cardiac carcinoid syndrome producing ascites secondary to heart failure. In stage one disease, unilateral oophorectomy does not appear to predispose to recurrence. There is the potential for a long progression-free interval of more than 10 years, with prolonged follow-up warranted. Survival in higher stage disease is poor; with a historical 33% 5-year survival reported [75].

Although CT scan of the chest, abdomen and pelvis is recommended for full staging, as for other advanced ovarian cancers, the majority of carcinoid tumours will have somatostatin receptors avid for Indium labelled Octreotide or pentreotide and uptake of these radiotracers can be used for localisation of the primary tumour and metastatic disease as well as targeted direct therapy with therapeutic doses of radioisotopes. Follow-up imaging can be prompted by a rise in urinary 5 hydroxy indole acetic acid (5 HIAA) and/or plasma serotonin. For non-functioning tumours, CT/PET is likely to localise metastases, although CT post-contrast, particularly in a late arterial phase, is likely to detect most deposits due to the hypervascular nature of this tumour.

In common with carcinoid tumours from lung and bowel, an unusual feature is the presence of sclerotic bone metastases, which can be easily overlooked (Fig. 4.34). These usually show intense uptake on isotopebone s cans.

4.5.10 Immature Teratomas

Malignant, immature ovarian teratomas or germ cell tumours, comprise approximately 2–3% of ovarian cancers. Apart from their usual presentation in the first three decades of life, these tumours, which contain immature or embryonic tissues, typically secrete a combination of human chorionic gonadotrophins, alpha fetoproteins, human placental lactogen and lactic dehydrogenase. Cross-sectional imaging, with either CT or MR in these young patients is often prompted by an abnormal tumour marker profile after a complex mass is initially seen on ultrasound. Occasionally, patients will present acutely with pain, secondary to torsion or haemorrhage and a diagnosis will only be made following emergency surgery. Five percent of these tumours are bilateral, predominantly dysgerminomas and less often yolk sac tumours, so pre-operative imaging is important to define the extent of disease so that fertility sparing surgery can be considered. In 10–15% of cases, CT or MR will identify a benign mature teratoma on the contralateralo vary.

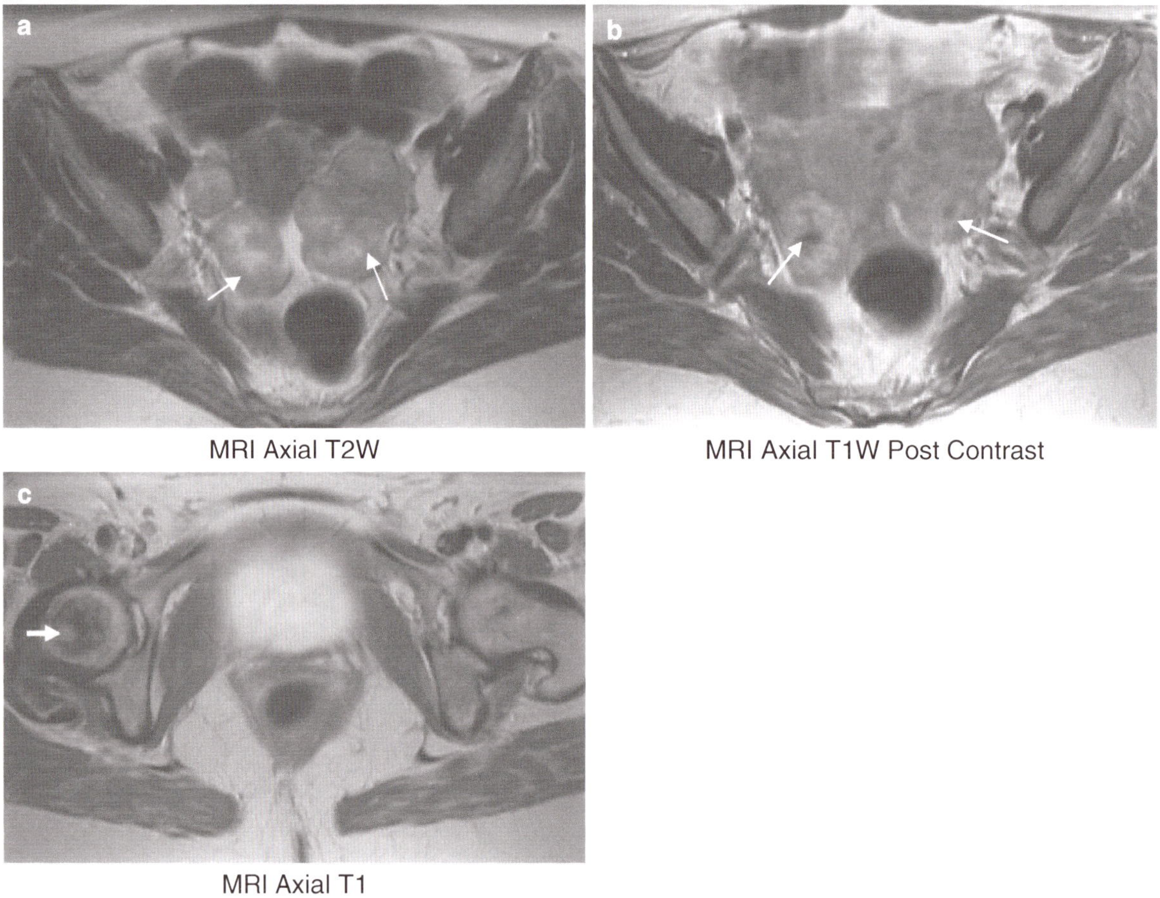

Fig. 4.34 Bilateral ovarian carcinoid tumours; 50 year old patient. Solid, well-defined, lobulated, hypervascular masses with areas of central necrosis (*arrows*).(**c**)S cleroticm etastasist or ightf emoralhe ad

Many of these tumours are aggressive, often with a poor prognosis, although treatment and survival has improved, particularly with dysgerminomas. Early haematogenous and lymphatic spread in most germ cell tumours requires full staging of chest, abdomen and pelvis. Initial CT of the chest is recommended to detect lung metastases. Although CT in the abdomen is more sensitive than MRI for the detection of calcification, MRI is often more appropriate for assessment of the abdomen and pelvis, to minimise radiation doses in these young patients, particularly when a malignant diagnosis has not been established.

On imaging, immature germ cell tumours can be differentiated from mature teratomas by their larger size, (mean diameter 12–25 cm) and by the larger proportion of solid tissue, often irregularly dispersed around the cystic mass. Fat and calcification also tend to be more irregularly dispersed within the cyst (Figs. 4.35 and 4.36). Metastatic disease within the peritoneal cavity may manifest not only as areas of solid enhancing tissue, but as foci of calcification and fat (Fig. 4.37). Ascites may or may not accompany metastatic peritoneal dissemination, but tends to be less prominent than in routine epithelial tumours.

At surgery, or on follow-up imaging, multiple small peritoneal implants may be seen. This condition is likely to represent benign gliomatosis peritonei. Some of these deposits may grow large enough to warrant surgical excision. However, they should be distinguished from the development of metastatic peritoneal deposits of tumour which may be distinguished by showing discrete foci of fat or calcification, best appreciated on CT rather than MRI on follow-up imaging (Fig. 4.37).

Dysgerminomas comprise approximately 50% of malignant germ cell tumours, occurring most often in the second to third decades. They are typically solid, with a propensity to spread to lymph nodes and up to 10% can be bilateral.

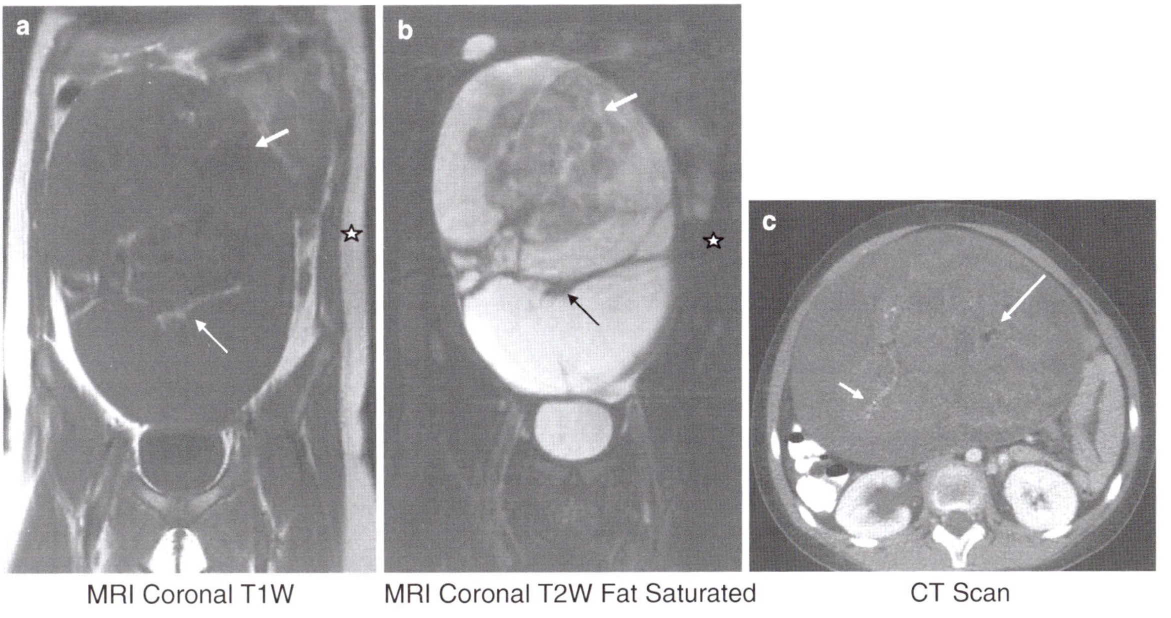

Fig. 4.35 Immature cystic teratoma, 13 year old: (**a**) Very large complex malignant cystic immature teratoma extending to the xiphisternum. The fat component (*arrow*) follows that of subcutaneous fat signal (*). (**b**) T2W fat saturated image; the fat follows the subcutaneous fat signal and the high signal fluid and solid tissue component (*short arrow*) is accentuated. (**c**) CT shows the fat (*arrow*), but also fine calcification (*small arrow*) and solid tissue within the cyst. Note right hydronephrosis secondaryt opr essuree ffect

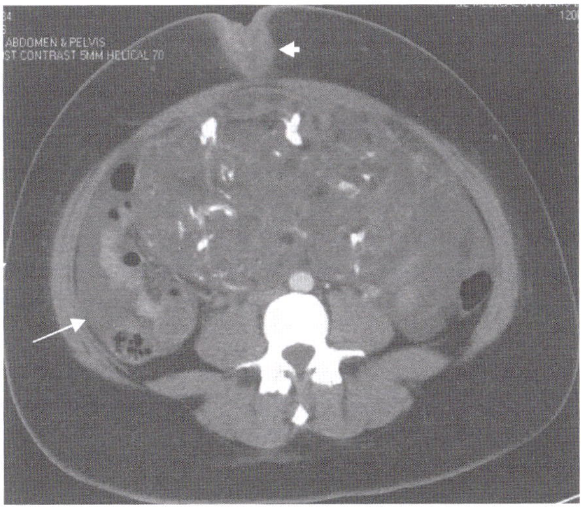

Fig. 4.36 CT: large Immature teratoma with foci of fat, calcification, solid tissue, ascites (*arrow*) and malignant umbilical nodule (*arrowhead*)

On imaging with CT or MR, there is often a large, solid, lobulated mass with areas of haemorrhage, central necrosis and on CT, speckles of calcification. Post-contrast, there is general enhancement of the tumour bulk but with prominent, characteristic enhancement of fibro vascular septae running through the mass. Ascites may be present, but nodal spread is more common than peritoneal dissemination (Figs. 4.38a nd 4.39) [47].

These tumours often present with stage one disease unlike other malignant germ cell tumours and generally have a better prognosis with 5-year survival for early stage of 95%, reducing to 65% for advanced stage disease. Fertility sparing surgery is therefore particularly important. In patients with dysgenetic gonads (containing a Y chromosome) there is a 50% chance of gonadal malignant degeneration. If bilateral oophorectomy is not performed, the contralateral ovary should be carefully assessed and followed up with both imaging and tumour markers (HCG and LDH) [76]. Although there is little supporting evidence, 6 monthly transvaginal ultrasound and tumour markers may be appropriate, in-line with patients at high genetic risk for development of epithelial ovarian cancer. In these young patients, surveillance of the abdomen and pelvis should preferably utilise MRI, but comprehensive imaging of abdomen and pelvis in early stage disease may only be necessary if triggered by a rise in tumour markers suggesting recurrence.

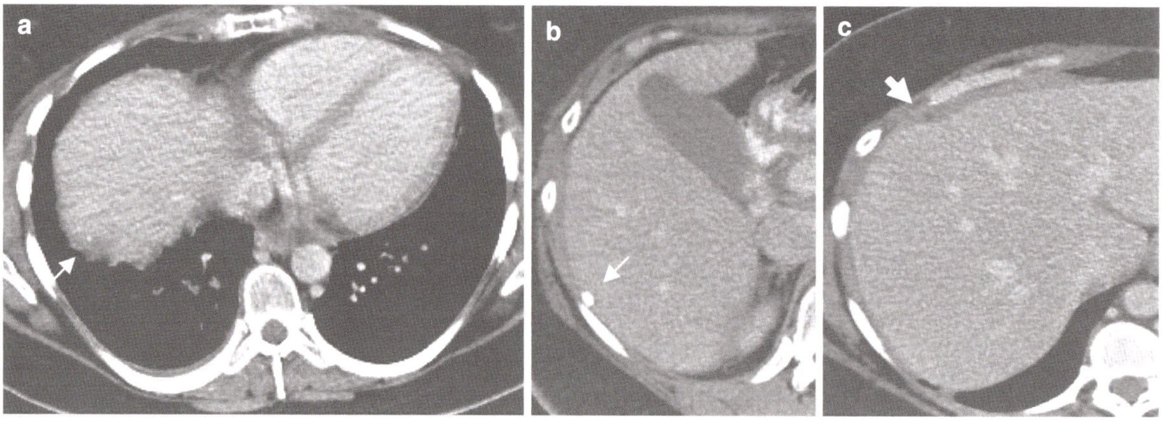

Fig. 4.37 Immature Teratoma recurrence: (**a**) CT: Follow-up, after hysterectomy and bilateral oophorectomy. Peritoneal thickening over the dome of the liver (*arrow*). (**b**) Six months later, there is increase in calcification within the hepatic pericapsular deposit (*arrow*) and (**c**) a deposit of fat (negative Hounsfield units on CT) appearing in an anterior subcapsular deposit (*arrowhead*)

4.5.11 Yolk Sac Tumours

Yolk sac tumours, or endodermal sinus tumours, comprise approximately 20% of malignant germ cell tumours; less than 1% of all malignant ovarian tumours, usually presenting in the second decade of life [77]. They often have mixed histology, occurring in combination with other tumour types, but these are usually aggressive tumours, rapidly increasing in size and often presenting with advanced stage disease.

They are usually large, greater than 10 cm solid/cystic, hypervascular masses, and frequently presenting with increasing girth, pain, haemorrhagic ascites or haemoperitoneum leading to emergency laparotomy. Pre-operative imaging and staging is often limited when there is an acute presentation, but as these tumours are almost always unilateral, bilateral oophorectomy is not generally indicated, although the prognosis is related to optimal surgical debulking. On CT [78], and MRI (Fig. 4.40) a complex, hypervascular mass with areas of cystic change/degeneration and prominent tumoural and feeding blood vessels is typically seen, with dense ascitic fluid corresponding to haemorrhage. A concurrent mature teratoma may be present which can contribute an area of focal fat and calcification. Peritoneal dissemination can occur with ascites and peritoneal implants. If acute cyst rupture occurs, these tumours may be mistaken for an ectopic pregnancy, presenting with haemoperitoneum and a complex adnexal mass, but as they secrete alpha fetoprotein rather than HCG, a complex ruptured luteal cyst is more likely to cause greater diagnostic confusion in the pre-operative differential diagnosis.

Prognosis is often poor with 5-year survival of 95% for stage 1, diminishing to 25% for stage 4 disease with frequent early local and peritoneal recurrence [48].

4.5.12 Sex Cord Stromal Tumours

Sex cord stromal tumours are uncommon, comprising approximately 8% of ovarian tumours. They arise from ovarian stromal cells, giving rise to thecomas, fibromas and Leydig tumours [88]. Primitive sex cords give rise to tumours of granulosa cell, steroid cell and Sertoli cell lines within ovarian tumours. These tumours affect all age groups and a large proportion of them give rise to oestrogenic or virilising effects. Hormonal effects prompt earlier presentation and unlike epithelial tumours, most (70%) of the malignant tumours present at FIGO stage 1, and therefore usually have a good prognosis following complete surgical excision. In contrast to epithelial and immature germ cell tumours, most sex cord tumours are predominantly solid(Fig. 4.41) [77, 80].

4.5.13 Granulosa Tumours

These tumours comprise between 2 and 5% of all ovarian neoplasms and are the commonest malignant sex cord stromal tumour. Most tumours are functional, secreting oestrogen, which results in approximately two thirds of patients presenting with endocrine manifestations of either pseudo precocity (early puberty without

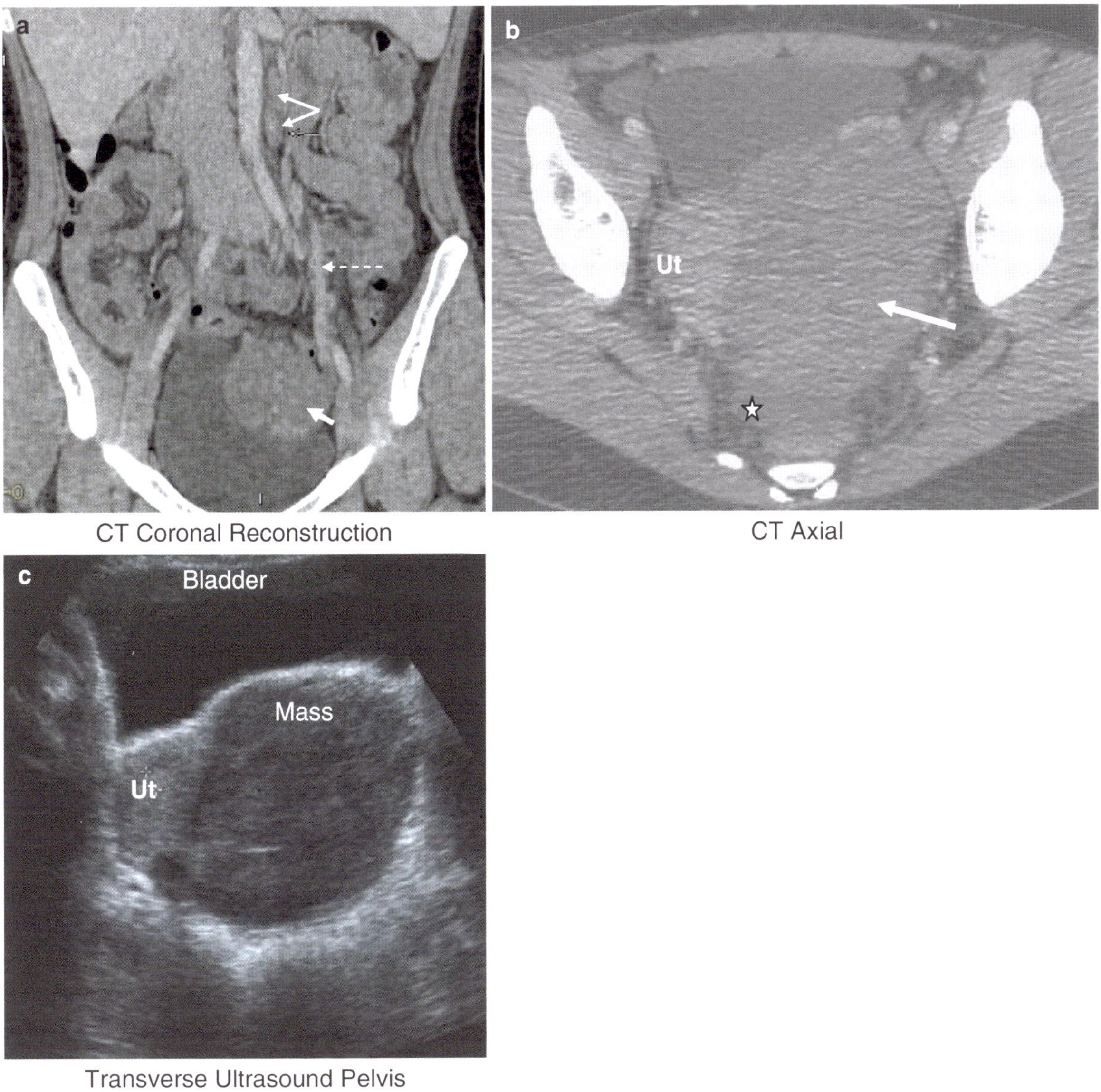

Fig. 4.38 Dysgerminoma of left ovary in a 25-year-old with abdominal pain and distension. (**a** and **b**) Large solid left adnexal mass (*broad arrow*) displacing uterus (Ut) with distended left ovarian vein (*broken arrow*), enlarged para-aortic lymph nodes (*small arrows*) and ascites (*). Corresponding initial ultrasound; (**c**)c onfirmss olidhom ogenousna ture

early ovulation), or post-menopausal or unscheduled bleeding secondary to endometrial hyperplasia or endometrial cancer. Due to the hypervascular nature of this tumour, patients can also present with an acute abdomen secondary to haemoperitoneum, mimicking an ectopic pregnancy in younger patients.

Granulosa cell tumours (GCT) are divided into juvenile and adult types, depending on histology. The juvenile type is associated with Ollier's disease (multiple enchondromatosis) and Mafucci syndrome (multiple enchondromatosis and haemangiomas)and should be considered in a young patient with stigmata of the disease, presenting with a pelvic mass or if enchondromata are seen on staging CT or MR scans.

Over 75% patients with GCT present with stage 1 disease, confined to the ovary. The juvenile form in particular tends to present early and have a more favourable prognosis, with less likelihood of recurrence. The more common adult type accounts for 95% of these tumours, with a peak prevalence around the menopause, 50–55 years, although it can occur at any age. These tumours are considered to be a low grade malignancy, but are characterised by unpredictable recurrence, more than 30 years after complete surgical resection [81] although

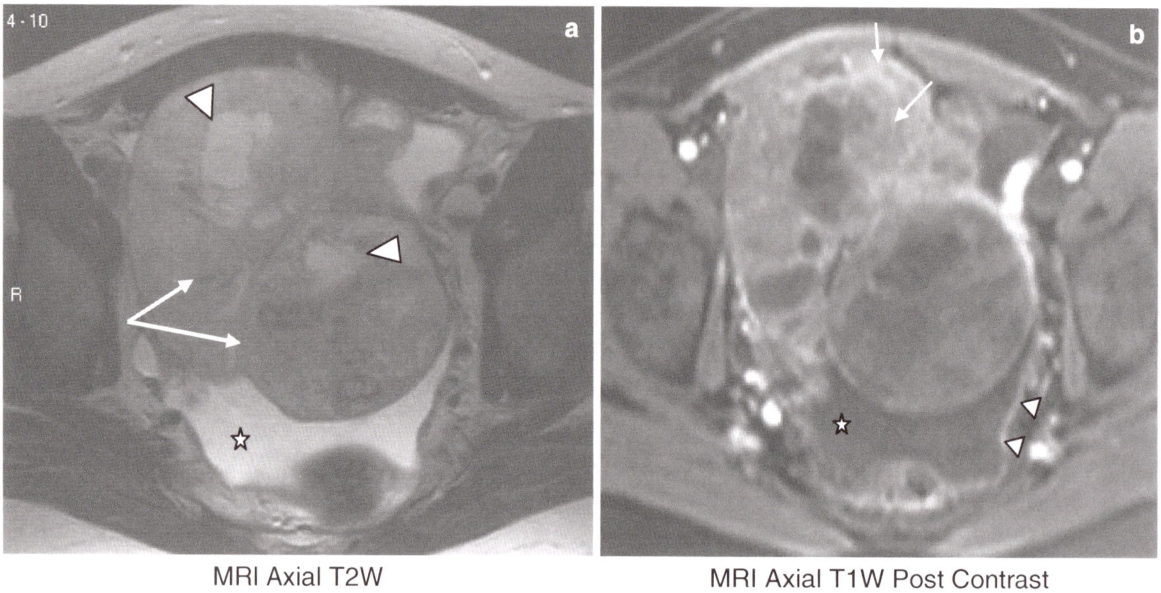

Fig. 4.39 (**a** and **b**) Dysgerminoma left ovary in a 19-year-old with abdominal pain and distension. MRI appearances confirm a largely solid, enhancing large lobulated mass (*arrows*) with areas of cystic degeneration (*arrowhead*) and foci of haemorrhage. Arterial phase post-contrast images (4.39b) demonstrate enhancing fibrovascular septae (*arrows*). Ascites (*) and widespread peritoneal dissemination (*arrowheads*) has occurred in additiont opa ra-aorticnoda lm etastasis(nots hown)

average recurrence times are between 5 and 10 years [80]. The likelihood of recurrence is most closely related to stage at presentation, but despite complete surgical resection, a significant number of patients with disease confined to the ovary will unexpectedly relapse [82, 83].

On imaging, GCT's have a spectrum of appearances, but are typically a unilateral, fairly slow growing, encapsulated multi-cystic mass with septations and a large proportion of solid tissue. They can also appear as completely solid masses. GCT's are hypervascular tumours, which can lead to, complex, haemorrhagic cysts (Fig. 4.42) and it is this tendency to haemorrhage which can result in rupture with an accompanying haemoperitoneum. A small proportion of these tumours will be almost completely cystic and these are more often associated with androgen secretion and virilisation. Unlike epithelial tumours, calcification and diffuse intraperitoneal and nodal dissemination is rare and accompanying ascites is more likely to reflect previous or recent haemorrhage.

MRI is the most useful imaging to diagnose these tumours pre operatively, due to its ability to display the cyst morphology and to detect haemorrhage (Figs. 4.42 and 4.43). On MRI, the tumour characteristically appears as a hypervascular mass with a myriad of small cysts [83]. The presence of secondary oestrogenic effects of endometrial thickening and hypertrophic endocervical mucous glands in a post-menopausal patient will also prompt suspicion that a complex adnexal mass may be a GCT.

Recurrrent GCT tumours share the same distribution pattern as epithelial tumours. Although deposits within the peritoneal cavity are the commonest site of recurrence (Fig. 4.44), involvement of the omentum or bowel mesentery is more unusual. Retroperitoneal recurrence also occurs frequently, although this probably relates to growth from a nodal deposit, but evidence of more generalised lymphadenopathy is rare. Haematogenous dissemination is rare, even with relapsed disease, but hepatic and lung metastases have been reported.

Recurrent tumour deposits tend to be slow growing, well circumscribed and ranging in size from 1 to 10 cm. They are usually solid but heterogenous, which reflects areas of necrosis and hypervascularity. The presentation of these masses, so long after treatment for the original tumour, not infrequently leads to an erroneous diagnosis of alternative pathology such as nerve sheath tumours or paragangliomas, depending on the site of recurrence.

Devising a follow-up approach for "at risk" patients is difficult due to this tumour's unpredictable behaviour. Metastatic disease is often localised, which unlike most epithelial cancers, can result in significant long-term survival following repeat surgery. Thus imaging follow-up for asymptomatic individuals may be justified.

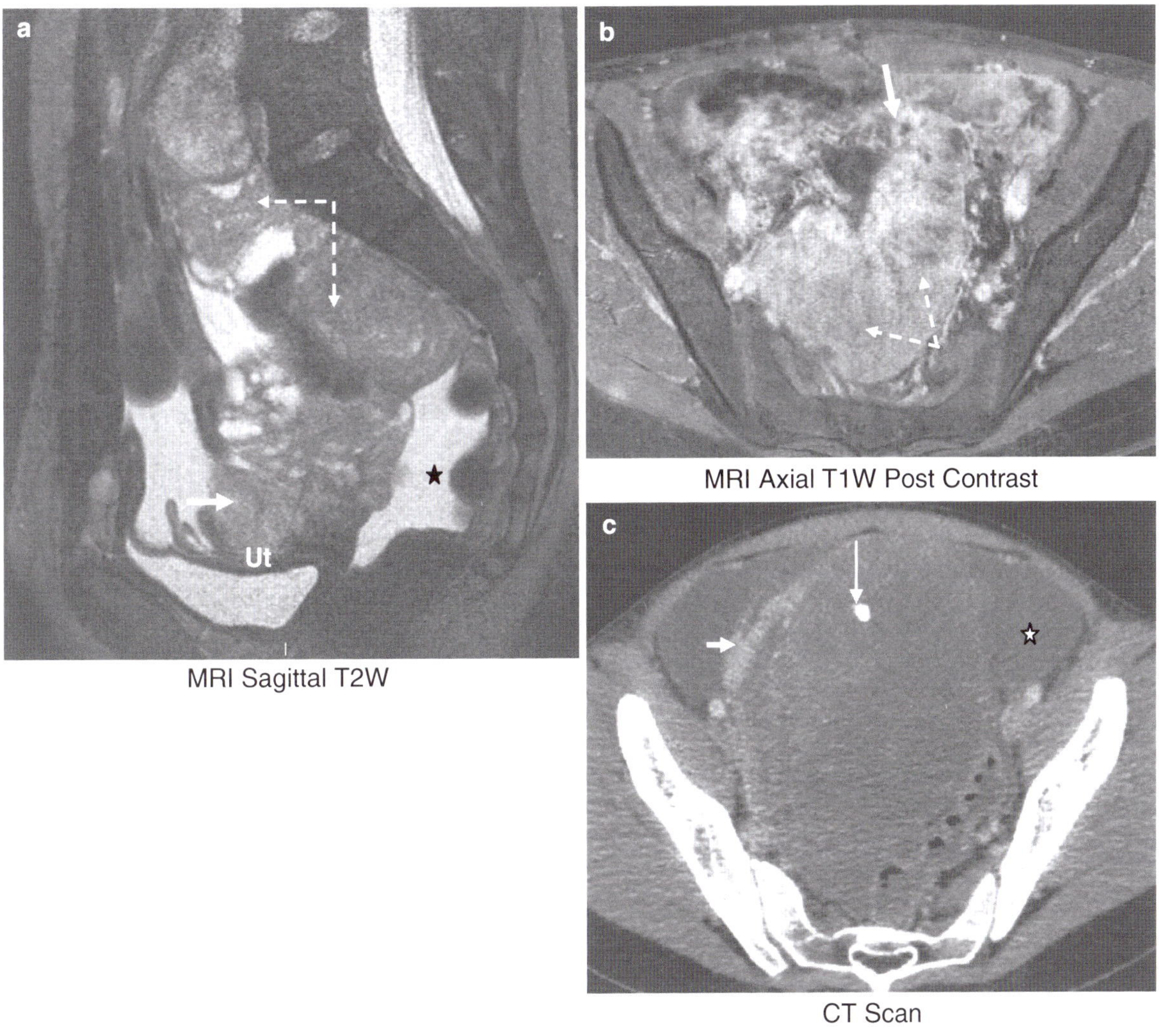

Fig. 4.40 Yolk sac tumour: Fifteen year old with abdominal pain and distension. (**a**) MRI largely solid adnexal mass (*solid arrow*) invading uterus (Ut), with ascites (*), extensive peritoneal deposits (*broken arrows*) and lymph node involvement. (**b**) MRI post-contrast: extensive and rapid enhancement of primary tumour, peritoneal deposits (*broken arrows*) and lymph nodes. (**c**) CT scan with foci of calcification, (*arrow*) in complex solid/cystic mass, dense ascites (*) and tortuous blood vessels in right ovarian pedicle (*short arrow*)

In common with many other rare tumours, there is no evidence recommending a sensible strategy. Tumour markers are not always reliable, but a rise in serum inhibin levels may prompt a repeat imaging survey. Follow-up with screening ultrasound and MRI is preferable to CT, to avoid cumulative radiation dose. Following a complete surgical resection, which may be limited to oophorectomy in selected cases, a follow-up of 2 yearly MRI scans, with interval annual ultrasound of abdomen and pelvis for 10 years should be considered, with symptomatic review subsequently. If recurrence occurs, more frequent MR scans may be indicated. CT/PET may not be reliable in detecting recurrence due to the variable growth-rate and heterogenousmorphologyofre currence [84].

4.5.14 Steroid Cell Tumours

Steroid cell tumours are particularly rare tumours, usually presenting in the fourth to fifth decade as virilising tumours, or occasionally presenting with Cushing's syndrome. Approximately, one third are malignant.

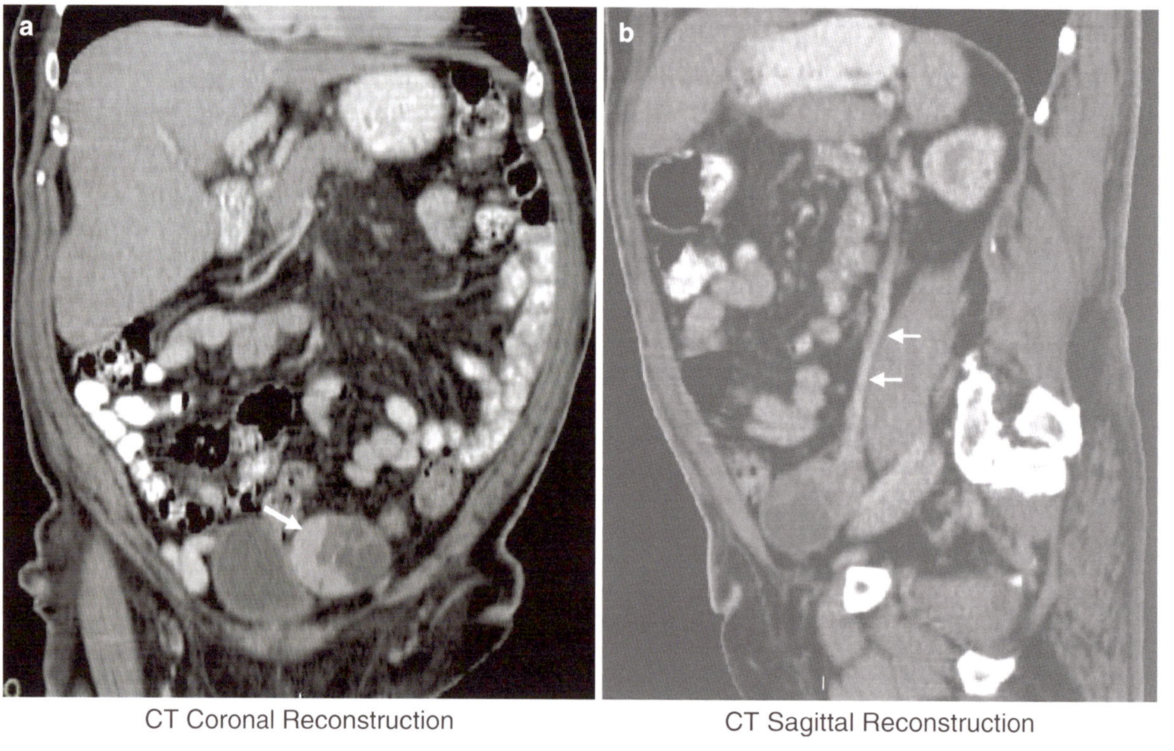

Fig. 4.41 Sertoli Leydig Tumour; High Grade, stage 1A: Fifty-six year old post-menopausal female. CT followed TV ultrasound for investigation of post-menopausal bleeding. (**a**) Note small well-defined and hypervascular solid area (*arrow*) adjacent to a few well-defined small cysts, within an enlarged left ovary. (**b**) A dilated left ovarian vein (*arrow*) reflects increased ovarian blood flow

They are usually unilateral, small tumours, less than 3 cm in size and on MR imaging, not only is there marked contrast enhancement, in common with other functioning sex cord stromal tumours, but the abundant intracellular fat deposits that are characteristic in this tumour can be detected on MR with appropriate fat saturated or in and opposed phase sequences. Small areas of cystic change or necrosis can also be seen but these are more often solid tumours. On transvaginal doppler ultrasound, intense vascularity can make these usually small tumours unusually conspicuous compared to other small, solid tumours such as Brenner tumoursorthe comas(Fig. 4.45).

4.5.15 Stromal Tumours

Thecomas and fibromas are derived from the stromal elements of the ovary. They range from pure thecomas, with oestrogenic activity and little fibrosis, to fibromas with little hormonal activity. There is usually a combination of these cell types and these benign tumours constitute 4–6% of all ovarian tumours and about half of all gonadal stromal tumours. The oestrogenic activity in thecomas is less than for GCT's and the peak age for presentation is a decade later at 59 years. The imaging appearances will depend to some extent on the proportion of thecoma to fibroma within the mass. Pure thecomas are slow growing, small, solid, well-defined tumours, which rarely calcify. Occasionally, it may be possible to detect foci of fat on MRI. However, there is often a non-specific imaging appearance of a small solid mass on ultrasound, CT or MRI. Contrast enhancement will depend on the proportion of functioning tissue, with fibrous tissue generally enhancing poorly and only late in the contrast phase (Fig. 4.46).

Fibromas are often larger asymptomatic masses, typically well-defined, with low/intermediate signal on T1 and T2W MRI sequences, reflecting the fibrous tissue content within the mass (Fig. 4.46). They can be

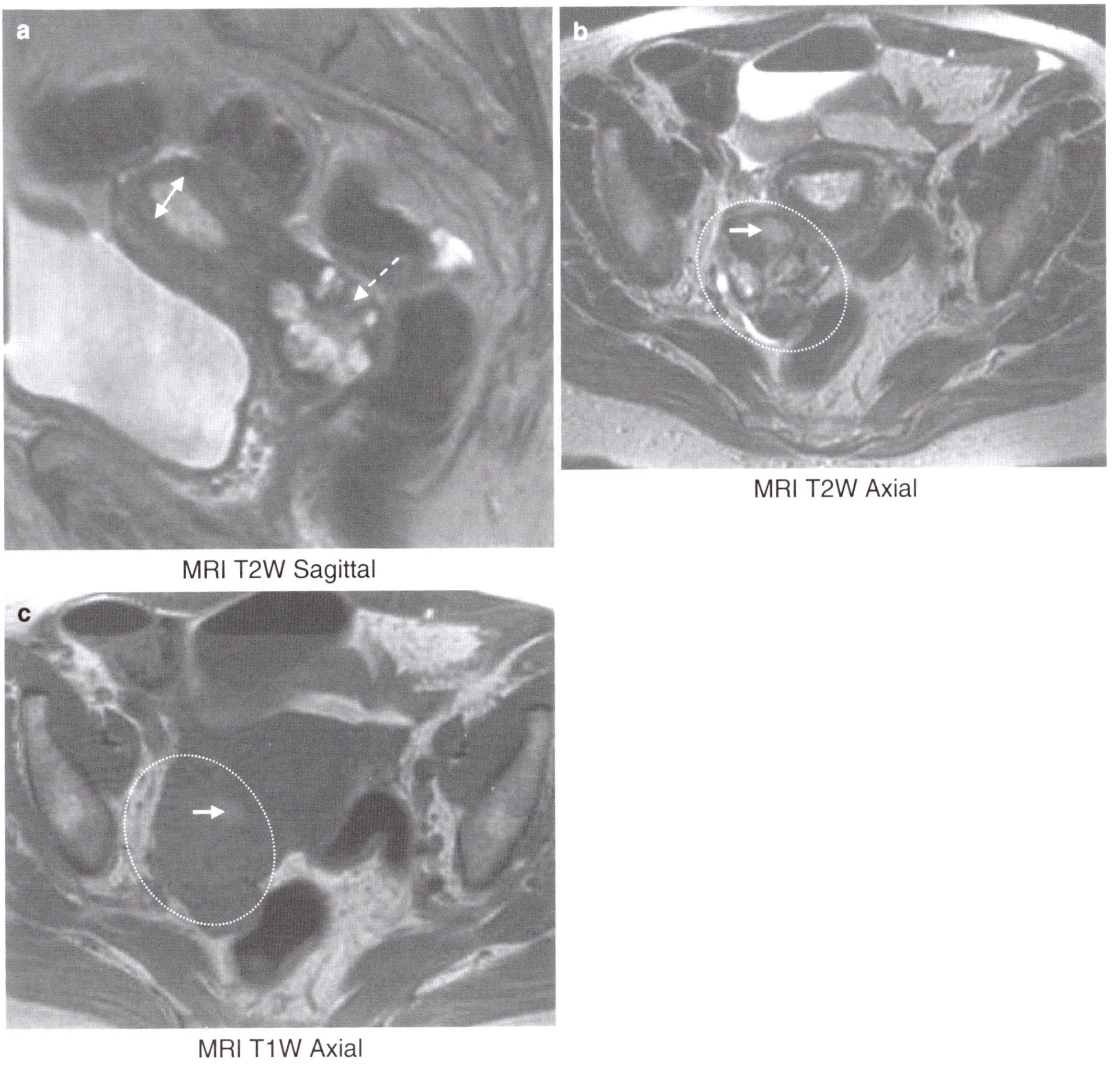

Fig. 4.42 Granulosa cell tumour. Post-menopausal patient with PMB. (**a**) endometrial thickening and hyperplasia (*double arrow*) with prominent endocervical glands (*broken arrow*). (**b**) Small complex right ovarian cyst, with multiple septations (*ellipse*). (**c**) T1W image shows intra cystic haemorrhage (*arrow*)

confused with serosal uterine leiomyomas, but areas of calcification are uncommon; and they also occasionally undergo cystic degeneration. Infrequently, they result in Meig's syndrome with benign, gross ascites and pleural effusions [85]. When associated with Gorlin's syndrome (Multiple basal naevus syndrome), they are usually multiple and occur at an earlier age. The main differential diagnosis of these consistently low signal masses on MRI are epithelial benign ovarian Brenner tumours.

Sarcomatous degeneration can rarely occur and is manifest by an increasing signal on T2W images [88].

4.5.16 Rare Epithelial Tumours

4.5.16.1 ClearC ellC arcinoma

Clear cell ovarian cancers are unusual, accounting for approximately 10% of epithelial ovarian cancer, usually presenting in a post-menopausal age group. Clear cell tumours are associated with endometriosis in approximately one third of cases; more than other types of epithelial cancer. This association with clear cell cancer is also increased in extra-ovarian sites of endometriosis.

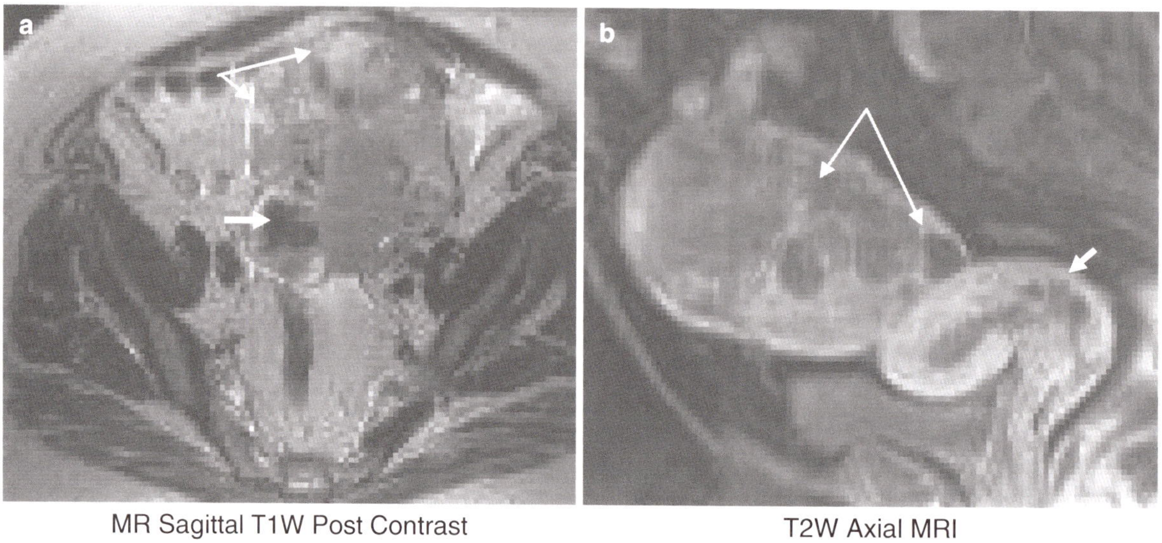

Fig. 4.43 (**a**) Post-menopausal patient shows multiple small cysts within a well-defined solid mass (*arrow*). Some of these are haemorrhagic (*broad arrow*) (**b**) Prominent post-contrast stromal enhancement outlines the multiple small cysts within the mass (*arrows*). Note also the thickened endometrium and prominent endocervical glands (*short arrow*)i nt heut erus.

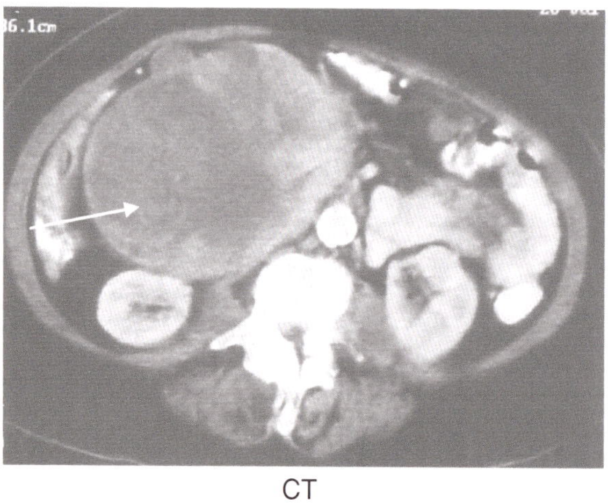

Fig. 4.44 CT recurrent GCT 30 years post-pelvic clearance. Large solid, intraperitoneal, hypervascular and partially necrotic heterogenousm ass

They generally present earlier, with stage 1 and 2 disease compared to other ovarian adenocarcinoma, due to initial slow growth and a more common presentation as a pelvic mass. But stage for stage, clear cell carcinoma has a worse prognosis, probably related to relative resistance to standard chemotherapy. It also has an increased presentation with thromboembolic phenomena and a higher incidence of paraneoplastic hypercalcaemiat hano there pithelialc ancers [49].

MR provides better characterization of the mass, and clues to the likely pathology may be present with evidence of endometriosis, which is more difficult to appreciate with CT. Typically, this cancer manifests as a large, unilateral cystic adnexal mass with one or more intraluminal, often well defined, solid protusions or vegetations (Figs.4.47 and 4.48). The cyst content can be haemorrhagic or proteinaceous.

Contrast is helpful, particularly in the setting of endometriosis to distinguish a chronic endometriotic cyst from the development of neoplasm. Unlike blood clot, the solid component of the cyst will enhance avidly, as will any nodular peritoneal implants. Elevation of CA 125 levels may not be discriminatory, as levels are variably elevated in both endometriotic cysts and clear cell tumours.

4.5.17 Brenner Tumours

Brenner tumours are generally benign epithelial tumours composed of transitional epithelium with dense stroma. They are often discovered as an incidental finding on ultrasound and are usually solid and small, less than 2 cm in size. The stromal component of a Brenner tumour can secrete oestrogens, so that secondary effects of endometrial hyperplasia may be

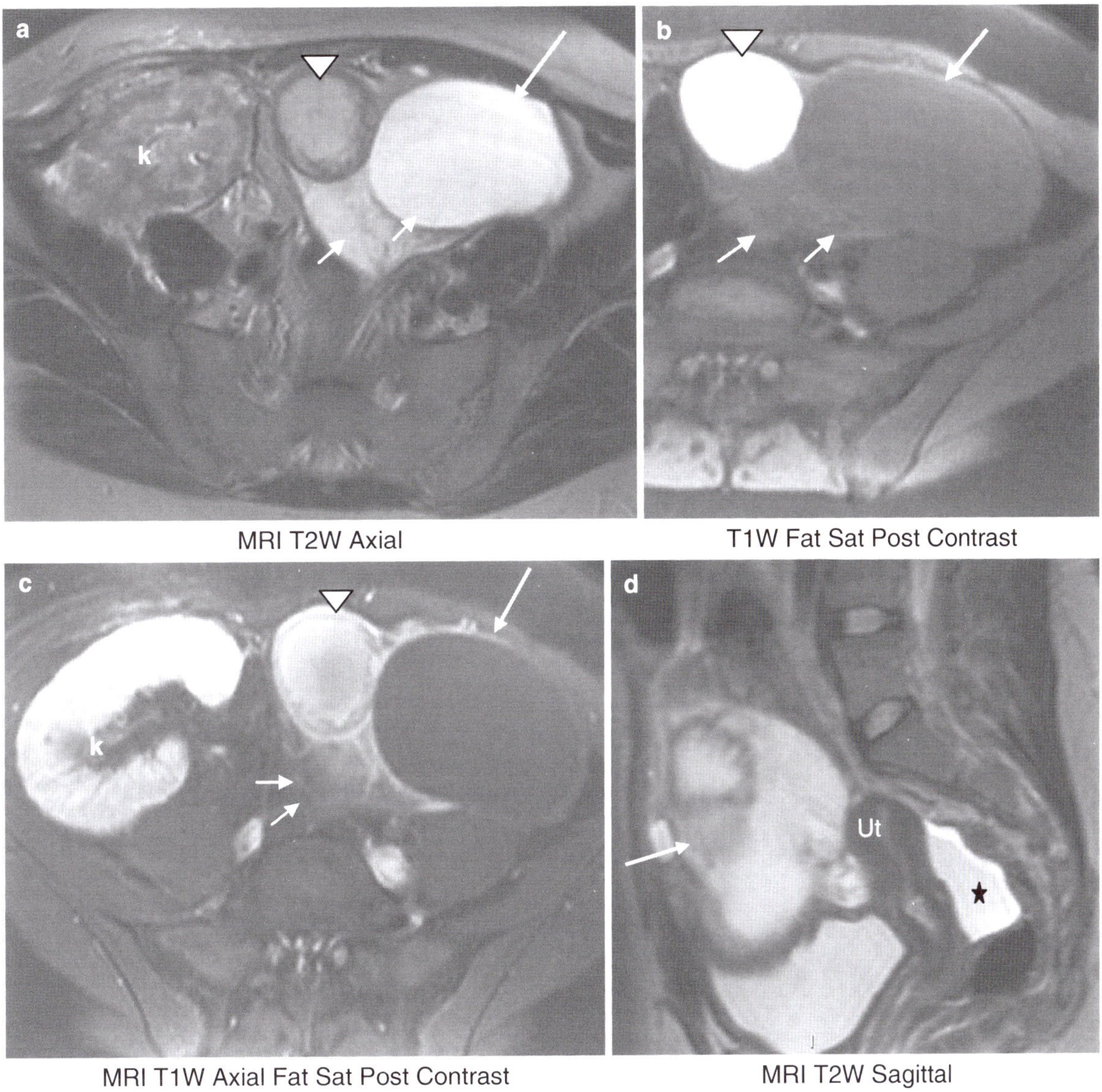

Fig. 4.45 Steroid cell stromal tumour in a teenager with precocious puberty and virilism. (Previous right renal transplant (k)) (**a**-**c**) Haemorrhagic/complex cystic (*arrowhead*) fluid component of mass (*long arrow*), prominent enhancing solid parenchyma containing small fatty foci (*short arrows*). (**d**) Premenarchal sized uterus (Ut). Ascitic fluid (*)

present. In 30% of cases, they are associated with other tumours, particularly mucinous epithelial ovarian tumours, but occasionally mature cystic teratomas. On CT or MRI, they can be either well-defined small, solid tumours, or larger cystic/solid tumours, particularly when in association with other tumours, with florid amorphous calcification of the solid component. There is only mild to moderate post-contrast enhancement of the solid component, depending on the fibrous content, so that on MRI, appearances can mimic a thecoma, with intense low signal on both T1 and T2 weighted sequences [86]. Although malignant Brenner tumours are extremely rare, (Fig. 4.49) there are no imaging features to discriminate organ confined disease from other suspect epithelial neoplasms with calcification e.g.s erousne oplasms [79, 85].

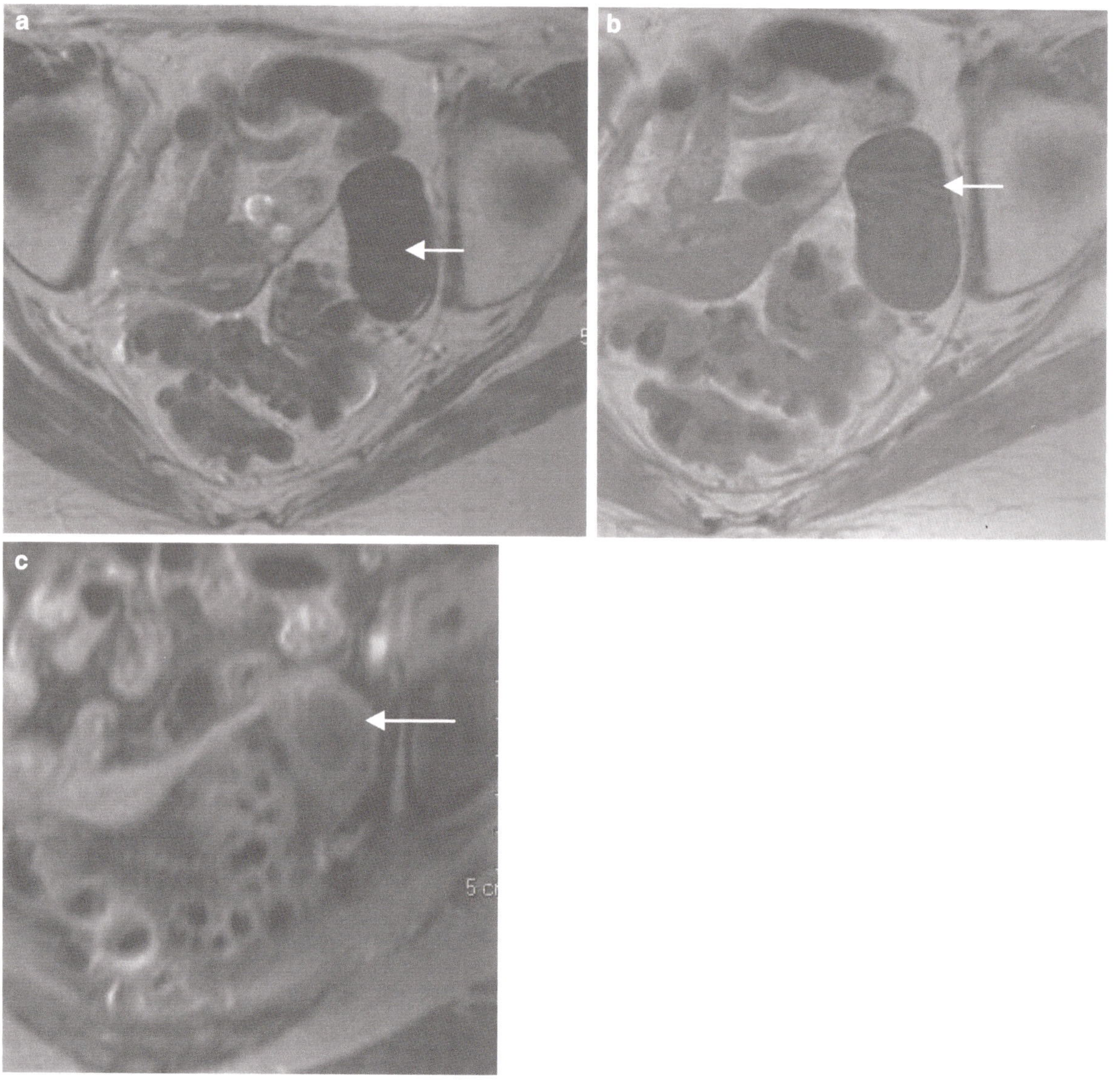

Fig. 4.46 Fibrothecoma in a post-menopausal patient with vaginal bleeding. MRI demonstrates a consistently low signal, well defined, homogenous left adnexal mass on both T2W (**a**) and (**b**) T1W images, (**c**) with only a thin rim of contrast enhancement at thec apsularm argin

4.5.18 *Small Cell Ovarian Cancer*

Small cell ovarian cancer is a rare, undifferentiated tumour with the majority occurring in young women. These are usually unilateral, mostly solid and hypervascular masses, greater than 10 cm (Fig. 4.50) which rapidly increase in size. More than fifty percent present with extra-ovarian disease. Particularly in younger women, with a non-pulmonary type of small cell tumour, there may be hypercalcaemia, hypoglycaemia or hyponatraemia at presentation with symptoms related to these biochemical abnormalities sometimes precipitating presentation. The prognosis is generally very poor, particularly in greater than stage 1 disease, with early relapse and metastasis. A 10% 5-year survivalis re portedins tage1C pa tients [87].

In common with most small cell tumours of the lung, these tumours appear to be hypervascular but in

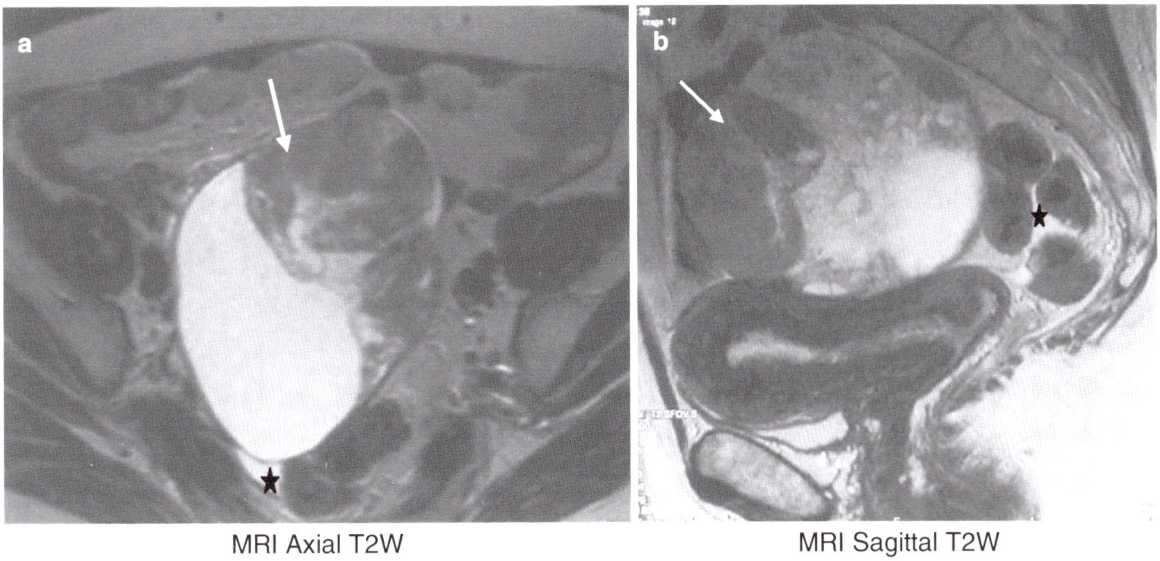

Fig. 4.47 Clear cell Ovarian Carcinoma. Stage1 in a premenopausal patient. Despite the size of the cyst, (**a**) and (**b**), it is well defined with a thin wall but with complex cystic/solid well defined masses protruding into the cyst (*arrow*). Solid areas enhance post contrast. (not shown) A trace of reactive ascites (*) isi nt heP ouchof D ouglas

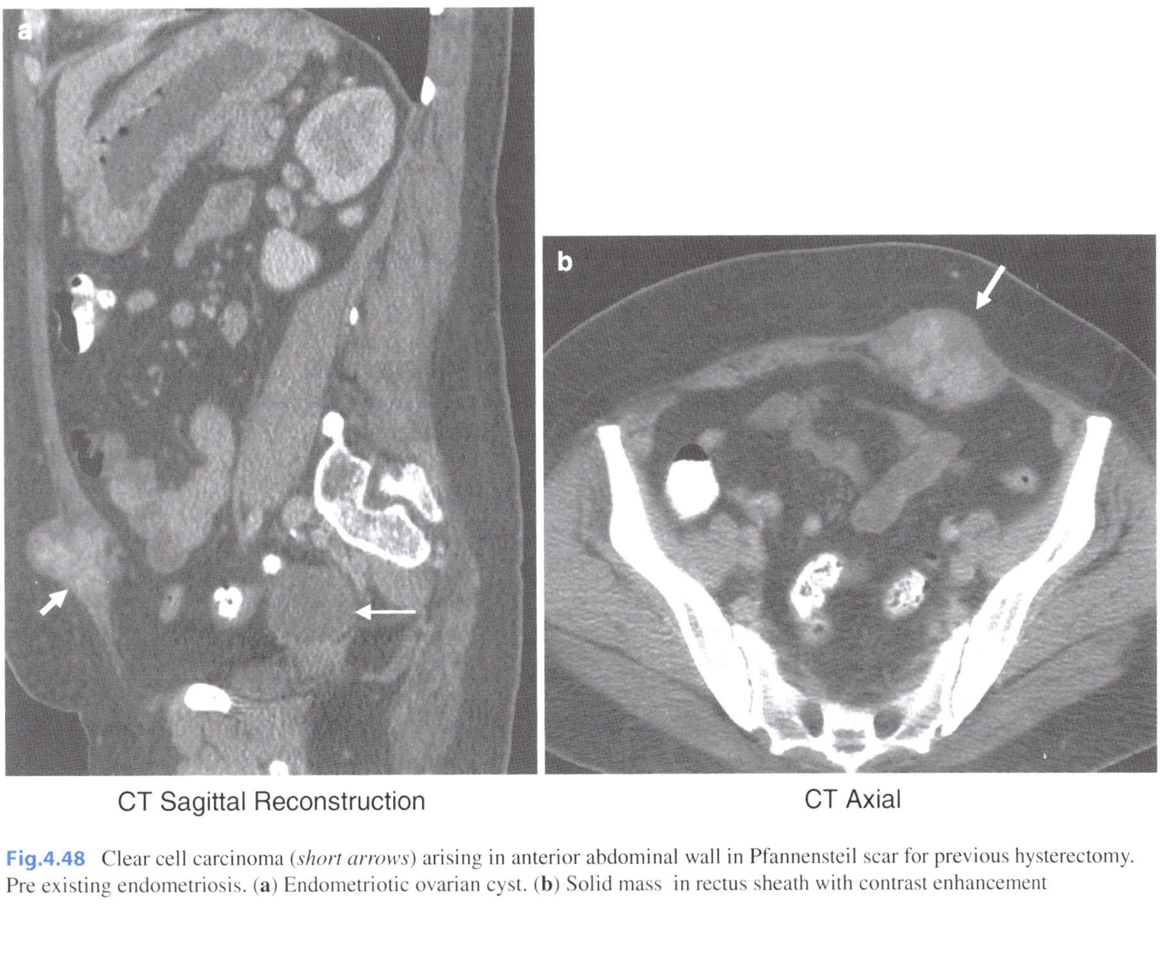

Fig.4.48 Clear cell carcinoma (*short arrows*) arising in anterior abdominal wall in Pfannensteil scar for previous hysterectomy. Pre existing endometriosis. (**a**) Endometriotic ovarian cyst. (**b**) Solid mass in rectus sheath with contrast enhancement

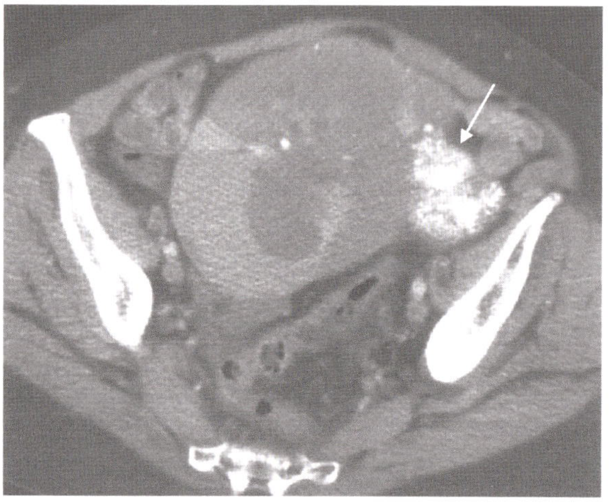

Fig. 4.49 Malignant Brenner tumour: typical florid amorphous calcification (*arrow*) within the solid component, with a much larger complex cyst than normally seen in a benign tumour

contrast to common ovarian epithelial neoplasms there is a propensity for early haematogenous and lymphatic dissemination. Their metastases may also be hypervascular (Fig. 4.50) [87]. Lymph node metastases are often bulky and confluent. This propensity for a hypervascular mass with bulky lymphadenopathy may help to differentiate the appearance pre-operatively from other hypervascular stromal tumours e.g. GCT.

As for other small cell tumours, staging requires to be comprehensive and CT or CT/PET is recommended. Small cell lung neoplasm with secondary ovarian metastases should be excluded and on CT imaging this will usually be apparent from the distribution of larger lymph node metastases in the thorax, rather than in the abdomen or pelvis.

4.5.19 Fallopian Tube Carcinoma

The classical presentation of this unusual tumour is the classical triad of profuse vaginal discharge, abdominal pain (sometimes relieved by watery or bloody vaginal discharge) and a pelvic mass, which constitutes the pathognomonic hydrops tubae profluens. Twenty per cent of cases are bilateral [89]. The diagnosis should be suspected in a post-menopausal woman with a serosanguinous vaginal discharge and a hydrosalpinx, often discovered at initial pelvic ultrasound.

Vaginal cytology is usually negative and more commonly, the diagnosis is confirmed post-operatively. Diagnosis is dependent on excluding spread from an adjacent ovarian epithelial adenocarcinoma. Tubal carcinoma results in increased secretions and tubal distension, producing a hydrosalpinx as tumour occludes the fimbrial end of the tube. Initial spread is to the uterus, and if the tube is not occluded, to the peritoneal cavity and adjacent ovary with dissemination via the peritoneal cavity to produce disseminated disease similar to that of ovarian cancer.

On MRI, there may be the tell-tale signs of profuse watery vaginal discharge producing vaginal distension and outlining the cervix. A hydrometra, with a hydrosalpinx and solid enhancing nodules studding the mucosal surface (Fig. 4.51) or a solid mass involving the tube, may also be apparent.

MR is preferable to CT, providing better soft tissue detail of the fallopian tube and more clearly excluding primary disease in the adjacent ovary.

Prognosis is worse; stage for stage, than in epithelial ovarian cancer and complete surgical resection provides the best prospect of survival. Treatment and follow up, including tumour markers is otherwise as fore pithelialo varianc ancers.

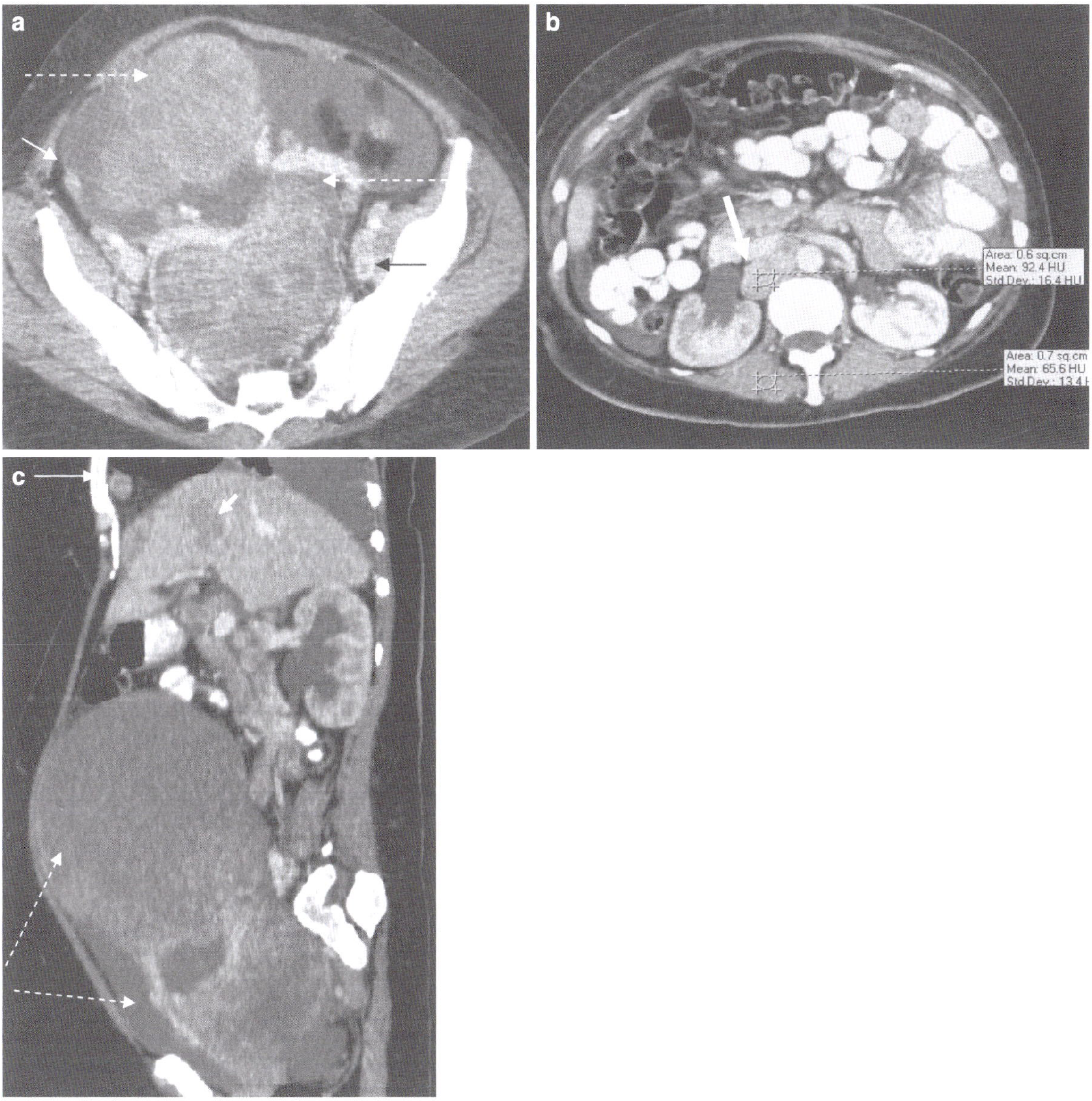

Fig. 4.50 Small cell carcinoma of ovary, stage 4, presenting with hypercalcaemia. (**a**) Bilateral hypervascular ovarian masses (*broken arrows*). Disseminated peritoneal and lymphatic metastases (*small arrows*) and ascites. (**b**) Vascular nodal metastases, with post-contrast density greater than adjacent muscle (*arrow*). (**c**) Haematogenous liver metastases (*solid arrow*) with right hydronephrosis and enlarged para cardiac nodes (*arrow*) within the chest

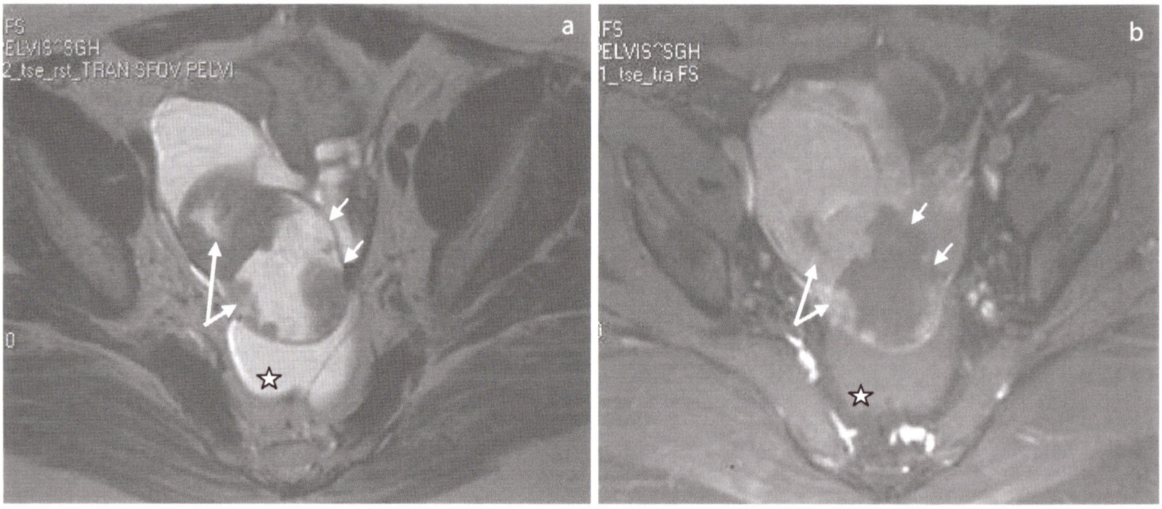

MRI Axial T2W

MRI Axial T1W Fat Sat Post Contrast

Fig. 4.51 Fallopian tube carcinoma. Patient with colectomy for Crohn's disease. Presentation with serosanguinous vaginal discharge and pain. (**a**) Fallopian tube carcinoma with solid nodules of tumour (*long arrows*) seeding the mucosal surface within a right hydrosalpinx (*small arrows*). (**b**) Post-contrast enhancement. Tumour nodules (*long arrows*) enhance avidly along enhancingm ucosals urfaceo fh ydrosalpinx

References

1. Scottish Intercollegiate Guidelines Network -SIGN guideline 61; 2002, Investigation of Post-Menopasal Bleeding A national clincal guideline.
2. Jacobs I et al. A risk of malignancy index incorporating CA125, ultrasound and menopausal status for the accurate preoperative diagnosis of ovarian cancer. Br J Obstet Gynaecol.1990;97(10):922–9.
3. Tingulstad S et al. Evaluation of a risk of malignancy index based on serum CA125, ultrasound findings and menopausal status in the pre-operative diagnosis of pelvic masses. Br J Obstet Gynaecol. 1996;103(8):826–31.
4. K.Kinkel et al. Indeterminate mass at US: incremental value of second imaging test for characterisation- meta-analysis and Bayesian analysis. Radiology. 2005;236:85–94
5. Kurtz AB et al. Diagnosis and staging of ovarian cancer: comparative values of Doppler and conventional US, CT, and MR imaging correlated with surgery and histopathologic analysis – Report of the Radiology Diagnostic Oncology Group. Radiology. 1999;212:19–27.
6. Tempany CM et al. Staging of advanced ovarian cancer: comparison of imaging modalities – Report from the Radiological Diagnostic Oncology Group. Radiology. 2000; 215:761–7.
7. American College of Radiology Appropriateness Criteria – Staging and Follow up of ovarian Cancer 2007.
8. Smith-Bindman R et al. Radiation associated with common computed tomography examinations and the associated lifetime attributable risk of cancer. Arch Intern Med. 2009;169: 2078–86.
9. Committee to Assess the Health Risks from Exposure to Low Levels of Ionizing Radiation, BEIR VII, National Research Council. Health Risks from Exposure to Low Levels of Ionizing Radiation. Washington: National Academies; 2006.
10. Amendola MA et al. Utilization of diagnostic studies in the pretreatment evaluation of invasive cervical cancer in the United States: results of intergroup protocol ACRIN 6651/GOG 183. J Clin Oncol. 2005;23(30):7454–9.
11. Ho K-C et al. 18F-fluorodeoxyglucose positron emission tomography in uterine carcinosarcoma. Eur J Nucl Med Mol Imaging.2008; 35:484–92.
12. Pecorelli S. Revised FIGO staging for carcinoma of the vulva, cervix, and endometrium. Int J Gynecol Obstet. 2009;105:103–4.
13. Whittaker CS et al. Diffusion-weighted MR imaging of female pelvic tumors: a pictorial review. Radiographics. 2009;29:759–74.
14. Hall TB et al. The role of ultrasound-guided cytology of groin lymph nodes in the management of squamous cell carcinoma of the vulva: 5-year experience in 44 patients. Clin Radiol.2003; 58(5):367–71.
15. Javadi M et al. FDG-CT/PET in assessing ovarian cancer recurrence and patient outcome: comparison to CA-125. J Nucl Med. 2009;50 Suppl 2:45.
16. Rockall AG et al. Diagnostic performance of nanoparticle-enhanced magnetic resonance imaging in the diagnosis of lymph node metastases in patients with endometrial and cervical cancer. J Clin Oncol. 2005;23:2813–21.
17. Choi HJ et al. MRI for pretreatment lymph node staging in uterine cervical cancer. Am J Roentgenol. 2006;187:W538–43.
18. Schwarz JK et al. The role of 18F-FDG PET in assessing therapy response in cancer of the cervix and ovaries. J Nucl Med. 2009;50(5 Suppl):64S–73S.
19. Sandro S et al. Lymph node metastasis in patients with clinical early-stage cervical cancer: detection with integrated FDG CT/PET. Radiology. 2006;238:272–9.

20. Kitajima K et al. Accuracy of integrated FDG-PET/contrast-enhanced CT in detecting pelvic and paraaortic lymph node metastasis in patients with uterine cancer. Eur Radiol. 2009; 16:1529–36.
21. Kim SK et al. Additional value of MR/PET fusion compared with CT/PET in the detection of lymph node metastases in cervical cancer patients. Eur J Cancer. 2009;45:2103–9.
22. Lewis JS et al. An imaging comparison of 64Cu-ATSM and 60Cu-ATSM in cancer of the uterine cervix. J Nucl Med. 2008;49:1177–82.
23. Levenback C. Lymphatic mapping and sentinel node identification in patients with cervix cancer undergoing radical hysterectomy and pelvic lymphadenectomy. J Clin Oncol. 2002;20(3):688.
24. Janssen M et al. The sentinel node procedure for detection of pelvic lymph node metastases of uterine cervical cancer: a systematic review. J Nucl Med. 2009;50 Suppl 2:1703.
25. Corrigendum to "FIGO staging for uterine sarcomas" [International Journal of Gynecology and Obstetrics (2009) 104:179.
26. Reznek R, Sohaib S. Cancer of the ovary. Cambridge University;2007.
27. Horowitz NS et al. Prospective evaluation of FDG-PET for detecting pelvic and para-aortic lymph node metastasis in uterine corpus cancer. Gynecol Oncol. 2004;95:546–51.
28. Van der Zee AGJ et al. Sentinel node dissection is safe in the treatment of early-stage vulvar cancer. J Clin Oncol. 2008;26(6):884–9.
29. Amant F et al. Seminar: endometrial cancer. Lancet. 2005; 366(9484):491–505.
30. Selman TJ et al. Diagnostic accuracy of tests for lymph node status in primary cervical cancer: a systematic review and meta-analysis. CMAJ. 2008;178(7):855–62.
31. Grubnic S et al. MR evaluation of normal retroperitoneal and pelvic lymph nodes. Clin Radiol. 2002;57(3):193–200.
32. Yang WT et al. Comparison of dynamic helical CT and dynamic MR imaging in the evaluation of pelvic lymph nodes in cervical carcinoma. AJR. 2000;175(3):759–66.
33. Heesakkers AM et al. MRI with a lymph-node-specific contrast agent as an alternative to CT scan and lymph-node dissection in patients with prostate cancer: a prospective multicohort study. Lancet Oncol. 2008;9(9):850–6.
34. Taylor A et al. An atlas of the pelvic lymph node regions to aid radiotherapy target volume definition. Clin Oncol. 2007; 19:542–50.
35. Heesakkers RA et al. Noninvasive detection of clinically occult lymph-node metastases in prostate cancer. N Engl J Med.2003;348:249 1–9.
36. Park JY et al. Comparison of the validity of magnetic resonance imaging and positron emission tomography/computed tomography in the preoperative evaluation of patients with uterine corpus cancer. Gynecol Oncol. 2008;108(3): 486–92.
37. Park JY et al. Role of PET or CT/PET in the post-therapy surveillance of uterine sarcoma. Gynecol Oncol. 2008;109(2): 255–62.
38. Szklaruk J et al. MR imaging of common and uncommon large pelvic masses. Radiographics. 2003;23:403–24.
39. Sironi S et al. Integrated FDG CT/PET in patients with persistent ovarian cancer: correlation with histologic findings. Radiology.2004; 233:433–40.
40. Rezvani M. Imaging of cervical pathology. Clin Obstet Gynecol.2009; 52(1):94–111.
41. Rustin GJ, et al. A randomized trial in ovarian cancer (OC) of early treatment of relapse based on CA125 level alone versus delayed treatment based on conventional clinical indicators (MRC OV05/EORTC 55955 trials. J Clin Oncol. 2009;27(18S) (Suppl;abstr 1):1.
42. Hiromura T et al. Clear cell adenocarcinoma of the uterine cervix arising from a background of cervical endometriosis. Br J Radiol. 2009;82:e20–2.
43. Arrastia C.D. et al. Uterine carcinosarcomas: incidence and trends in management and survival. Gynecol Oncol. 1997; 65(1):158–63.
44. Ohguri T et al. MRI findings including gadolinium-enhanced dynamic studies of malignant, mixed mesodermal tumors of the uterus: differentiation from endometrial carcinomas. Eur Radiol.2002; 12(11):2737–42.
45. Koyama T et al. MR imaging of endometrial stromal sarcoma: correlation with pathologic findings. Am J Roentgenol. 1999;173:767–72.
46. Hricak H, et al. In: Diagnostic imaging: gynaecology. Amirsys; 2007. p. 163–5.
47. Hricak H, et al. Diagnostic imaging gynaecology. Amirsys; 2007. p. 3:26-28.
48. Hricak H, et al. Diagnostic imaging gynaecology. Amirsys; 2007. p. 3:30-33.
49. Hricak H, et al. Diagnostic imaging gynaecology. Amirsys; 2007. p. 3:44-47.
50. Umesaki N et al. Positron emission tomography with 18F-fluorodeoxyglucose of uterine sarcoma: a comparison with magnetic resonance imaging and power Doppler imaging. Gynecol Oncol. 2001;80:372–7.
51. Sala E et al. American college of radiology: appropriateness criteria; endometrial cancer of the uterus. AJR. 2007;188: 1087–97.
52. Kinkel K et al. Radiologic staging in patients with endometrial cancer: a metaanalysis. Radiology. 1999;212: 711–8.
53. Brooks JJ. Malignancy arising in extragonadal endometriosis: a case report and summary of the world literature. Cancer.1977; 40(6):3065–73.
54. Major FJ et al. Prognostic factors in early-stage uterine sarcoma: A Gynecologic Oncology Group Study. Cancer. 1993; 71:1702–9.
55. Ueda M et al. MR imaging findings of uterine endometrial stromal sarcoma: differentiation from endometrial carcinoma. Eur Radiol. 2001;11:28–33.
56. Sahdev A et al. MR imaging of uterine sarcomas. Am J Roentgenol. 2001;177:1307–11.
57. Parker WH et al. Uterine sarcoma in patients operated on for presumed leiomyoma and rapidly growing leiomyoma. Obstet Gynecol. 1994;83:414–8.
58. Tanaka YO et al. Smooth muscle tumors of uncertain malignant potential and leiomyosarcomas of the uterus: MR findings. J Magn Reson Imaging. 2004;20(6): 998–1007.
59. Tamai K et al. The utility of diffusion-weighted MR imaging for differentiating uterine sarcomas from benign leiomyomas. Eur Radiol. 2008;18:723–30.
60. Ozols R, et al. American cancer society, atlas of clinical oncology: ovarian cancer. 2003. p. 235.

61. Doi T et al. Adenoma malignum: MR imaging and pathologic study. Radiology. 1997;204:39–42.
62. Sugiyam K et al. MR findings of pseudoneoplastic lesions in the uterine cervix mimicking adenoma malignum. Br J Radiol.2007;80:878–83.
63. Lotocki RJ et al. Glassy cell carcinoma of the cervix: a bimodal treatment strategy. Gynecol Oncol. 1992;44:254–9.
64. Yang DH et al. MRI of small cell carcinoma of the uterine cervix with pathologic correlation. Am J Roentgenol. 2004;182:1255–8.
65. Husband JE, Reznek RH, editors. Imaging in oncology, vol. 2. 2nd ed. 2004. p. 850.
66. Yoshikazu O et al. MR imaging of the uterine cervix: imaging – pathologic correlation. Radiographics. 2003;23:425–45.
67. Parikh J et al. MR imaging features of vaginal malignancies. Radiographics.200 8;28(1):49–63.
68. Taylor MB et al. Magnetic resonance imaging of primary vaginal carcinoma. Clin Radiol. 2007;62(6):549–55.
69. López C et al. MRI of vaginal conditions. Clin Radiol. 2005;60(6):648–66.
70. Kim KA et al. Benign ovarian tumours with solid and cystic components that mimic malignancy. Am J Roentgenol. 2004;182:1259–65.
71. Park SB et al. Imaging findings of complications and unusual manifestations of ovarian teratomas. Radiographics. 2008; 28:969–83.
72. Outwater EK et al. Ovarian teratomas: tumor types and imaging characteristics. Radiographics. 2001;21:475–90.
73. Comerci Jr JT et al. Mature cystic teratoma: a clinicopathologic evaluation of 517 cases and review of the literature. Obstet Gynecol. 1994;84:22–8.
74. Diaz-Montes TP et al. Primary insular carcinoid of the ovary. Gynecol Oncol. 2006;101:175–8.
75. Davis KP et al. Primary ovarian carcinoid tumours. Gynecol Oncol.1996;61:259 –65.
76. Ozols R, et al. American cancer society atlas of clinical oncology: ovarian cancer. BC Decker; 2003. p. 224.
77. Ozols R, et al. American cancer society atlas of clinical oncology: ovarian cancer. BC Decker; 2003. p. 226.
78. Levitin AE et al. Endodermal sinus tumor of the ovary: imaging evaluation. Am J Roentgenol. 1996;167:791–3.
79. Jung SE et al. CT and MR imaging of ovarian tumors with emphasis on differential diagnosis. Radiographics. 2002;22: 1305–25.
80. Jung SE et al. CT and MRI findings of sex cord stromal tumor of the ovary. Am J Roentgenol. 2005;185:207–15.
81. Hines JF et al. Recurrent granulose cell tumor of the ovary 37 years after initial diagnosis: a case report and review of the literature. Gynecol Oncol. 1996;60:484–8.
82. Rha SE et al. Recurrent ovarian granulosa cell tumors: clinical and imaging features. Abdom Imaging. 2008;33: 119–25.
83. Schumer ST. Granulosa cell tumor of the ovary. J Clin Oncol. 2003;21:1180–9.
84. Huang YT et al. Variable F-18 fluorodeoxyglucose avidity of metastatic recurrent adult granulosa cell tumor. Clin Nucl Med.2009; 34(10):710–2.
85. Outwater EK et al. Sex cord-stromal and steroid cell tumors of the ovary. Radiographics. 1998;18:1523–46.
86. Won Jin M et al. Brenner tumor of the ovary: CT and MR findings. J Comput Assist Tomogr. 2000;24(1):72–6.
87. Young RH et al. Small cell carcinoma of the ovary, hypercalcemic type. A clinicopathological analysis of 150 cases. Am J Surg Pathol. 1994;18(11):1102–16.
88. Shanbhogue A. et al Clinical syndromes associated with ovarian Neoplasms: A Comprehensive Review. Radiographics 2010 30, 903-919.
89. Hosokawa C et al. Bilateral fallopian tube carcinoma: findings on sequential MRI. AJR. 2006;186:1046–50.
90. Saba L et al. Mature and immature ovarian teratomas: CT, US and MR imaging characteristics. Eur Jou Radiol 2009 72(3):454- 63

Part II

Ovarian Rare Cancers

MucinousC ancers:Ovar y

5

Jonathan A. Ledermann and Fharat A. Raja

5.1 IntroductionandEp idemiology

Mucinous tumours of the ovary are uncommon. Approximately, 75% are benign and the remainder are either "borderline" tumours or malignant (about 12% [1]). Overall, malignant mucinous tumours are rare and are estimated from the SEER registry to be 11.6% of all invasive ovarian tumours. Only a small proportion of these present at an advanced stage (FIGO III or IV) [2]. Historical data may have overcalled the number of malignant mucinous tumours, and in some cases primary tumours may not have been distinguished from secondary cancers. It is partly because of their rarity that accurate data on incidence are hard to find. While patients entered into clinical trials often have their pathology reviewed, patients with mucinous cancers in these studies may not reflect the true incidence of the disease. Firstly, most patients with invasive mucinous cancer have early stage disease, managed by surgery alone. Secondly, patients with advanced disease who entered into chemotherapy trials may under-represent the true incidence of this histological subtype. From an analysis of 1,895 patients with stage III ovarian cancer entered into six GOG trials over a 13-year period, only 1.8% of cases were classified as mucinous-type [3].

In this chapter, we will discuss the controversies that exist about the diagnosis of primary invasive mucinous cancers of the ovary, and the management of early and advanced invasive disease.

5.2 Pathology

Mucinous tumours may be of "intestinal-type" or "endocervical-type" (Müllerian). Amongst borderline tumours the vast majority are "intestinal-type". These have a much lower incidence of bilaterality than the less common "endocervical-type" that may be bilateral in up to 40% of cases. However, invasive tumours may be of either type. A minority of these patients with early disease (15–20%) have bilateral tumours. Stromal invasion may be infiltrative or expansile, or a mixture of the two [4]. The key challenge is differentiating primary ovarian tumours from metastatic cancers involving the ovary. Most women present with early stage disease, and the mean age of women is generally younger (36–50 years) than for the more common types of invasive ovarian cancer. Symptoms are usually due to an expanding pelvic mass. In early stage disease, these cystic masses can be large, averaging 16–19 cm in diameter [5].

For all mucinous tumours, and particularly those that have spread beyond the ovary the differential diagnosis includes tumours of the gastrointestinal tract – large intestine, appendix and pancreas in particular, and less commonly metastases from the stomach or biliary tract. Rarely, endocervical mucinous cancer may metastasise to the ovary. In a series of 52 cases reported by Seidman et al. [1] 40 (77%) were metastatic, and tumours of the pancreas, colon, stomach and cervix were the four most common sites (25 out of 40). Features, such as bilaterality or deposits on the surface of the ovaries increase the

J.A.Le dermann(✉)
CR-UK and UCL Cancer Trials Centre, 90 Tottenham Court Road, London W1T4T J, UKa nd
UCLC ancerIns titute, UniversityC ollegeLondon, London W1T4TJ , UK
e-mail:j.le dermann@ctc.ucl.ac.uk

F.A.R aja
UCLC ancerIns titute, UniversityC ollegeLondon, London W1T4TJ , UK

N. Reed et al. (eds.), *Rare and Uncommon Gynecological Cancers*,
DOI: 10.1007/978-3-642-13492-0_5, © Springer-Verlag Berlin Heidelberg 2011

index of suspicion of metastatic carcinoma. Microscopic features, such as nodular growth, hilar involvement and presence of signet-ring cells and surface microscopic mucin, are also more in keeping with the possibility of a metastatic tumour [6]. A co-existing Brenner tumour or teratoma is more in keeping with a primary mucinous tumour. An algorithm has been developed by Seidman et al. to help distinguish primary from secondary tumours. This is based chiefly on size, and bilaterality. Bilateral tumours and those with a diameter <10 cm are usually metastatic; conversely unilateral tumours >10 cm in diameter are generally primary ovarian tumours [1].

5.3 Biomarkers and Immunophenotyping

Immunophenotyping is commonly used to distinguish primary ovarian neoplasms from metastatic tumours but the ability of immunoprofiling mucinous tumours to make these distinctions has been less valuable than in other types of ovarian neoplasms. Serum carcinoembryonic antigen (CEA) levels may distinguish a primary colorectal cancer from an ovarian cancer. Serum CA125 levels are generally higher in ovarian cancers, and a ratio of CA125: CEA of greater than 25 has been used to distinguish primary ovarian cancer from colorectal neoplasms [7]. However, mucinous ovarian cancers of intestinal-type frequently stain positive for CEA. Primary ovarian tumours are characteristically cytokeratin (CK) 7 positive and CK 20 negative, which helps to distinguish the tumour from colorectal cancers that are characteristically CK 20 positive. However, primary mucinous tumours of the ovary may also be CK 20 positive [8]. Similarly, other mucinous tumours of the upper GI tract and elsewhere may also be CK 7 positive and CK 20 negative. The differential expression of cytokeratins has been reviewed in detail by Chu and Weiss [9]. The distinction of primary mucinous ovarian cancer from pancreatic cancers may be particularly challenging. In pancreatic cancers Dpc4 is lost in approximately half of all the cases but it is preserved in mucinous ovarian cancer [10]. CDX2 is expressed in almost all colonic cancers, most gastric cancers and some pancreatic tumours. Expression of CDX2 in primary mucinous ovarian cancer occurs less commonly than CK20, and it may therefore have some advantage in discriminating a primary mucinous ovarian cancer from upper gastrointestinal cancer metastases [11].

Genetic alterations other than mutations in K-ras have not been reported in mucinous ovarian tumours. Mutations are typically at codon 12 and have been reported in 46% of mucinous carcinomas but only 6% of serous carcinomas [12]. Unlike other solid tumours, such as colorectal cancer, mucinous ovarian cancers without K-ras mutations do not have alternative pathway signalling through a BRAF mutation [13]. However, gene-expression profiling has demonstrated significant differences between mucinous cystadenomas, borderline mucinous tumours and adenocarcinomas compared with their serous counterparts [14]. These findings could provide opportunities to develop drugs targeted to specific gene products or pathways.

5.4 Clinical Features: Primary vs. Secondary Cancer

The practical guide to differentiate primary mucinous ovarian cancer from metastatic tumours developed by Seidman et al. using unilaterality and tumour size ≥10 cm for primary tumours correctly predicted a primary ovarian origin in 82% of cases. For bilateral tumours, a diameter <10 cm, was predictive of a metastatic mucinous tumour in 95% of cases [1]. These and additional helpful features are summarised in Table 5.1. When metastatic cancer can be excluded on clinical assessment the remaining number of cases is

Table 5.1 Primary vs. metastatic mucinous tumours

	Primary	Metastatic	Reference
Unilateral	✓		[1]
Size ≥ 10 cm	✓		[1]
Smooth surface	✓		[1]
Vascular invasion		✓	[6]
CK 7 > CK20	✓		[9]
CA125/CEA > 25	✓		[7]
Co-existing borderline tumour/ Brenner	✓		[1]
Retained Dpc4 Expression	✓		[10]
Destructive stromal invasion		✓	[1]
CDX2		✓	[11]

small, and in most instances these are localised to the ovary. Thus, the incidence of advanced stage primary mucinous cancer is small, but nevertheless a challenge for clinical management. Currently, mucinous ovarian cancers are treated similarly to serous ovarian cancers.

5.5 ClinicalMa nagement

5.5.1 Imaging

Preoperative imaging can be useful in distinguishing benign from malignant tumours, and in assessing the extent of disease. This is particularly important in the investigation of mucinous tumours, most of which are either benign or tumours of low malignant potential, and confined to the ovary. Radiological investigations are crucial in the diagnosis and staging of malignant ovarian tumours and ultrasonography is a particularly useful first investigation. It may aid in the differentiation of primary and secondary tumours of the ovary and give some indication about whether the tumour is a mucinous-type or not. The precision of ultrasonography is improved with Doppler studies that are able to detect neovascularity associated with malignant ovarian tumours. Computed Tomography (CT) is essential for pre-operative staging and may provide valuable information about the spread of disease and whether there is a likely primary site other than the ovary. From a large single institution series of 553 patients, about 17.4% of ovarian tumours were secondary deposits to the ovary [15]. Imaging of the upper gastrointestinal tract is particularly relevant as primary mucinous tumours of the pancreas or biliary tract may present with ovarian masses. In the case of mucinous ovarian cancers, the size of the tumour is often large and may even be enormous. Mucinous ovarian tumours are multi-locular cystic structures and have relatively few solid components. This appearance is less common in tumours metastatic to the ovary. Magnetic Resonance Imaging (MRI) is sometimes used for staging but less commonly than CT. It is able to provide greater morphological information about the ovary than CT, but has little advantage over CT and ultrasound. PET scanning has been useful in diagnosing and staging many different types of benign and malignant conditions. However, in the case of mucinous tumours, high false negative rates have been reported due to lack of FDG uptake by mucin [16].

5.6 TumourMar kers

CA125 is routinely measured in women with ovarian masses. However, it is not always raised in mucinous tumours even when they are advanced. CA19-9, a carbohydrate antigen related to the Lewis blood group antigen may be helpful in the diagnosis and monitoring of mucinous tumours. In a study from the Netherlands over a 15 year period, 46% of 44 women with borderline ovarian tumours were found to have a raised CA 19-9 compared to 24% who had a raised CA125 and 9% who had an elevated CEA [17]. CA19-9 has also been used to follow up patients after treatment, and like CA125 it may rise before clinical relapse [18]. Marker profiles have not been systematically studied in mucinous carcinomas, but in the author's experience, monitoring of CA19-9 changes in response to chemotherapy or follow-up after treatment has been helpful in many cases.

5.7 Endoscopy/Colonoscopy

Endoscopic examination of the gastrointestinal tract is one of the most commonly debated investigations in patients with mucinous ovarian cancer. As a proportion of patients will have tumours of the gastrointestinal tract some clinicians routinely request these investigations. However with improvements in histological assessment of tumours, and in particularly immunophenotyping, the routine use of oesophago-gastro-duodenoscopy and colonoscopy is diminishing. However, small tumours or tumours in the appendix, or rarely small bowel may be missed on endoscopy. There are no definitive recommendations; judgement about these investigations should be on an individual case and following review in a multidisciplinary clinical environment.

5.8 Treatmento fMuc inousEp ithelial Ovarian Cancer

The prognosis of early stage mucinous ovarian cancer is excellent with a 5-year survival of greater than 90% following surgery. The risk of recurrence was lower than for other histological subtypes (HR 0.37 95% CI 0.25–0.53) [19]. There is no evidence that additional treatment with chemotherapy is beneficial. The ICON1 and ACTION studies were two parallel and complementary trials in early stage ovarian cancer that were analysed together. The trial randomised 925 patients between adjuvant platinum-based chemotherapy and observation, with deferred chemotherapy at relapse [20]. The majority of patients in both trials (93%) had stage I ovarian cancer, and of these 180 (20%) had a mucinous type. Subgroup analyses revealed 10 patients with mucinous ovarian cancer relapsed in the adjuvant arm compared with 22 patients in the observation group, comprising a total of 18% of all relapses. These differences were not statistically significant, and with the small number of patients in each arm of this subset, it is not possible to conclude that patients with early stage mucinous ovarian cancer benefit from adjuvant chemotherapy.

5.9 Treatmento fA dvanced Mucinous Ovarian Cancer

The results of treatment of stage I disease contrast greatly with the survival of patients who have advanced mucinous tumours. Their outcome is worse than those patients with the more common types of ovarian histology. Primary surgical intervention is usually performed as in other types of ovarian cancer, so it is unusual to have a pre surgical histological diagnosis unless the tumour is very advanced and therefore unlikely to be successfully debulked at primary surgery. Staging and maximal cytoreduction is undertaken before chemotherapy. In cases where a biopsy has been performed first, tests to exclude a non-ovarian primary tumour should be performed before surgery. If the preoperative imaging or clinical appearances suggest a tumour of mucinous origin, most surgeons will also perform an appendicectomy, as this may be the site of origin in some cases.

Chemotherapy with carboplatin and paclitaxel, the standard of care for ovarian cancer [21] is generally given irrespective of the histological subtype. Case-controlled studies have provided information on the poor prognosis of advanced mucinous ovarian cancer. The Royal Marsden Hospital, London, UK performed a retrospective case-controlled study in women with advanced mucinous and non-mucinous ovarian cancer (FIGO stage III and IV) undergoing first-line platinum-based chemotherapy [22]. Controls were matched for stage of disease and date of diagnosis. Eighty-one patients (27 cases and 54 controls) fulfilling the study criteria were identified and analysed. The response rate to chemotherapy was 26% in mucinous tumours and 65% for non-mucinous tumours ($p=0.01$). The median progression-free survival (PFS) was 5.7 months compared to 14.1 months ($p<0.001$), and median overall survival (OS) 12 months in patients with mucinous tumours compared to 36.7 ($p<0.001$) months in the case-controls. These data are supported by the pooled analysis of six GOG trials of 1,895 patients. There were 34 patients with mucinous ovarian cancer. All patients received platinum/paclitaxel combinations, and the progression-free and overall survival of patients with mucinous tumours was significantly worse that those with serous cancers (10.5 v 16.9 and 14.8v45.1months ,re spectively) [3].

A second retrospective study performed by the Hellenic Cooperative group analysed 141 advanced ovarian cancer patients (47 patients with mucinous carcinoma and 94 matched controls), treated with platinum-based chemotherapy [23]. The response rate was 38.5 and 70% ($p=0.001$) in mucinous and non-mucinous tumours respectively. In this study, the time to progression and overall survival were not significantly different in the two groups though there was a trend to worse median time to tumour progression in patients with mucinous tumours (11.8 vs. 20 months, $p=0.18$).

A third small retrospective study from Italy reviewed the outcome of patients with "platinum-sensitive" relapse (greater than 6 months platinum-free interval) disease. Twenty patients with mucinous tumours and 388 patients with other histological subtypes were studied. At initial diagnosis, patients with mucinous tumours had a lower tumour grade than in other subgroups ($p=0.0056$) and FIGO stage was less advanced ($p=0.025$). At the time of recurrence, patients with mucinous tumours had a statistically significant poorer performance status ($p=0.024$). Patients with mucinous tumours frequently were treated with single agent platinum rather than combination treatment, and received fewer subsequent lines of treatment. The tumour response rate was 36% for the mucinous sub-type and 62% ($p=0.04$) for other histological types. The median PFS and OS were also poorer in the mucinous tumour group. This study has limitations as it is small, but nevertheless, the data are informative as there are no other reports on the outcome of mucinous ovarian cancer afters econd-linec hemotherapy [24].

5.10 NewSt udiesf orMu cinous Ovarian Cancer

Improvements in the treatment of advanced disease are urgently needed. As mucinous tumours of the ovary resemble the histological appearance of mucinous tumours from the bowel, stomach and pancreas, some clinicians have used "gastrointestinal-type" chemotherapy. This is not an evidence-based approach to the management of mucinous ovarian cancer and clinical trials are needed to evaluate these therapies. There is a good rationale for taking this approach forward. Sato et al., [25] examined the effect of a variety of chemotherapy agents in vitro, using five human ovarian mucinous cell lines. They found that two of the five cell lines were sensitive to oxaliplatin, 5-fluorouracil (5-FU) and etoposide. Interestingly, all cell lines were resistant to cisplatin and paclitaxel. A second series of experiments involved testing chemotherapy drugs in a murine mucinous ovarian cancer model. Mice treated with the combination of oxaliplatin plus 5-FU survived significantly longer compared to either oxaliplatin or 5-FU alone, suggesting a

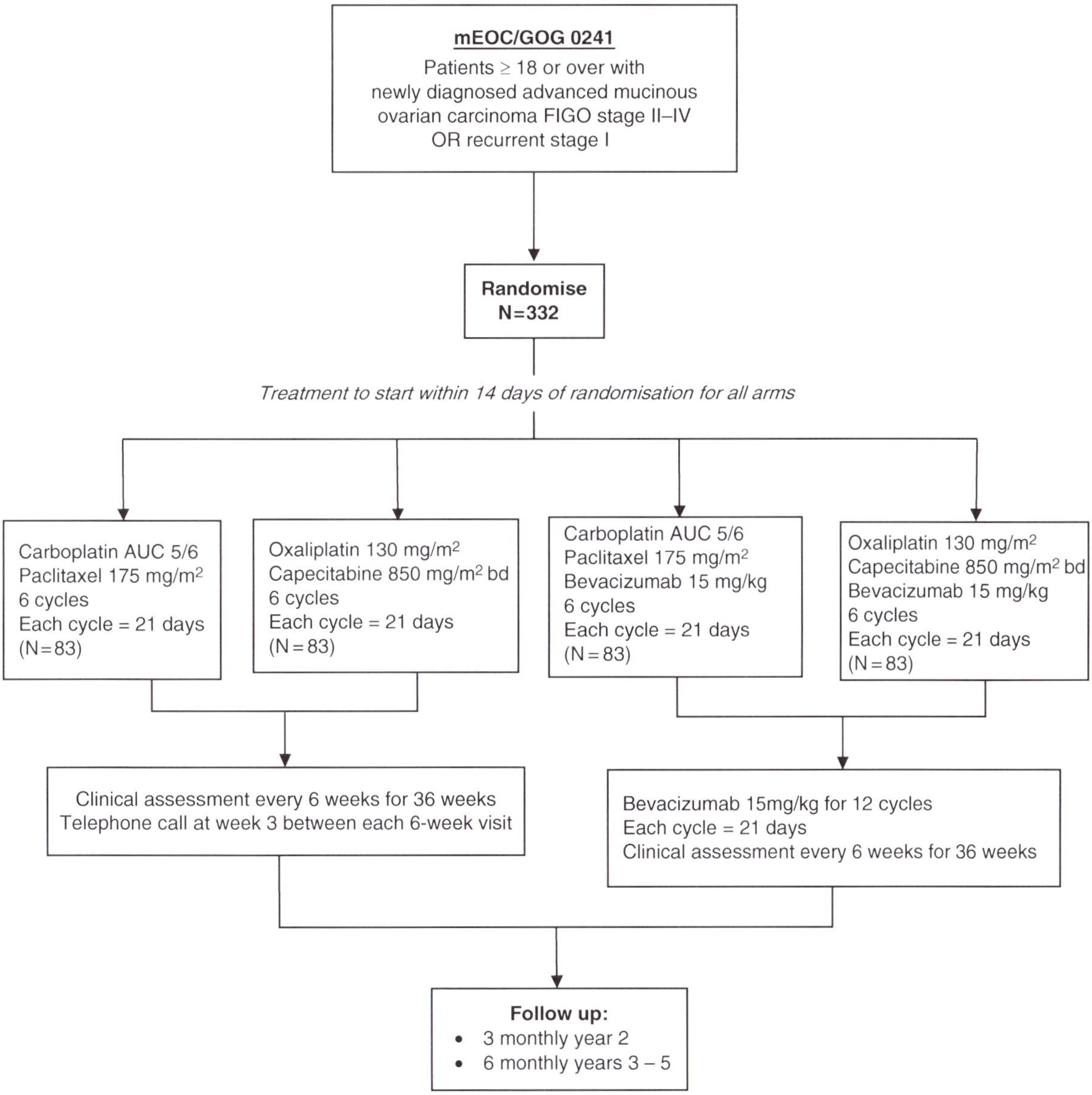

Fig. 5.1 Trial schema: GCIG study (GOG 0241- NCRI mEOC) for mucinous ovarian cancer

synergistic or additive effect of this combination, as is the case when these two drugs are used together in patients with advanced colorectal cancer [26].

Both oxaliplatin and 5-FU have activity in ovarian cancer. In a platinum-resistant population, a response rate of 29% has been reported with the FOLFOX-4 regimen [27]. It therefore seems reasonable to examine oxaliplatin and 5-FU, or the increasingly commonly used oral fluoropyrimidine, capecitabine for the first-line therapy in advanced mucinous ovarian cancer. A randomised phase III trial, comparing oxaliplatin and capecitabine with carboplatin and paclitaxel has now been set up. This type of study is challenging, as the disease is rare. It requires international collaboration and academic sponsorship, as treatment of this group of women is not a high priority for the pharmaceutical industry. Through the Gynaecological Cancer Inter Group (GCIG), a trial with two parallel and identical protocols has been developed and it will be conducted by many of the GCIG collaborative groups. Many centres within the GCIG groups will need to participate as only a few patients will be recruited by an individual centre each year. This makes the trial more complex and more expensive to run. One protocol, GOG 0241 will enrol patients in the USA and Korea and the other, mEOC, run by the NCRI in the UK will co-ordinate the trial in the UK, Europe and Australia.

The trial will recruit 332 patients over a period of 5 years with a further follow up of 5 years. To make the trial as efficient and informative as possible the investigators are also examining the role of bevacizumab in combination with chemotherapy in a 2×2 factorial design (Fig. 5.1). This is particularly relevant, as phase III studies with bevacizumab in conjunction with chemotherapy have demonstrated an improvement in the survival of patients with metastatic bowel cancer [28,29]. Furthermore, in ovarian cancer, the results of phase II studies with bevacizumab, given as a single agent, have been encouraging [30,31]. The progression-free survival results of two large trials of bevacizumab in combination with first-line chemotherapy (ICON 7 and GOG 218) are due in 2010.

The new first-line study will provide an opportunity to collect a large number of tissue samples and associated clinical data. Molecular analysis of these tumours will provide valuable information that could be used to design further studies, initially in those women relapsing after first-line therapy. The current randomised clinical trial acknowledges the biologically distinct behaviour of mucinous tumours and represents the first global effort needed to explore new treatments, targeted at the biological characteristics of the tumour.

References

1. Seidman JD, Kurman RJ, et al. Primary and metastatic mucinous adenocarcinomas in the ovaries: incidence in routine practice with a new approach to improve intraoperative diagnosis. Am J Surg Pathol. 2003;27(7):985–93.
2. McGuire V, Jesser CA, et al. Survival among U.S. women with invasive epithelial ovarian cancer. Gynecol Oncol. 2002;84(3):399–403.
3. Winter III WE, Maxwell GL, et al. Prognostic factors for stage III epithelial ovarian cancer: a Gynecologic Oncology Group Study. J Clin Oncol. 2007;25(24):3621–7.
4. Hart WR. Mucinous tumors of the ovary: a review. Int J Gynecol Pathol. 2005;24(1):4–25.
5. Hoerl HD, Hart WR. Primary ovarian mucinous cystadenocarcinomas: a clinicopathologic study of 49 cases with long-term follow-up. Am J Surg Pathol. 1998;22(12): 1449–62.
6. Lee KR, Young RH. The distinction between primary and metastatic mucinous carcinomas of the ovary: gross and histologic findings in 50 cases. Am J Surg Pathol. 2003;27(3): 281–92.
7. Yedema CA, Kenemans P, et al. Use of serum tumor markers in the differential diagnosis between ovarian and colorectal adenocarcinomas. Tumour Biol. 1992;13(1–2):18–26.
8. Wauters CC, Smedts F, et al. Keratins 7 and 20 as diagnostic markers of carcinomas metastatic to the ovary. Hum Pathol. 1995;26(8):852–5.
9. Chu PG, Weiss LM. Keratin expression in human tissues and neoplasms. Histopathology. 2002;40(5):403–39.
10. Ji H, Isacson C, et al. Cytokeratins 7 and 20, Dpc4, and MUC5AC in the distinction of metastatic mucinous carcinomas in the ovary from primary ovarian mucinous tumors: Dpc4 assists in identifying metastatic pancreatic carcinomas. Int J Gynecol Pathol. 2002;21(4):391–400.
11. Vang R, Gown AM, et al. Immunohistochemical expression of CDX2 in primary ovarian mucinous tumors and metastatic mucinous carcinomas involving the ovary: comparison with CK20 and correlation with coordinate expression of CK7. Mod Pathol. 2006;19(11):1421–8.
12. Ichikawa Y, Nishida M, et al. Mutation of K-ras protooncogene is associated with histological subtypes in human mucinous ovarian tumors. Cancer Res. 1994;54(1):33–5.
13. Gemignani ML, Schlaerth AC, et al. Role of KRAS and BRAF gene mutations in mucinous ovarian carcinoma. Gynecol Oncol. 2003;90(2):378–81.
14. Wamunyokoli FW, Bonome T, et al. Expression profiling of mucinous tumors of the ovary identifies genes of clinicopathologic importance. Clin Cancer Res. 2006;12(3 Pt 1): 690–700.
15. Demopoulos RI, Touger L, et al. Secondary ovarian carcinoma: a clinical and pathological evaluation. Int J Gynecol Pathol.1987; 6(2):166–75.

16. Berger KL, Nicholson SA, et al. FDG PET evaluation of mucinous neoplasms: correlation of FDG uptake with histopathologic features. AJR Am J Roentgenol. 2000;174(4):1005–8.
17. Engelen MJ, de Bruijn HW, et al. Serum CA 125, carcinoembryonic antigen, and CA 19-9 as tumor markers in borderline ovarian tumors. Gynecol Oncol. 2000;78(1):16–20.
18. Fioretti P, Gadducci A, et al. The concomitant determination of different serum tumor markers in epithelial ovarian cancer: relevance for monitoring the response to chemotherapy and follow-up of patients. Gynecol Oncol. 1992;44(2):155–60.
19. Vergote I, De Brabanter J, et al. Prognostic importance of degree of differentiation and cyst rupture in stage I invasive epithelial ovarian carcinoma. Lancet. 2001;357(9251):176–82.
20. Trimbos JB, Parmar M, et al. International Collaborative Ovarian Neoplasm trial 1 and Adjuvant ChemoTherapy In Ovarian Neoplasm trial: two parallel randomized phase III trials of adjuvant chemotherapy in patients with early-stage ovarian carcinoma. J Natl Cancer Inst. 2003;95(2):105–12.
21. du Bois A, Quinn M, et al. 2004 consensus statements on the management of ovarian cancer: final document of the 3rd International Gynecologic Cancer Intergroup Ovarian Cancer Consensus Conference (GCIG OCCC 2004). Ann Oncol. 2005;16 Suppl 8:viii 7–12.
22. Hess V, A'Hern R, et al. Mucinous epithelial ovarian cancer: a separate entity requiring specific treatment. J Clin Oncol. 2004;22(6):1040–4.
23. Pectasides D, Fountzilas G, et al. Advanced stage mucinous epithelial ovarian cancer: the Hellenic Cooperative Oncology Group experience. Gynecol Oncol. 2005;97(2):436–41.
24. Pignata S, Ferrandina G, et al. Activity of chemotherapy in mucinous ovarian cancer with a recurrence free interval of more than 6 months: results from the SOCRATES retrospective study. BMC Cancer. 2008;8:252.
25. Sato S, Itamochi H, et al. Combination chemotherapy of oxaliplatin and 5-fluorouracil may be an effective regimen for mucinous adenocarcinoma of the ovary: a potential treatment strategy. Cancer Sci. 2009;100(3):546–51.
26. deBraud F, Munzone E, et al. Synergistic activity of oxaliplatin and 5-fluorouracil in patients with metastatic colorectal cancer with progressive disease while on or after 5-fluorouracil. Am J Clin Oncol. 1998;21(3):279–83.
27. Pectasides D, Pectasides M, et al. Oxaliplatin plus high-dose leucovorin and 5-fluorouracil (FOLFOX 4) in platinum-resistant and taxane-pretreated ovarian cancer: a phase II study. Gynecol Oncol. 2004;95(1):165–72.
28. Hurwitz H, Fehrenbacher L, et al. Bevacizumab plus irinotecan, fluorouracil, and leucovorin for metastatic colorectal cancer. N Engl J Med. 2004;350(23):2335–42.
29. Saltz LB, Clarke S, et al. Bevacizumab in combination with oxaliplatin-based chemotherapy as first-line therapy in metastatic colorectal cancer: a randomized phase III study. J Clin Oncol. 2008;26(12):2013–9.
30. Burger RA. Experience with bevacizumab in the management of epithelial ovarian cancer. J Clin Oncol. 2007;25(20):2902–8.
31. Cannistra SA, Matulonis UA, et al. Phase II study of bevacizumab in patients with platinum-resistant ovarian cancer or peritoneal serous cancer. J Clin Oncol. 2007;25(33):5180–6.

Pseudomyxoma Peritonei

6

Faheez Mohamed and Brendan J. Moran

6.1 Introduction

Pseudomyxoma peritonei (PMP) is an uncommon disease with an estimated incidence of 1–2 per million per year [1]. PMP is characterised by diffuse intra-abdominal gelatinous collections with mucinous implants on peritoneal surfaces and the omentum, manifesting clinically as "jelly belly" [2]. PMP commonly simulates ovarian cancer clinically, radiologically and at surgery. Whilst most cases are now considered to originate from a perforated mucinous appendiceal tumour, ovarian masses are one of the commonest clinical presenting features of PMP in women. Many cases present unexpectedly at laparoscopy or laparotomy, or may be suspected at cross-sectional imaging during the investigation, or staging, of another pathological entity.

Although PMP has generally been considered benign, its behaviour suggests that it should, at best, be considered a borderline malignancy with disease progression, over time, to massive abdominal distension and nutritional compromise in most cases. The long-term survival remains poor with reported five- and ten-year survival rates of 50 and 10–30%, respectively [3]. Over the last 10 years there has been increasing global interest in the management of PMP, particularly in macroscopic removal of tumour by complex surgical techniques combined with heated intraperitoneal chemotherapy [4].

F. Mohamed and B. J. Moran (✉)
Pseudomyxoma Peritonei Centre, Basingstoke and North Hampshire Hospital Foundation Trust, Aldermaston Road, Basingstoke, Hampshire RG24 9NA, UK
e-mail: brendan.moran@bnhft.nhs.uk

6.2 Origin of PMP

Werth [5] in 1884 coined the term, describing pseudomyxoma peritonei in association with a mucinous tumour of the ovary. In 1901 Frankel [6] described a case associated with a cyst of the appendix. Since these early reports there has been ongoing debate as to the primary origin of PMP, particularly in women. Most acknowledge that PMP predominantly originates in the appendix in men and increasingly, evidence suggests a similar site of origin in women [7, 8]. In women, synchronous ovarian and appendiceal disease is common, and PMP appears more prevalent. However immunohistochemistry and molecular genetic techniques support the hypothesis that in the majority of women, the ovarian tumour is metastatic from a perforated appendiceal mucinous tumour [9–15]. Recently MUC 2 overexpression has been suggested as a molecular marker for PMP of intestinal rather than ovarian origin [16, 17]. From a clinical perspective, whilst many have reported that PMP is more common in women, Moran and colleagues [7] have proposed that it is unlikely that the male and female appendices behave in a different manner with an expected similar number of appendiceal PMP cases in women.

Personal experience suggests that some of the reported increased female incidence may represent a "Will Rogers" phenomenon [18] with earlier and more precise diagnosis in women [3]. Women with non-specific symptoms are more likely to have cross-sectional imaging, particularly to rule out ovarian cancer.

Undoubtedly a proportion of cases arise from other organs, [19] with an ovarian primary being the commonest in this diverse group. In particular, low grade mucinous ovarian neoplasms are often indistinguishable clinically, radiologically or at operation from PMP of appendiceal origin [16]. Personal experience

N. Reed et al. (eds.), *Rare and Uncommon Gynecological Cancers*,
DOI: 10.1007/978-3-642-13492-0_6, © Springer-Verlag Berlin Heidelberg 2011

has shown that ovarian mucinous tumours with widespread dissemination have much worse prognosis compared with PMP of appendiceal origin despite complete tumour removal (unpublished data). PMP has been reported originating from the colon and rectum, the stomach, gallbladder and bile duct, small intestine, urinary bladder, lung, breast, fallopian tube and pancreas.

6.3 Pathophysiologyo f PMP

The sequence of events culminating in PMP is thought to involve growth of an appendiceal adenoma progressing to occlude the appendiceal lumen with distension of the appendix by mucus and mucinous tumour cells (Fig. 6.1). The appendix eventually ruptures, often initially by a "blow out" and subsequent slow leak of mucus containing epithelial cells from the adenoma. In most cases appendicular perforation is an occult event and it is notable that the appendix can be macroscopically normal, following rupture and resealing, such that the appendix should be removed, if feasible, in all patients with "jelly belly".

The distinctive feature of PMP is its characteristic "redistribution" within the peritoneal cavity [20]. In contrast to most carcinoma cells of gastrointestinal tract origin that implant in a random fashion near the site of perforation, PMP demonstrates a nomadic pattern of migration with epithelial cells accumulating at specific abdominal and pelvic sites.

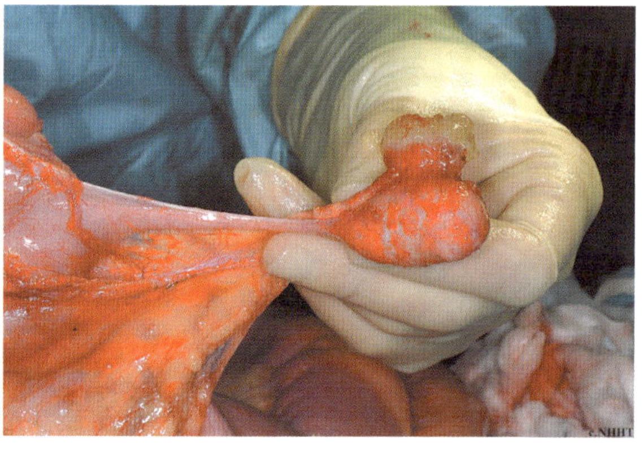

Fig.6.1 Ruptureofa ppendixw ithe xtravasationof m ucin

6.3.1 The Redistribution Phenomenon

The intraperitoneal distribution of PMP is determined by physical factors, namely the movement and absorption of peritoneal fluid and gravity. Normally peritoneal fluid migrates upwards, particularly in the right paracolic gutter towards the main sites of peritoneal fluid absorption on the undersurface of the right hemidiaphragm, the greater and lesser omentum. The open lymphatic lacunae on the undersurface of the right hemidiaphragm, and the lymphoid aggregates in the omentum, absorb fluid leading to bulky accumulations as the mucus is absorbed and epithelial cells "filtered out" and concentrated. From a clinical perspective, the concentrated tumour masses result in an omental cake (Fig. 6.2).

Gravity also plays a role, especially in the early stages, as mucus and cells concentrate in dependent portions of the abdomen and pelvis such as the rectovesical pouch, the right retrohepatic space and the paracolicgutte rs [20].

A pathognomic feature of favourable PMP is the complete, or nearly complete, absence of tumour masses on the freely mobile intestinal surfaces, especially the small bowel. Normal peristalsis, together with poor adherence properties of the tumour cells results in "bowel sparing". In contrast the parts of the gastrointestinal tract fixed to the retroperitoneum, such

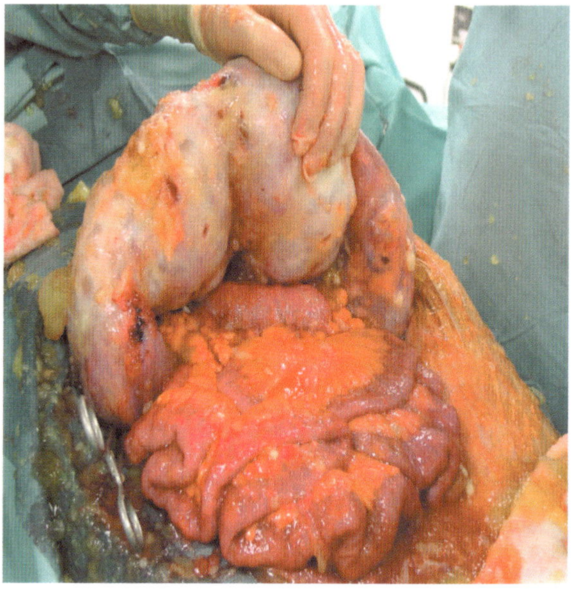

Fig. 6.2 Omentalc akea ssociatedw ithP MP

as the gastric pylorus and antrum and the ileocaecal and rectosigmoid regions, are often heavily diseased and commonly require resection to remove macroscopictumourin volvingthe bo wel [21].

6.4 PathologicalC lassification

Controversy persists over the classification of epithelial appendiceal neoplasms and their relationship to PMP. High-grade colonic mucinous neoplasms, adenocarcinomas of the appendix and mucinous adenocarcinomas originating from any other intra-abdominal organ, particularly the colon, can mimic the clinical, radiological and pathological features of PMP [13]. Additionally, there appears to be a spectrum of disease from low- to high-grade, though the pathological appearances may not correlate with clinical behaviour ofthe tumour [22].

Ronnett and colleagues, in a retrospective review of a series of patients who had undergone complete cytoreduction by Sugarbaker's group, reported a pathological system commonly quoted in the literature [23]. They classified low-grade tumours as disseminated peritoneal adenomucinosis (DPAM) and high-grade tumours as peritoneal mucinous carcinomatosis (PMCA), with an intermediate group (IG) demonstrating a mixture of DPAM and PMCA. Survival was significantly higher in the low-grade (DPAM) as compared with the high-grade tumours (IG and PMCA). They were unable to show a statistically significant difference between the IG and PMCA groups and subsequently grouped these together [13, 24]. Dichotomous categorisations of mucinous tumours of the appendix have been adopted elsewhere and what is emerging is that optimal outcomes result from the management of PMP originating from low-grade appendiceal mucinous tumours [25].

6.5 Diagnosis

The majority of patients are diagnosed during, or after, a laparotomy or laparoscopy for suspected appendicitis, peritonitis or gynaecological cancer.

In a series of 410 patients with appendiceal tumours, 217 had the diagnosis of PMP with histological confirmation [26]. Overall, 27% presented with suspected appendicitis, 23% with increasing abdominal distension and 14% with a new onset hernia. In women, PMP was most commonly diagnosed during investigation of an ovarian mass (39%) (Fig. 6.3).

Computed Tomography (CT) is currently the optimal imaging modality for the diagnosis and staging of PMP [27]. Classically "scalloping" of visceral surfaces, particularly of the liver and spleen, distinguishes mucinous from fluid ascites (Fig. 6.4) [28]. Contrast-enhanced CT can assist in predicting the likelihood of

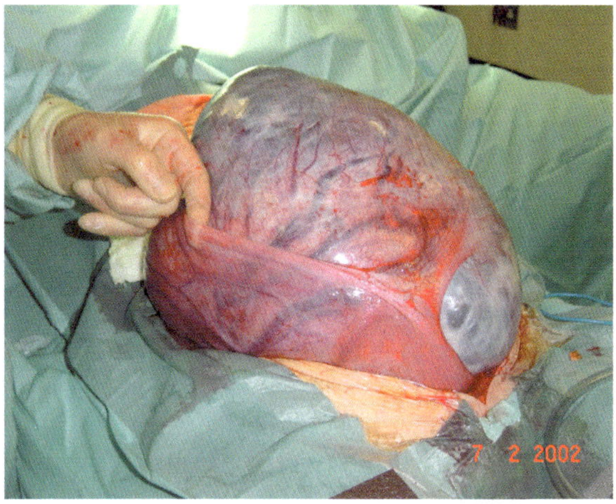

Fig. 6.3 Ovarian mass of primary intestinal origin presenting 3 years after right hemicolectomy for cystadenoma of the appendix

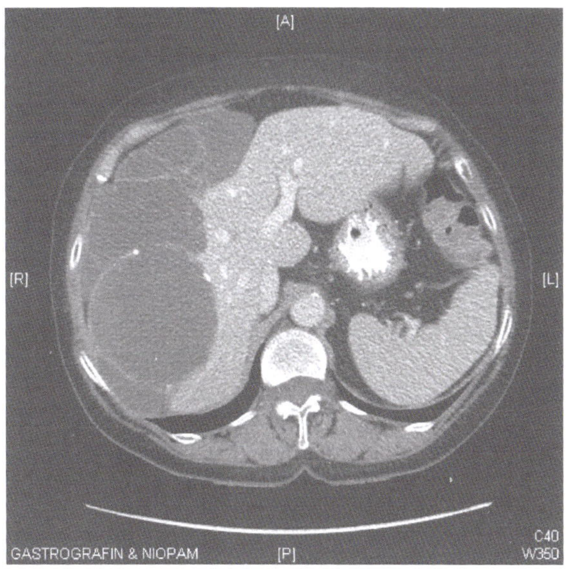

Fig. 6.4 AbdominalC Ts howing" scalloping"of t hel iver

complete cytoreduction [28]. A recent report on the use of delayed gadolinium enhanced MRI seems promising in staging and patient selection for cytoreductive surgeryb utre quiresfurthe re valuation [29].

6.5.1 Preop Assessment: Tumour Markers – CEA, CA125, CA19.9 and Laparoscopy

Elevated markers indicate more aggressive disease [30] with increased risk of recurrence [31–33]. When a patient presents with increasing abdominal girth as a result of presumed malignant ascites, the diagnosis is usually established with paracentesis, or laparoscopy and biopsy. If possible, paracentesis or laparoscopy should be performed through the midline as these sites can be excised by a midline abdominal incision [34].

6.5.2 Operative Strategy in Unexpected Case

It has been reported that extensive prior attempts to debulk PMP significantly impacts on subsequent attempts at complete tumour removal [35]. It is advisable, therefore, that the referring team perform the minimum surgery required to establish a histological diagnosis prior to specialist centre referral. In this context if one suspects that PMP in a female is of appendiceal origin, and is likely to be suitable for complete tumour removal (due to the relative sparing of the small bowel), surgery should comprise an appendicectomy and bilateral oophorectomy with the uterus and omentum left in place to facilitate subsequent surgery.

6.6 Treatment

The indolent behaviour of PMP led some to advocate no active treatment [36], although it is increasingly accepted that most patients with PMP, untreated, will progress to terminal starvation through intestinal obstructionbymuc inousa scites [37].

6.6.1 Surgical Treatment of PMP

Traditionally surgery involved repeated interval debulking with limited expectation of long-term survival and no prospect of cure. Gough reported ten-year survival in 32% of 56 patients who underwent serial debulking and selectively, intra-peritoneal radiotherapy, or chemotherapy, between 1957 and 1983 in the Mayo clinic [38]. In 2005, Miner reported a ten-year survival of 21% (12% disease free) in 97 patients treated by serial debulking, systemic chemotherapy and/or delayed intermittent intraperitoneal 5-fluorouracil over a 22-year period at Memorial Sloan Kettering [39]. All agree that over time, debulking becomes more difficult, less effective and more dangerous due to the risk of bowel injury and subsequent fistulaforma tion [2].

Sugarbaker introduced and popularised an approach combining cytoreductive surgery (CRS) (aiming for macroscopic complete tumour removal) with heated intraperitoneal chemotherapy (HIPEC) [40, 41]. This involves up to six different peritonectomy procedures in combination with visceral resections as required, to remove all visible tumour, or if not possible, to leave tumour deposits less than 2.5 mm. Surgery includes a greater omentectomy and splenectomy, left upper quadrant peritonectomy, right upper quadrant peritonectomy, lesser omentectomy and cholecystectomy, appendicectomy or right hemicolectomy, total colectomy, partial or total gastrectomy, and pelvic peritonectomy with anterior resection of the rectosigmoid colon. In addition most female patients require hysterectomy and bilateral salpingo-oophorectomy. Patients must be medically fit to safely undergo CRS with HIPEC due to the associated morbidity and mortality [42].

6.6.2 Rationale for Hyperthermic Intraperitoneal Chemotherapy (HIPEC)

The major advantage of intraperitoneal therapy is regional dose intensity [43]. The penetration of intraperitoneal chemotherapy into peritoneal carcinomatosis nodules is limited to between 2 and 5 mm, even when combined with heat [44] making reduction of intraperitoneal tumour volume essential [45]. Hyperthermia alone is cytotoxic at cellular and tissue levels [46] and studies in cultured mammalian cells, and in animal tumours, show that hyperthermia can enhance cytotoxicity of some chemotherapeutic agents [47]. Combining hyperthermia with intraperitoneal chemotherapy optimisesc ytotoxicity.

6.6.3 Survival Following CRS and HIPEC

The single most important factor in survival has been the ability to achieve complete tumour removal [24, 48]. No clear strategy exists for patients identified at preoperative assessment or intraoperatively to have disease not amenable to complete resection due to tumour extent and distribution, serious co-morbidity or age. There is increasing evidence that these patients benefit from a major palliative resection with reasonable intermediate-term survival of 43% at two years and 15% at five years and improved quality of life [49, 50].

6.6.4 Morbidity and Mortality of CRS with HIPEC

There have been a number of reports addressing the morbidity and mortality associated with CRS and HIPEC [51]. Major morbidity includes anastomotic leakage, enteric and pancreatic fistulation, cardiopulmonary events, thromboembolism and intra-abdominal abscesses.

Recent reports suggest that the initial high morbidity and mortality seen with CRS and HIPEC decreases with increasing experience [52, 53]. Experience results in improvements in patient selection, surgical expertisea ndpos toperativema nagement [54].

6.7 Conclusion

PMP, though uncommon, can present unexpectedly at laparotomy or laparoscopy and in women commonly simulates ovarian cancer clinically, radiologically and at operation. Accumulating evidence suggests that optimal surgical resection (complete cytoreduction if possible) combined with HIPEC is an effective strategy for treating PMP. The treatment is complex, associated with significant morbidity and mortality and a substantial institutional, and individual, "learning curve" [55].

All surgeons who operate in the abdomen will occasionally encounter a patient with PMP. In this unexpected event the best strategy to facilitate subsequent attempts at complete cytoreduction is to take generous biopsies, remove the appendix if accessible and refrain from major resectional interventions. Following recovery and histological confirmation of the clinical diagnosis, an opinion should be sought from a specialised assessmenta ndtre atmentc entre [56].

PMP is at best a "borderline" peritoneal malignancy despite the indolent pathology and slow progression in some cases. Other mucinous tumours, including aggressive adenocarcinomas may simulate PMP and caution is required before labelling such cases as PMP to avoid the false hopes of favourable outcomes increasingly reported from management of true PMP.

References

1. Smeenk RM, van Velthuysen ML, Verwaal VJ, Zoetmulder FA. Appendiceal neoplasms and pseudomyxoma peritonei: a population based study. Eur J Surg Oncol. 2008;34: 196–201.
2. Moran BJ, Cecil TD. The etiology, clinical presentation, and management of pseudomyxoma peritonei. Surg Oncol Clin N Am. 2003;12:585–603.
3. Hinson FL, Ambrose NS. Pseudomyxoma peritonei. Br J Surg.1998; 85:1332–9.
4. Moran B, Baratti D, Yan TD, Kusamura S, Deraco M. Consensus statement on the loco-regional treatment of appendiceal mucinous neoplasms with peritoneal dissemination (pseudomyxoma peritonei) J Surg Oncol 2008;98:277-282
5. Werth R. Klinische and Anastomische Untersuchungen Zur Lehre von der Bauchgeswullsten und der laparotomy. Arch Gynecol Obstet. 1884;84:100–18.
6. Frankel E. Uher das sogenaute pseudomyxoma peritonei. Med Wochenschr. 1901;48:965–70.
7. Mukherjee A, Parvaiz A, Cecil TD, Moran BJ. Pseudomyxoma peritonei usually originates from the appendix: a review of the evidence. Eur J Gynaecol Oncol. 2004;25:411–4.
8. Sherer DM, Abulafia O, Eliakim R. Pseudomyxoma peritonei: a review of current literature. Gynecol Obstet Invest. 2001;51:73–80.
9. Chuaqui RF, Zhuang Z, Emmert-Buck MR, Bryant BR, Nogales F, Tavassoli FA, et al. Genetic analysis of synchronous mucinous tumors of the ovary and appendix. Hum Pathol.1996; 27:165–71.
10. Guerrieri C, Franlund B, Fristedt S, Gillooley JF, Boeryd B. Mucinous tumors of the vermiform appendix and ovary, and pseudomyxoma peritonei: histogenetic implications of cytokeratin 7 expression. Hum Pathol. 1997;28:1039–45.

11. Prayson RA, Hart WR, Petras RE. Pseudomyxoma peritonei. A clinicopathologic study of 19 cases with emphasis on site of origin and nature of associated ovarian tumors. Am J Surg Pathol. 1994;18:591–603.
12. Ronnett BM, Shmookler BM, Diener-West M, Sugarbaker PH, Kurman RJ. Immunohistochemical evidence supporting the appendiceal origin of pseudomyxoma peritonei in women. Int J Gynecol Pathol. 1997;16:1–9.
13. Sugarbaker PH, Ronnett BM, Archer A, Averbach AM, Bland R, Chang D, et al. Pseudomyxoma peritonei syndrome. Adv Surg. 1996;30:233–80.
14. Szych C, Staebler A, Connolly DC, Wu R, Cho KR, Ronnett BM. Molecular genetic evidence supporting the clonality and appendiceal origin of Pseudomyxoma peritonei in women. Am J Pathol. 1999;154:1849–55.
15. Young RH, Gilks CB, Scully RE. Pseudomyxoma peritonei. Am J Surg Pathol. 1993;17:1068–71.
16. Ferreira CR, Carvalho JP, Soares FA, Siqueira SA, Carvalho FM. Mucinous ovarian tumors associated with pseudomyxoma peritonei of adenomucinosis type: immunohistochemical evidence that they are secondary tumors. Int J Gynecol Cancer.20 08;18:59–65.
17. O'Connell JT, Hacker CM, Barsky SH. MUC2 is a molecular marker for pseudomyxoma peritonei. Mod Pathol. 2002;15:958–72.
18. Feinstein AR, Sosin DM, Wells CK. The Will Rogers phenomenon. Stage migration and new diagnostic techniques as a source of misleading statistics for survival in cancer. N Engl J Med. 1985;312:1604–8.
19. Smeenk RM, Bex A, Verwaal VJ, Horenblas S, Zoetmulder FA. Pseudomyxoma peritonei and the urinary tract: involvement and treatment related complications. J Surg Oncol. 2006;93:20–3.
20. Sugarbaker PH. Pseudomyxoma peritonei. A cancer whose biology is characterized by a redistribution phenomenon. Ann Surg. 1994;219:109–11.
21. Carmignani CP, Sugarbaker TA, Bromley CM, Sugarbaker PH. Intraperitoneal cancer dissemination: mechanisms of the patterns of spread. Cancer Metastasis Rev. 2003;22: 465–72.
22. Mohamed F, Gething S, Haiba M, Brun EA, Sugarbaker PH. Clinically aggressive pseudomyxoma peritonei: a variant of a histologically indolent process. J Surg Oncol. 2004;86:10–5.
23. Ronnett BM, Zahn CM, Kurman RJ, Kass ME, Sugarbaker PH, Shmookler BM. Disseminated peritoneal adenomucinosis and peritoneal mucinous carcinomatosis. A clinicopathologic analysis of 109 cases with emphasis on distinguishing pathologic features, site of origin, prognosis, and relationship to "pseudomyxoma peritonei". Am J Surg Pathol. 1995; 19:1390–408.
24. Sugarbaker PH, Chang D. Results of treatment of 385 patients with peritoneal surface spread of appendiceal malignancy. Ann Surg Oncol. 1999;6:727–31.
25. Bradley RF, Stewart 4th JH, Russell GB, Levine EA, Geisinger KR. Pseudomyxoma peritonei of appendiceal origin: a clinicopathologic analysis of 101 patients uniformly treated at a single institution, with literature review. Am J Surg Pathol. 2006;30:551–9.
26. Esquivel J, Sugarbaker PH. Clinical presentation of the Pseudomyxoma peritonei syndrome. Br J Surg. 2000;87: 1414–8.
27. Jacquet P, Jelinek JS, Chang D, Koslowe P, Sugarbaker PH. Abdominal computed tomographic scan in the selection of patients with mucinous peritoneal carcinomatosis for cytoreductive surgery. J Am Coll Surg. 1995;181:530–8.
28. Sulkin TV, O'Neill H, Amin AI, Moran B. CT in pseudomyxoma peritonei: a review of 17 cases. Clin Radiol. 2002;57: 608–13.
29. Low RN, Barone RM, Gurney JM, Muller WD. Mucinous appendiceal neoplasms: preoperative MR staging and classification compared with surgical and histopathological findings. AJR Am J Roentgenol 2008;190: 656 -665
30. Baratti D, Kusamura S, Martinetti A, Seregni E, Laterza B, Oliva DG, et al. Prognostic value of circulating tumor markers in patients with pseudomyxoma peritonei treated with cytoreductive surgery and hyperthermic intraperitoneal chemotherapy. Ann Surg Oncol. 2007;14:2300–8.
31. Alexander-Sefre F, Chandrakumaran K, Banerjee S, Sexton R, Thomas JM, Moran B. Elevated tumour markers prior to complete tumour removal in patients with pseudomyxoma peritonei predict early recurrence. Colorectal Dis. 2005;7: 382–6.
32. Carmignani CP, Hampton R, Sugarbaker CE, Chang D, Sugarbaker PH. Utility of CEA and CA 19-9 tumor markers in diagnosis and prognostic assessment of mucinous epithelial cancers of the appendix. J Surg Oncol. 2004;87:162–6.
33. van Ruth S, Hart AA, Bonfrer JM, Verwaal VJ, Zoetmulder FA. Prognostic value of baseline and serial carcinoembryonic antigen and carbohydrate antigen 19.9 measurements in patients with pseudomyxoma peritonei treated with cytoreduction and hyperthermic intraperitoneal chemotherapy. Ann Surg Oncol. 2002;9:961–7.
34. Sugarbaker PH. New standard of care for appendiceal epithelial neoplasms and pseudomyxoma peritonei syndrome? Lancet Oncol. 2006;7:69–76.
35. Harmon RL, Sugarbaker PH. Prognostic indicators in peritoneal carcinomatosis from gastrointestinal cancer. Int Semin Surg Oncol. 2005;2:3.
36. Friedland JS, Allardice JT, Wyatt AP. Pseudomyxoma peritonei. J R Soc Med. 1986;79:480–2.
37. Sugarbaker PH. Pseudomyxoma peritonei. Cancer Treat Res.1996; 81:105–19.
38. Gough DB, Donohue JH, Schutt AJ, Gonchoroff N, Goellner JR, Wilson TO, et al. Pseudomyxoma peritonei. Long-term patient survival with an aggressive regional approach. Ann Surg.1994; 219:112–9.
39. Miner TJ, Shia J, Jaques DP, Klimstra DS, Brennan MF, Coit DG. Long-term survival following treatment of pseudomyxoma peritonei: an analysis of surgical therapy. Ann Surg. 2005;241:300–8.
40. Sugarbaker PH. Surgical treatment of peritoneal carcinomatosis: 1988 Du Pont lecture. Can J Surg. 1989;32:164–70.
41. Sugarbaker PH, Kern K, Lack E. Malignant pseudomyxoma peritonei of colonic origin. Natural history and presentation of a curative approach to treatment. Dis Colon Rectum. 1987;30:772–9.
42. Stewart 4th JH, Shen P, Levine EA. Intraperitoneal hyperthermic chemotherapy for peritoneal surface malignancy: current status and future directions. Ann Surg Oncol. 2005; 12:765–77.
43. Dedrick RL. Theoretical and experimental bases of intraperitoneal chemotherapy. Semin Oncol. 1985;12:1–6.

44. Glehen O, Beaujard AC, Arvieux C, Huber O, Gilly FN. Peritoneal carcinomatosis. Surgical treatment, peritonectomy and intraperitoneal chemohyperthermia. Gastroentérol Clin Biol. 2002;26:210–5.
45. Barakat RR, Sabbatini P, Bhaskaran D, Revzin M, Smith A, Venkatraman E, et al. Intraperitoneal chemotherapy for ovarian carcinoma: results of long-term follow-up. J Clin Oncol. 2002;20:694–8.
46. Oleson JR, Calderwood SK, Coughlin CT, Dewhirst MW, Gerweck LE, Gibbs Jr FA, et al. Biological and clinical aspects of hyperthermia in cancer therapy. Am J Clin Oncol. 1988;11:368–80.
47. Urano M, Kuroda M, Nishimura Y. For the clinical application of thermochemotherapy given at mild temperatures. Int J Hyperthermia. 1999;15:79–107.
48. Gonzalez-Moreno S, Sugarbaker PH. Right hemicolectomy does not confer a survival advantage in patients with mucinous carcinoma of the appendix and peritoneal seeding. Br J Surg.2004;91:304–11.
49. Glehen O, Mohamed F, Sugarbaker PH. Incomplete cytoreduction in 174 patients with peritoneal carcinomatosis from appendiceal malignancy. Ann Surg. 2004;240:278–85.
50. Stewart 4th JH, Shen P, Russell GB, Bradley RF, Hundley JC, Loggie BL, et al. Appendiceal neoplasms with peritoneal dissemination: outcomes after cytoreductive surgery and intraperitoneal hyperthermic chemotherapy. Ann Surg Oncol.2006; 13:624–34.
51. Yan TD, Black D, Savady R, Sugarbaker PH. A systematic review on the efficacy of cytoreductive surgery and perioperative intraperitoneal chemotherapy for pseudomyxoma peritonei. Ann Surg Oncol. 2007;14:484–92.
52. Smeenk RM, Verwaal VJ, Zoetmulder FA. Learning curve of combined modality treatment in peritoneal surface disease. Br J Surg. 2007;94:1408–14.
53. Yan TD, Links M, Fransi S, Jacques T, Black D, Saunders V, et al. Learning curve for cytoreductive surgery and perioperative intraperitoneal chemotherapy for peritoneal surface malignancy – a journey to becoming a Nationally Funded Peritonectomy Center. Ann Surg Oncol. 2007;14: 2270–80.
54. Moran BJ. Decision-making and technical factors account for the learning curve in complex surgery. J Public Health (Oxf).2006; 28:375–8.
55. Moran BJ. Establishment of a peritoneal malignancy treatment centre in the United Kingdom. Eur J Surg Oncol. 2006;32:614–8.
56. Murphy EM, Farquharson SM, Moran BJ. Management of an unexpected appendiceal neoplasm. Br J Surg. 2006;93: 783–92.

OvarianC learC ell Carcinoma

7

Amy Ford and John A. Green

7.1 Introduction

Clear cell carcinoma is a distinct entity from other epithelial ovarian carcinomas, not simply because of its characteristic histology, but because of its specific biological and clinical behaviour. It is the second most common histological subtype of ovarian cancer, after serous carcinoma, accounting for 4–12% of ovarian epithelial cancers in Western countries [1, 2]. It comprises a greater proportion of ovarian epithelial cancers in Japan, up to 20% [1], where the incidence is rising [3]. Even in the West, clear cell carcinoma accounts for a significantly higher proportion of ovarian cancers in people of Japanese descent, compared to all other ethnicgroups [2].

The median age of presentation with clear cell carcinoma is nearly 10 years younger than for all other ovarian epithelial cancers, at 55 years [2]. Common presenting symptoms include a firm, unilateral palpable pelvic mass, the development or exacerbation of dysmenorrhea or dyspareunia, gastrointestinal symptoms, pelvic pain, and less commonly, abdominal distension [4]. Clear cell carcinoma is significantly more likely to be diagnosed at FIGO Stage I or II than other ovarian epithelial cancers, but after adjusting for stage, outcomesa res tillw orse [2].

Protective factors against the development of clear cell cancer appear to be hormonal contraceptive use in excess of 5 years, increased parity, and possibly smoking [5]. The former two factors result in decreased ovulation, but it is not clear if this is the mechanism of risk reduction. Obesity is associated with a twofold increased risk of developing clear cell carcinoma [5, 6], but the most well established and widely recognised risk is the presence of endometriosis [7] which is associated with a threefold increase in the risk of clear cell ovarian cancer [5]. Despite this, a recently reported prospective Japanese study revealed that less than 1% of patients with endometriosis go on to develop ovarian cancer, although among these, clear cell was the commonest histology [8]. This risk appears to increase with age, post-menopausal status and with endometrioma exceeding 9 cm in diameter. However, among those with endometriosis, increasing parity and smoking status did not appear to influence the risk of developing ovarian cancer [8]. Presenting symptoms do not appear to differ between those patients with and without concurrent endometriosis, although those patients with clear cell carcinoma arising within endometriosis are reported as presenting at a significantly younger age than other clear cell carcinomas [9]. As these are not dissimilar to the presenting symptoms of ovarian cancer, these patients may be investigated earlier. The presence of endometriosis does not appear to alter initial resectability [9]. Disease recurrence and death were significantly lower among optimally resected patients with endometriosis, compared to those without, and their median overall survival was significantly longer, but this may be a result of the earlier stage of presentation in this group of patients and could be explained by the symptoms accompanying the endometriosis leadingt oe arlieri nvestigation [4, 9].

In addition to the association with endometriosis, clear cell carcinoma of the ovary is less frequently associated with clear cell adenofibromas. It has been suggested that this may represent an alternative clonal

A.F ord(✉)
ClatterbridgeC entrefo rO ncology, Merseyside, UK
e-mail:a my_ford@talktalk.net

J.A.G reen
School of Cancer Studies, University of Liverpool,
LiverpoolL693B X, UK

N. Reed et al. (eds.), *Rare and Uncommon Gynecological Cancers*,
DOI: 10.1007/978-3-642-13492-0_7, © Springer-Verlag Berlin Heidelberg 2011

precursor for clear cell carcinoma [10]. To date, few studies have examined their behaviour in detail and the results have been conflicting. Some suggest these tumours are less aggressive in comparison to non-adenofibromatous clear cell carcinoma [11, 12], whereas others link them with poorer outcomes [13]. Compared to non-adenofibromatous clear cell carcinoma, fewer ofthe sea rea ssociatedw ithe ndometriosis [11].

Clear cell carcinomas are associated with paraneoplastic phenomena. In particular, they have been shown to be the most common gynaecological histology associated with parathyroid hormone-related protein excretion. This correlates with serum hypercalcaemia, which appears to respond well to treatment [14]. Clear cell carcinoma is also associated with a 2.5-fold risk of venous thrombo-embolism compared to other epithelial ovarian cancers, even when prophylactic anticoagulation is used, and a role for therapeutic anticoagulation has been proposed [15]. Those patients with recurrent disease appear to be at greater risk [16]. It has been postulated that tissue factor expression, which shows significant correlation with both venous thromboembolism and clear cell ovarian cancer, may be a contributing factor to this phenomenon [17].

7.2 Management

Since 1988, the International Federation of Gynaecology and Obstetrics has recommended that surgical staging for ovarian cancer includes pelvic and para-aortic lymph node sampling or lymphadenectomy. This provides prognostic information and helps determine the need for adjuvant treatment. However, there is yet to be a sound evaluation of its impact, if any, on survival in clear cell carcinoma. Retrospective studies of Stage I clear cell carcinomas to date have involved a variety of adjuvant chemotherapies between, and sometimes within, the lymphadenectomy and non-lymphadenectomy groups and have produced conflicting results. One of the earlier studies suggested superior outcomes for those who underwent lymphadenectomy, but this group received adjuvant chemotherapy with paclitaxel in addition to carboplatin, whereas those in the non-lymphadenectomy group received cisplatin-based chemotherapy [18]. Data from the Surveillance, Epidemiology and End Results programme has been analysed for all ovarian cancer patients, revealing a significant improvement in 5-year survival in all epithelial ovarian cancer groups who underwent lymphadenectomy, with the exception of clear cell carcinomas [19]. A further study of clear cell carcinoma alone showed no improvement in disease-free or overall survival with lymphadenectomy [20]. Any apparent survival benefit from lymphadenectomy may be attributable to more accurately staged patients in this group being compared against under-staged patients, with an intrinsically poorer prognosis in the non-lymphadenectomy group.

There are no established international guidelines for fertility sparing surgery in clear cell ovarian carcinoma, despite the frequency of presentation at an early stage. In epithelial ovarian carcinoma fertility sparing surgery is usually reserved for stage IA disease. In a small retrospective series, ten patients with clear cell carcinoma who would normally have undergone radical surgery, but who instead underwent fertility sparing surgery, were reviewed. All but one received adjuvant chemotherapy irrespective of stage. Nine were alive and five pregnancies had occurred in four patients [21]. Larger studies are needed to evaluate the longer term risks of this approach.

In early stage disease, it has been shown that adjuvant platinum-based chemotherapy significantly increased disease-free survival, compared to no adjuvant chemotherapy, in patients with serous adenocarcinoma, but not in patients with clear cell carcinoma [22]. In advanced disease, first-line treatment with carboplatin and paclitaxel is the current standard for epithelial ovarian cancer [23, 24], but it has been shown that response rates to this combination in clear cell carcinoma are significantly lower than in serous adenocarcinoma [25]. There is emerging evidence that irinotecan, in combination with cisplatin, achieves superior outcomes in both early and advanced clear cell carcinoma [26–29] and a phase III trial of irinotecan and cisplatin combination therapy vs. paclitaxel and carboplatin therapy as first-line treatment for clear cellc arcinomais inprogre ss [30].

There are few reported studies of second-line treatment in clear cell carcinoma and those published highlight extreme chemoresistance in this context. Even when a treatment-free period of greater than 6 months has been achieved, response rates to second-line chemotherapy are less than 10% [31, 32], much lower than that seen in other ovarian epithelial cancers.

7.3 Histopathologyand Mo lecular Characterisation

Ovarian cancers are a heterogeneous group of tumours conventionally subdivided by grade and degree of differentiation. Molecular studies have shown specific genetic defects to be present in certain histologic subtypes, and cell line and mouse models have helped establish new insights into pathogenesis and indicate useful targets for preclinical testing of new treatments [34]. The general model for the development of ovarian cancer by Shih and Kurman in 2004 [35] was based largely on data from serous tumours, and the subdivision into type 1 and 2 serous tumours first proposed by them has been generally accepted, although not based on category 1 evidence. Type 1 serous tumours are typically associated with KRAS or BRAF tumours, while type 2 tumours show p53 mutations. Much less well categorised were endometrioid tumours, although a series of 29 cases has suggested a similar dual pathogenetic pathway with β-catenin, KRAS mutations and MSI associated with low-grade endometrioid carcinoma, and p53 mutations associated with high-grade tumours [34].

Clear cell tumours characteristically have large, cuboidal, hobnail or flattened epithelial cells containing abundant clear cytoplasm lining tubules and cysts and growing in solid, tubular or glandular elements. An oncocytic form exists where the tumour cells have eosinophilicra thertha nc learc ytoplasm [36].

Immunohistochemical studies have usually demonstrated positive staining for the pro-apoptotic protein BAX, p21 and cyclin E [37–39]. HNF-1beta expression levels are significantly higher in CCC than non-CCC ovarian cancer [40]. Weak staining for TP53, HER2 and cyclin A may also be seen, although TP53 mutations are rare [37]. A study by Maeda [41] found 28% of CCC positive for glypican 3 (GPC3) staining, higher than the serous, endometrioid and mucinous tumours.

Loss of PTEN expression is seen in 40% of early stage clear cell tumours [42]. Mutation in PTEN has been suggested to be a key event in the progression from benign endometrial to endometrial tumours and clear cell carcinoma [43]. This lipid phosphatase in the AKT pathway inhibits cyclin D1 (CCND1) and p27, thus blocking cell cycle progression. In contrast to serous tumours, expression of the zinc finger transcription factor protein WT1 is usually absent in clear cell tumours [44], and the mechanism may be promoter methylation. E-cadherin is a cell adhesion molecule which is a transcriptional target of WT1 and whose expression is reduced in clear cell tumours [45]. CD44-10v splice variant expression has also been demonstrated in clear cell tumours to be associated with adverse outcome. However, examination of multiple simultaneous factors has not been carried out in these small series to determine the independent contribution to prognosis, and it is not clear the extent to which they play a central part in development.

Molecular genetic features show copy number changes at 8q11–q13, 8q21–q22, 8q23, 8q24-qter, 17q25-qter, 20q13-qter and 21q22-qter and reduced copy number on 19p [46], while another investigator found amplifications on 3 and 13q [47]. Deletions were also found at 9p, which is the known location of the cyclin-dependent kinase inhibitor 2(CDKN2) genes which encode the proteins p16 (INK4A), p15 (INK4B), and p14 (ARF) which are known tumour suppressors by regulating pathways interacting with Rb and p53. Interestingly, 9p deletions have also been noted in clear cellc arcinomasofthe kidne y [48].

There is significant intraobserver variation in the diagnosis of mixed ovarian surface epithelial carcinoma, with consequences for data collection on chemoresistance and prognosis. Mixed serous epithelial cancer with clear cell and serous components shows similar stage, mitotic activity and immunoreactivity to those of pure serous carcinoma and is likely to represent serous carcinoma with clear cell changes [49]. A commonly accepted criterion is that the clear cell component must be 50% or greater for the diagnosis of clear cell cancer.

Occasionally, distinguishing serous low malignant potential (S-LMP) from CCC with prominent papillary architecture may prove difficult, and also unilaterality, non-hierarchical branching, monomorphous cell population, and the presence of more typical CCC patterns elsewhere in the tumour may be found to be helpful. The presence of endometriosis is not specific, but should prompt for consideration of papillary CCC. Increased number of mitotic figures may not be present and high-grade cytologic atypia may be focal, requiring careful examination of multiple tumour sections for detection. CCC and S-LMP exhibit significantly different immunoreactivity for Wilm's Tumour one (WT1) and oestrogen receptor; these markers may be useful adjunctive tests in problematic cases [49]. Metachronous metastases from clear cell renal carcinoma need to be differentiated from primary CCC, using histopathology and imaging.

7.4 Biomarkers

The chemoresistance of clear cell carcinoma is well recognised, although the mechanisms underlying this are not fully understood. Decreased drug accumulation, increased drug detoxification, increased DNA repair activity and low cell proliferation are all thought to contribute [1]. Glutathione peroxidase 3 (GPX3) has been identified to be a gene highly expressed in CCC. Since GPX3 suppression increased the cisplatin sensitivity of CCC in vitro, GPX3 may be a candidate gene associated with the low cisplatin sensitivity of CCC [56]. Gene deletion of GPC-3 in clear cell carcinoma may render these tumours more sensitive to the taxol [51].

The Ki-67 labelling index in CCC tumours was significantly lower than in serous ovarian cancer. The Ki-67 labelling index for responders was significantly higher than that for non-responders in both tumour types. A multivariable analysis revealed that Ki-67 labelling index and residual tumour size were independent prognostic factors in CCC. Therefore, lower proliferation of the tumour cells may contribute to their resistance to chemotherapy [1]. Hypoxia-inducible factor 1 alpha (HIF-1alpha) was significantly higher in CCC than in other histological subtypes ($P=0.001$) and maybe a factor contributing to chemoresistance [52]. Expression of annexin A4 is elevated in ovarian CCC and is associated with chemoresistance in ovarian cancer cells, in part by enhancing drug efflux [59].

The expression in CCC of the genes involved in transcription, signalling, cell cycle, adhesion, matrix degradation and drug detoxification differs from other epithelial subtypes of ovarian cancer [54, 55]. Up-regulation of the hepatocyte nuclear factor-1 beta (HNF-1beta) and Polo-like kinase (PLK)-Early mitotic inhibitor-1 (Emi 1) as well as their downstream targets is found in most CCC [55, 56]. Early mitotic inhibitor-1 (Emi 1) is a key cell cycle regulator, which promotes S-phase and mitotic entry by inhibiting the anaphase promoting complex. Significant overexpression of EM1 protein was present in 82% (27/33) of CCC, independent of patient age, presence of ovarian/pelvic endometriosis and FIGO stage, while the corresponding figures were 0/10 for mucinous carcinomas and19%(6/32)e ndometrialc arcinomas [57].

Several significant common pathways observed in CCC of the ovary overlap the datasets identified in CCC of the kidney. Inhibitors of HNF-1beta and PLK-Emi 1 and their downstream signalling molecules are promising therapeutic targets which need evaluation [47].

CCC exhibit higher levels of hENT1, dCK, 5'NT and RRM1 compared to serous ovarian tumours. A statistically significant direct association of RRM2 expression levels and the relative risk of death was observed (Chi=8.18, $P=0.0043$). Cases with high RRM2 expression had a shorter OS than cases with low RRM2 levels ($P=0.05$), and this marker may deserve further investigation in a larger series. Osteopontin expression is elevated in CCC and is closely associated with transcription factor hepatocyte nuclear factor (HNF)-1 beta overexpression, which upregulatedinC CC [56, 58].

Loss of phosphate and tensin homolog (PTEN) expression is more in CCC, but PTEN mutations are not often observed. The mechanism of PTEN gene silencing in CCC is still not clear. Neither PTEN promoter methylation nor LOH at 10q23 locus is significantly related to PTEN inactivation and is not an adverse prognostic factor in CCC [59, 60]. Similarily, TP53 overexpression and mutation is more in CCC, andnota us efulprognos ticf actor [61].

Weak nm23-H1 and high AKT and pAKT expression was observed in ovarian serous adenocarcinoma and CCC. The expression of nm23-H1 was negatively correlated with tumour stage and grade and lymph node metastasis, whereas the expression of AKT/pAKT was positively correlated with these clinical factors. Oestrogen up-regulated pAKT expression and reduced nm23-H1 expression, which inhibited cell migration. The PIK3 kinase inhibitor LY 294002 antagonised the effect of oestrogen, yet reinforced the effect of progestin. The data suggested that AKT and pAKT are unfavourable prognostic factors for ovarian serous adenocarcinoma and CCC, whereas nm23-H1 expressionpre dictsf avourablepa tientpr ognosis [56].

7.5 TherapeuticT argets

GPC3 is a heparin sulphate proteoglycan overexpressed in some neoplasms and currently regarded as a tumour marker and potential target for immunotherapy. It was found in 44% of CCC, but rarely found in other histological subtypes (mucinous 4%, endometriod 5%, serous 11%; $P<0.0001$), apart from yolk sac tumour (100%). GPC3 expression was significantly associated with poor overall survival in Stage III/IV CCC, suggesting it may be related to the development and aggressive behaviour of CCC [41]. mTOR is frequently activated in CCC (86.6 vs. 50% of serous adenocarcinomas) and could be a promising therapeutic target in thema nagementofC CC [63].

Endometriosis serves as precursor of both CCC and endometrioid tumours of the ovary. Molecular events including p53 alteration, PTEN silencing, KRAS mutations and HNF-1 activation have been implicated in this transition, but the exact mechanisms remains unclear as do the optimum targets needing evaluation [64].

The need for further research into targeted agents with greater activity in both the first- and second-line treatment of CCC is paramount. Many studies have been small and few biomarkers have been validated in separate series. Sequence mutations of PIK3CA, TP53, KRAS, PTEN and CTNNB1 and BRAF occurred in 33, 15, 7, 5, 3 and 1% of CCC cases, respectively as shown in Fig 7.2. Drugs targeting PIK3CA may offer a more effective therapeutic approach compared with current chemotherapeutic agents for patients with advanced stage and recurrent CCC [62] Fig. 7.2. Yoshida et al. [66] in a review of genes highly expressed in clear cell tumours focussed on HNF-1 and its downstream targets, polo-like kinases/early mitotic inhibitor-1 (PLK-Emi 1), KRAS and their downstream targets,a nds ummarisedinFig. 7.1.

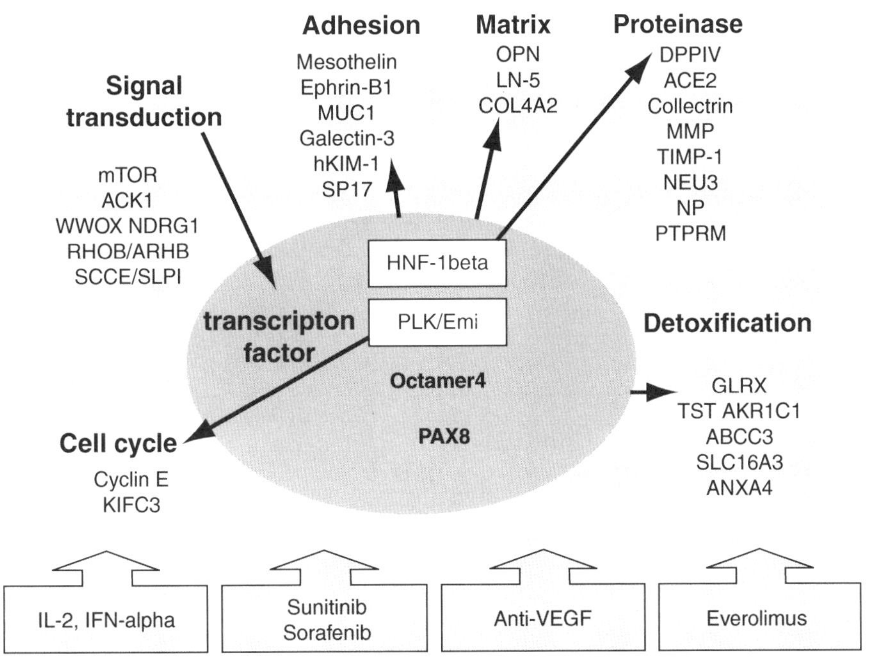

Fig. 7.1 Proposed model for treatment strategies of CCC based on possible target genes. This figure shows signal transduction pathway predominantly found in CCC and the designing strategies to treat CCC using a new model. These genes are mainly related to proliferation, invasion and metastasis. Other effects include adhesion, ECM remodelling, and detoxification. Several significant common pathways observed in CCC of the ovary overlap the datasets identified in RCC. Therefore, proposed inhibitors of this pathway are cytokines (IL-2, IFN-alpha), antibodies (anti-VEGF), and small molecules (sunitinib, sorafenib) that currently used for treatment of RCC. From Yoshida et al. [66]r eprintedw ithpe rmission

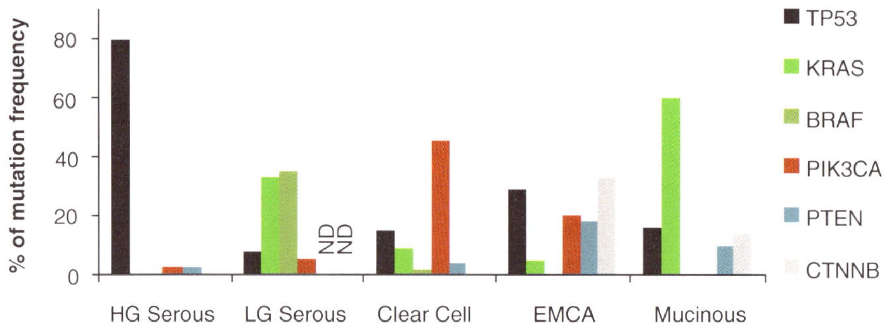

Fig. 7.2 The mutation profile of TP53, KRAS, BRAF, PIK3CA, PTEN, and CTNNB1 in different histological types of ovarian epithelial neoplasms. The frequency of individual mutations is shown in the bar chart in various types of ovarian carcinoma including high-grade (HG) serous carcinoma, low-grade (LG) serous carcinoma, clear cell carcinoma, endometrioid carcinoma (EMCA), and mucinous carcinoma. The mutation frequency is estimated from several studies based on a sizable sample size. The frequency of PIK3CA mutation in clear cell carcinoma is based on the current study showing 46% in purified tumours and cell lines. The mutation frequency of PTEN and CTNNB1 has not been determined (ND) in LG serous carcinomas. Mutation spectrum in clear cell tumours compared to other histological subtypes of ovarian cancer from collected series – reprinted with permissionf romK uoe ta l. [65]

References

1. Itamochi H, Kigawa J, Terakawa N. Mechanisms of chemoresistance and poor prognosis in ovarian clear cell carcinoma. Cancer Sci. 2008;99(4):653–8.
2. Chan JK, Teoh D, Hu JM, Shin JY, Osann K, Kapp DS. Do clear cell ovarian carcinomas have poorer prognosis compared to other epithelial cell types? A study of 1411 clear cell ovarian cancers. Gynecol Oncol. 2008;109(3):370–6.
3. Ushijimi K. Current status of gynecologic cancer in Japan. J Gynecol Oncol. 2009;20(2):67–71.
4. Lim MC, Lee DO, Kang S, Seo SS, Lee BY, Park SY. Clinical manifestations in patients with ovarian clear cell carcinoma with or without co-existing endometriosis. Gynecol Endocrinol. 2009;25(7):435–40.
5. Nagle CM, Olsen CM, Webb PM, Jordan SJ, Whiteman DC, Green AC, et al. Endometrioid and clear cell ovarian cancers: a comparative analysis of risk factors. Eur J Cancer. 2008;44(16):2477–84.
6. Olsen CM, Nagle CM, Whiteman DC, Purdie DM, Green AC, Webb PM, et al. Body size and risk of epithelial ovarian and related cancers: a population-based case-control study. Int J Cancer. 2008;123(2):450–6.
7. Ness RB, Cramer DW, Goodman MT, Kjaer SK, Mallin K, Mosgaard BJ, et al. Infertility, fertility drugs, and ovarian cancer: a pooled analysis of case-control studies. Am J Epidemiol.2002;155(3):217–24.
8. Kobayashi H, Sumimoto K, Kitanaka T, Yamada Y, Sado T, Sakata M, et al. Ovarian endometrioma–risks factors of ovarian cancer development. Eur J Obstet Gynecol Reprod Biol.2008;138(2):187–93.
9. Orezzoli JP, Russell AH, Oliva E, Del Carmen MG, Eichhorn J, Fuller AF. Prognostic implication of endometriosis in clear cell carcinoma of the ovary. Gynecol Oncol. 2008; 110(3):336–44.
10. Yamamoto S, Tsuda H, Takano M, Hase K, Tamai S, Matsubara O. Clear-cell adenofibroma can be a clonal precursor for clear-cell adenocarcinoma of the ovary: a possible alternative ovarian clear-cell carcinogenic pathway. J Pathol. 2008;216(1):103–10.
11. Veras EMD, Mao T-LMDP, Ayhan AMDP, Ueda SMD, Lai HPM, Hayran MMD, et al. Cystic and adenofibromatous clear cell carcinomas of the ovary: distinctive tumors that differ in their pathogenesis and behavior: a clinicopathologic analysis of 122 cases. Am J Surg Pathol. 2009;33(6):844–53.
12. Yamamoto S, Tsuda H, Yoshikawa T, Kudoh K, Kita T, Furuya K, et al. Clear cell adenocarcinoma associated with clear cell adenofibromatous components: a subgroup of ovarian clear cell adenocarcinoma with distinct clinicopathologic characteristics. Am J Surg Pathol. 2007;31(7):999–1006.
13. Roth LM, Langley FA, Fox H, Wheeler JE, Czernobilsky B. Ovarian clear cell adenofibromatous tumors. Benign, of low malignant potential, and associated with invasive clear cell carcinoma. Cancer. 1984;53(5):1156–63.
14. Savvari P, Peitsidis P, Alevizaki M, Dimopoulos MA, Antsaklis A, Papadimitriou CA. Paraneoplastic humorally mediated hypercalcemia induced by parathyroid hormone-related protein in gynecologic malignancies: a systematic review. Onkologie. 2009;32(8–9):517–23.
15. Duska LR, Garrett L, Henretta M, Ferriss JS, Lee L, Horowitz N. When 'never-events' occur despite adherence to clinical guidelines: The case of venous thromboembolism in clear cell cancer of the ovary compared with other epithelial histologic subtypes. Gynecol Oncol. 2010;116(3):374–7.
16. Lim MC, Lee HS, Kang S, Seo SS, Lee BY, Park SY. Minimizing tumor burden by extensive cytoreductive surgery decreases postoperative venous thromboembolism in ovarian clear cell carcinoma. Arch Gynecol Obstet. 2010;281(2):329–34.
17. Uno K, Homma S, Satoh T, Nakanishi K, Abe D, Matsumoto K, et al. Tissue factor expression as a possible determinant of thromboembolism in ovarian cancer. Br J Cancer. 2007; 96(2):290–5.
18. Ho C-M, Chien T-Y, Shih B-Y, Huang S-H. Evaluation of complete surgical staging with pelvic and para-aortic

lymphadenectomy and paclitaxel plus carboplatin chemotherapy for improvement of survival in stage I ovarian clear cell carcinoma. Gynecol Oncol. 2003;88(3):394–9.
19. Chan JK, Munro EG, Cheung MK, Husain A, Teng NN, Berek JS, et al. Association of lymphadenectomy and survival in stage I ovarian cancer patients. Obstet Gynecol. 2007;109(1):12–9.
20. Suzuki S, Kajiyama H, Shibata K, Ino K, Nawa A, Sakakibara K, et al. Is there any association between retroperitoneal lymphadenectomy and survival benefit in ovarian clear cell carcinoma patients? Ann Oncol. 2008;19(7):1284–7.
21. Kajiyama H, Shibata K, Suzuki S, Ino K, Yamamoto E, Mizuno K, et al. Is there any possibility of fertility-sparing surgery in patients with clear-cell carcinoma of the ovary? Gynecol Oncol. 2008;111(3):523–6.
22. Timmers PJ, Zwinderman AH, Teodorovic I, Vergote I, Trimbos JB. Clear cell carcinoma compared to serous carcinoma in early ovarian cancer: same prognosis in a large randomized trial. Int J Gynecol Cancer. 2009;19(1):88–93.
23. du Bois A, Luck H-J, Meier W, Adams H-P, Mobus V, Costa S, et al. A randomized clinical trial of cisplatin/paclitaxel versus carboplatin/paclitaxel as first-line treatment of ovarian cancer. J Natl Cancer Inst. 2003;95(17):1320–9.
24. Ozols RF, Bundy BN, Greer BE, Fowler JM, Clarke-Pearson D, Burger RA, et al. Phase III trial of carboplatin and paclitaxel compared with cisplatin and paclitaxel in patients with optimally resected stage iii ovarian cancer: a gynecologic oncology group study. J Clin Oncol. 2003; 21(17):3194–200.
25. Enomoto T, Kuragaki C, Yamasaki M, Sugita N, Otsuki Y, Ikegami H, et al. Is clear cell carcinoma and mucinous carcinoma of the ovary sensitive to combination chemotherapy with paclitaxel and carboplatin? Proc Am Soc Clin Oncol. 2003;22:abstr1797 .
26. Takano M, Kita T, Kikuchi Y, Yaegashi N, Kuzuya K, Tsuda H, et al. Clinical characteristics of clear cell adenocarcinoma of the ovary -Japan Clear Cell Carcinoma Study Group. J Clin Oncol (Meeting Abstracts). 2005;23(16 Suppl):5123.
27. Sugiyama T, Yakushiji M, Kamura T, Ikeda M, Umesaki N, Hasegawa K, et al. Irinotecan (CPT-11) and cisplatin as first-line chemotherapy for advanced ovarian cancer. Oncology. 2002;63(1):16–22.
28. Takano M, Kikuchi Y, Yaegashi N, Suzuki M, Tsuda H, Sagae S, et al. Adjuvant chemotherapy with irinotecan hydrochloride and cisplatin for clear cell carcinoma of the ovary. Oncol Rep. 2006;16(6):1301–6.
29. Takano M, Sugiyama T, Yaegashi N, Suzuki M, Tsuda H, Sagae S, et al. Progression-free survival and overall survival of patients with clear cell carcinoma of the ovary treated with paclitaxel-carboplatin or irinotecan-cisplatin: retrospective analysis. Int J Clin Oncol. 2007;12(4):256–60.
30. http://www.gcig.igcs.org/files/JGOG3017_Protocol.pdf. Accessed 3 september 2010.
31. Takano M, Sugiyama T, Yaegashi N, Sakuma M, Suzuki M, Saga Y, et al. Low response rate of second-line chemotherapy for recurrent or refractory clear cell carcinoma of the ovary: a retrospective Japan Clear Cell Carcinoma Study. Int J Gynecol Cancer. 2008;18(5):937–42.
32. Crotzer DR, Sun CC, Coleman RL, Wolf JK, Levenback CF, Gershenson DM. Lack of effective systemic therapy for recurrent clear cell carcinoma of the ovary. Gynecol Oncol. 2007;105(2):404–8.
33. Pectasides D, Fountzilas G, Aravantinos G, et al. Advanced stage clear-cell epithelial ovarian cancer: the Hellenic cooperative oncology group experience. Gynecol Oncol. 2006; 102(2):285–91.
34. Geyer JT, Lopez-Garcia M, Sanches-Estevez C, Sarrio D, Moreno-Bueno G, Franceschetti I, et al. Pathogenic pathways in ovarian endometrioid adenocarcinoma. A molecular study of 29 cases. Am J Surg Pathol. 2009;33(8):1157–63.
35. Shih I-M, Kurman RJ. Ovarian tumorigenesis: a proposed model based on morphological and molecular genetic analysis. Am J Pathol. 2004; 164(5):1511-8
36. Young RH, Scully RE. Oxyphilic clear cell carcinoma of the ovary. A report of nine cases. Am J Surg Pathol. 1987; 11(9):661–7.
37. Skirnisdottir I, Seidal T, Karlsson MG, Sorbe B. Clinical and biological characteristics of clear cell carcinomas of the ovary in FIGO stages I-II. Int J Oncol. 2005;26(1):177–83.
38. Iwamoto H, Fukasawa H, Honda T, Hirata S, Hoshi K. HER-2/neu expression in ovarian clear cell carcinomas. Int J Gynecol Cancer. 2003;13(1):28–31.
39. Shimizu M, Nikaido T, Toki T, Shiozawa T, Fujii S. Clear cell carcinoma has an expression pattern of cell cycle regulatory molecules that is unique among ovarian adenocarcinomas. Cancer. 1999;85(3):669–77.
40. Kato N, Sasou S, Motoyama T. Expression of hepatocyte nuclear factor-1beta (HNF-1beta) in clear cell tumors and endometriosis of the ovary. Mod Pathol. 2006;19(1):83–9.
41. Maeda D, Ota S, Takazawa Y, Aburatani H, Nakagawa S, Yano T, et al. Glypican-3 expression in clear cell adenocarcinoma of the ovary. Mod Pathol. 2009; 22(6):824-32.
42. Hashiguchi Y, Tsuda H, Inoue T, Berkowitz RS, Mok SC. PTEN expression in clear cell adenocarcinoma of the ovary. Gynecol Oncol. 2006;101(1):71–5.
43. Sato N, Tsunoda H, Nishida M, et al. Loss of heterozygosity on 10q23.3 and mutation of the tumor suppressor gene PTEN in benign endometrial cyst of the ovary: possible sequence progression from benign endometrial cyst to endometrioid carcinoma and clear cell carcinoma of the ovary. Cancer Res. 2000;60(24):7052–6.
44. Kaneuchi M, Sasaki M, Tanaka Y, et al. WT1 and WT1-AS genes are inactivated by promoter methylation in ovarian clear cell adenocarcinoma. Cancer. 2005;104(9):1924–30.
45. Holcomb K, Delatorre R, Pedemonte B, McLeod C, Anderson L, Chambers J. E-cadherin expression in endometrioid, papillary serous, and clear cell carcinoma of the endometrium. Obstet Gynecol. 2002;100(6):1290–5.
46. Suehiro Y, Sakamoto M, Umayahara K, et al. Genetic aberrations detected by comparative genomic hybridization in ovarian clear cell adenocarcinomas. Oncology. 2000;59(1): 50–6.
47. Dent J, Hall GD, Wilkinson N, et al. Cytogenetic alterations in ovarian clear cell carcinoma detected by comparative genomic hybridisation. Br J Cancer. 2003;88(10):1578–83.
48. Cairns P, Tokino K, Eby Y, Sidransky D. Localization of tumor suppressor loci on chromosome 9 in primary human renal cell carcinomas. Cancer Res. 1995;55(2):224–7.
49. Köbel M, Kalloger SE, Carrick J, Huntsman D, Asad H, Oliva E, et al. A limited panel of immunomarkers can reliably distinguish between clear cell and high-grade

serous carcinoma of the ovary. Am J Surg Pathol. 2009; 33(1):14-21
50. Saga Y, Ohwada M, Suzuki M, Konno R, Kigawa J, Ueno S, et al. Glutathione peroxidase 3 is a candidate mechanism of anticancer drug resistance of ovarian clear cell adenocarcinoma. Oncol Rep. 2008;20(6):1299–303.
51. Umezu T, Shibata K, Shimaoka M, Kajiyama H, Yamamoto E, Ino K, et al. Gene silencing of glypican-3 in clear cell carcinoma of the ovary renders it more sensitive to the apoptotic agent paclitaxel in vitro and in vivo. Cancer Sci. 2010; 101(1):143–8.
52. Lee S, Garner EI, Welch WR, Berkowitz RS, Mok SC. Over-expression of hypoxia-inducible factor 1 alpha in ovarian clear cell carcinoma. Gynecol Oncol. 2007;106(2): 311–7.
53. Kim A, Enomoto T, Serada S, Ueda Y, Takahashi T, Ripley B, et al. Enhanced expression of Annexin A4 in clear cell carcinoma of the ovary and its association with chemoresistance to carboplatin. Int J Cancer. 2009;125(10): 2316–22.
54. Ferrandina G, Mey V, Nannizzi S, Ricciardi S, Petrillo M, Ferlini C, et al. Expression of nucleoside transporters, deoxycitidine kinase, ribonucleotide reductase regulatory subunits, and gemcitabine catabolic enzymes in primary ovarian cancer. Cancer Chemother Pharmacol. 2010;65(4):679–86.
55. Zorn KK, Bonome T, Gangi L, Chandramouli GV, Awtrey CS, Gardner GJ, et al. Gene expression profiles of serous, endometrioid, and clear cell subtypes of ovarian and endometrial cancer. Clin Cancer Res. 2005; 11(18):6422-30
56. Tsuchiya A, Sakamoto M, Yasuda J, et al. Expression profiling in ovarian clear cell carcinoma: identification of hepatocyte nuclear factor-1 beta as a molecular marker and a possible molecular target for therapy of ovarian clear cell carcinoma. Am J Pathol. 2003;163(6):2503–12.
57. Gütgemann I, Lehman NL, Jackson PK, Longacre TA. Emi1 protein accumulation implicates misregulation of the anaphase promoting complex/cyclosome pathway in ovarian clear cell carcinoma. Mod Pathol. 2008; 21(4):445-54.
58. Kato N, Motoyama T. Overexpression of osteopontin in clear cell carcinoma of the ovary: close association with HNF-1beta expression. Histopathology. 2008;52(6):682–8.
59. Ho CM, Lin MC, Huang SH, Huang CJ, Lai HC, Chien TY, et al. PTEN promoter methylation and LOH of 10q22-23 locus in PTEN expression of ovarian clear cell adenocarcinomas. Gynecol Oncol. 2009;112(2):307–13.
60. Furnari FB, Huang HJ, Cavenee WK. The phosphoinositol phosphatase activity of PTEN mediates a serum-sensitive G1 growth arrest in glioma cells. Cancer Res. 1998;58(22): 5002–8.
61. Okuda T, Otsuka J, Sekizawa A, et al. p53 mutations and overexpression affect prognosis of ovarian endometrioid cancer but not clear cell cancer. Gynecol Oncol. 2003;88(3): 318–25.
62. Hua K, Feng W, Cao Q, Zhou X, Lu X, Feng Y. Estrogen and progestin regulate metastasis through the PI3K/AKT pathway in human ovarian cancer. Int J Oncol. 2008;33(5):959–67.
63. Mabuchi S, Kawase C, Altomare DA, Morishige K, Sawada K, Hayashi M. et al. mTOR is a promising therapeutic target both in cisplatin-sensitive and cisplatin-resistant clear cell carcinoma of the ovary. Clin Cancer Res. 2009; 15(17): 5404-13.
64. Tan DS, Kaye S. Ovarian clear cell adenocarcinoma: a continuing enigma. J Clin Pathol. 2007; 60(4):355-60.
66. Kuo KT, Mao TL, Jones S, Veras E, Ayhan A, Wang TL, et al. Frequent activating mutations of PIK3CA in ovarian clear cell carcinoma. Am J Pathol. 2009;174(5):1597–601.
65. Yoshida S, Furukawa N, Haruta S, Tanase Y, Kanayama S, Noguchi T, et al. Theoretical model of treatment strategies for clear cell carcinoma of the ovary: focus on perspectives. CancerT reatR ev.2009; 35(7):608–15.

8 Clear Cell Carcinoma of the Ovary

Toru Sugiyama and Hiroshi Tsuda

Clear cell carcinoma of the ovary (CCC) was initially termed as "mesonephroid" by Schiller in 1939 because it was believed to originate from mesonephric structures and resembled renal carcinoma. Since 1973, CCC has been recognized by the World Health Organization's classification of ovarian tumors as a distinct histologic entity [1]. Recently, CCC, which frequently appears during stage I, has been considered resistant to platinum-based chemotherapy and to have a poorer prognosis with respect to other subtypes of epithelial ovarian cancer (EOC). Recent clinical and molecular studies support the hypothesis that CCC and mucinous cystadenocarcinoma (MAC) are rare and refractory cancers that are biologically distinct from other EOCs.

8.1 Incidence and Clinical Behavior

The proportion of CCC is higher in Japanese population (>20%) than that in the Western countries or other Asian countries (3–12%), though the reason for this remains unknown [2–4]. Recently, Chen et al. reported that patients with CCC were more likely to be Asian; the proportion of Asian, Whites, and Black with clear cell histology was 11.1, 4.8, and 3.1%, respectively [5].

CCC of the ovary is a histologic subtype of EOC showing a different clinical behavior. CCC frequently presents as a large pelvic mass, rarely occurs bilaterally, and occasionally associated hypercalcemia and/or thromboembolic vascular complication [2, 3, 6–9]. Development and proliferation of CCC differ from SAC, which is supported by in vitro studies [10].

T. Sugiyama (✉)
Department of Obstetrics and Gynecology, Iwate Medical University, 19-1 Uchimaru, Morioka, Iwate 020-8505, Japan
e-mail: sugiyaa@iwate-med.ac.jp

H. Tsuda
Department of Obstetrics and Gynecology, School of Medicine, Keio University, 35 Shinanomachi, Shinjuku-ku, Tokyo 160-8582, Japan

8.2 Histopathological Issues

8.2.1 Histopathological Characteristics

CCC has specific histologic subtype of EOC composed of glycogen-containing clear cells and hobnail cell, and occasionally, other cell types as follows; (1) The tumor invades ovarian stroma, manifested by stromal destruction, desmoplasia, hyalinization, and/or confluence of epithelial elements. (2) The tumor growth pattern is tubulocystic, papillary (Fig. 8.1a), solid (Fig. 8.1b), or a combination of two or all of these. (3) The tumor cells contain cytoplasm which is optically clear with hematoxylin staining (Fig. 8.1b), or project in a hobnail (Fig. 8.2a) or peglike pattern into neoplastic lumens, or display a combination of the clear and hobnail patterns. Occasional tumors may be partially or predominantly oncocytic (Fig. 8.2b). (4) Tumor cell nuclei are pleomorphic but mitotic figures are rarely numerous. (5) Less than ten percent of another epithelial carcinoma pattern (endometrioid, serous.etc.) is present. If more than 10%, the diagnosis is mixed type carcinoma.

The assessment of malignancy and the differentiation of primary and metastatic carcinoma in CCC patients can be performed more easily than in other EOC patients; however, it is possible for CCC to be misdiagnosed as high-grade serous adenocarcinoma (SAC). It is known that histological differentiation is a

N. Reed et al. (eds.), *Rare and Uncommon Gynecological Cancers*,
DOI: 10.1007/978-3-642-13492-0_8, © Springer-Verlag Berlin Heidelberg 2011

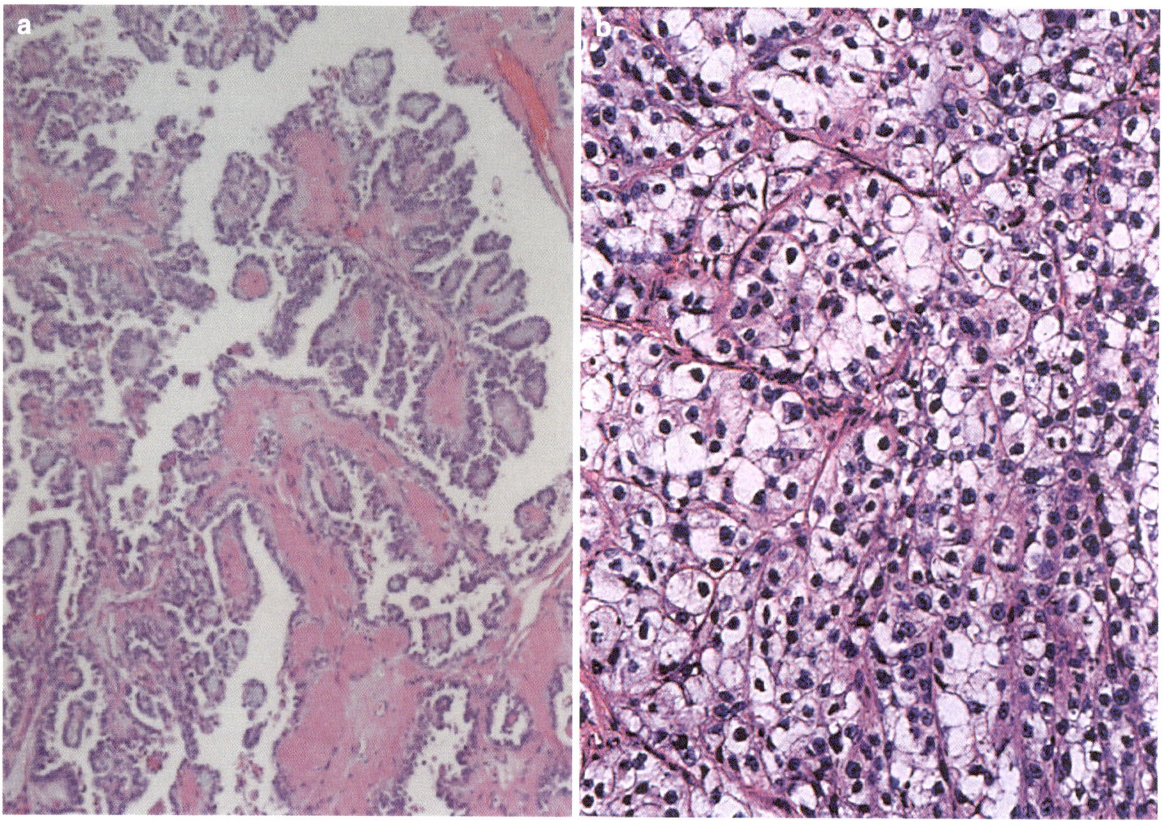

Fig. 8.1 The growth pattern of clear cell carcinoma is tubulocystic, papillary (**a**, H.E. stain, ×33), solid (**b**, H.E. stain, ×66), or a combinationof t woor a llof t hese

good prognostic factor for EOC. However, the pathology manual by the Gynecologic Oncology Group (GOG) does not recommend CCC grading due to its many associated problems.

8.2.2 Origin of CCC

It was reported that endometriosis frequently showed a sequential change to CCC and endometrioid adenocarcinoma (EAC), therefore, atypical endometriosis is considered as a precancerous change [11]. In addition, it was reported that the CCC arising in endometriosis has good prognosis [12]. Endometriosis causes gene mutation including loss of heterozygosity (LOH), suggesting that tumor suppressor gene inactivation is involved in development of peritoneal endometriosis [13]. It has also been reported that *K-ras* mutation is involved in transformation from endometriosis to CCC [14], and *p53* and *phosphatase and tensin homologue* (*PTEN*) mutation are often found in EAC [15]. The possibility of aggravation of endometriosis is estimated as 2.5% or more. A 9-year follow-up cohort study was carried out in 6,398 patients with endometrial cyst and 57,165 control patients in Japan, and 46 patients (0.72%) and seven patients (0.012%) developed EOC, respectively. The relative risk of aggravation of endometrial cyst was 12.4 (95% confidence interval: 7.9–17.3). Most EOCs from endometrial cyst are CCC and EAC, and when the incidence in 20s is considered 1.00, the incidences in 40s and 50s are 3.60 and 10.7, respectively, indicating that endometrial cyst can turn cancerousa roundme nopause [11].

Another origin of CCC is clear cell adenofibroma (CCAF). Yamamoto et al. conducted allelotype analysis of CCC and CCAF in 14 cases of CCC associated with benign CCAF and/or borderline CCAF, and demonstrated that the concordance rate in allelic patterns at all informative loci was 74% between benign CCAF

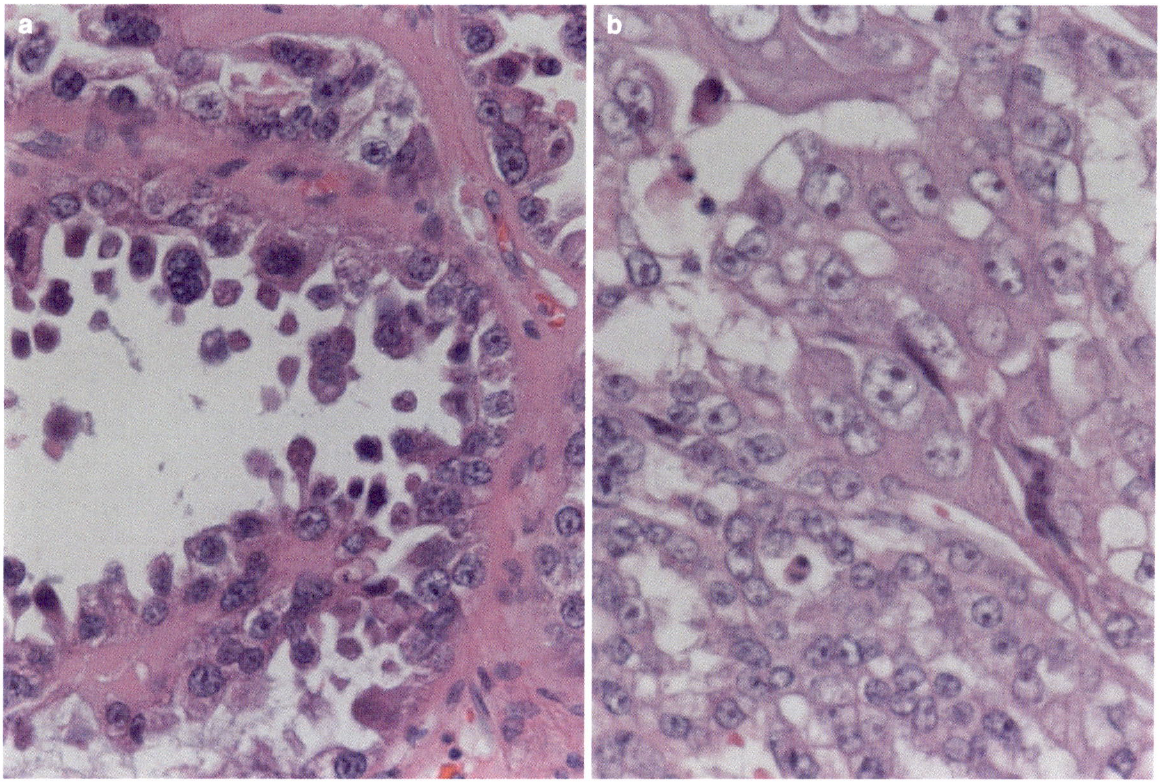

Fig. 8.2 The tumor cells contain cytoplasm which is optically clear with hematoxylin staining (Fig. 8.1b), or project in a hobnail (**a**, H.E.stain, ×100) or peglike pattern into neoplastic lumens, or display a combination of the clear and hobnail patterns. Occasional tumors may be partially or predominantly oncocytic (**b**,H .E.stain,× 100)

and adenocarcinoma components, 81%. Between borderline CCAF and adenocarcinoma components, and LOHs on 5q, 10q and 22q were frequent in both CCAF and adenocarcinoma components, whereas LOHs on 1p and 13q were rare in CCAF components but frequent in adenocarcinoma components [16]. They concluded that CCAF can be a clonal precursor for CCC.

8.3 Molecular Biology

EOC is usually divided into four histological types including SAC, mucinous adenocarcinoma (MAC), clear cell adenocarcinoma (CCC), and EAC and the origins of these four types are different, and genetic status is thought to be different among them. It was reported that the frequent distinct region of loss detected was 9p21 (41%), 1p (28%), 11q (22%), 16 (28%), and common region of amplification was 3 (33%), 13q (22), 15 (17%) in CCC [17]. Suehiro et al. reported that increased copy numbers of 8q11-q13, 8q21-q22, 8q23, 8q24-qter, 17q25-qter, 20q13-qter and 21q22-qter and reduced copy numbers of 19p are frequent and increased copy numbers of 17q25-qter and 20q13-qter occurred more frequently in recurrent/non-surviving patients than in disease-free patients in CCC ($p<0.05$). They finally concluded that CCC can be classified into two subtypes, one being cancer with an increase in copy numbers of 8q and the other being cancer with increase in copy numbers of 17q25-qter [18]. Okada et al. compared CCC and SAC using allelotype analysis and showed that LOH was detected on 1p (69%), 19p (45%) and 11q (43%) and the incidences of LOH on 5q, 12q, 13q and 17p were significantly lower in CCC than SAC [19]. Hirasawa et al. reported that gain of 17q21-q24 showed significantly negative correlation with disease-free and overall survival in CCC ($p=0.0012$ and 0.0039) [20]. In contrast, it was reported that gains of 2p22p25, 20q12q13 and loss of 5q14q22 were related with prognosis of other histologictype s [21–23].

Schwartz et al. analyzed expression profile in 113 EOCs and showed that MAC and CCC can be readily distinguished from SAC [24]. In addition, Zorn et al. compared the expression profile among SAC, EAC, CCC subtypes of ovarian and endometrial cancer, and kidney cancer and demonstrated that CCC showed a remarkable similarity in gene expression profiles across organs (including kidney) [25]. From these findings, gene expression is thought to be different among histological types. Generally, it was recognized that women with SAC has high p53 abnormalities rate and low PTEN abnormality rate [26, 27]. It was reported that women with CCC has lower expression or mutation rate of p53 compared with SAC [28, 29]. We previously showed that loss of PTEN expression is relatively common in CCC and cyclin E expression is significantlyhighe rinC CCtha ninSA C [30, 31].

8.4 Surgeryan dSur gicalSt aging

8.4.1 Cytoreductive Surgery

The residual tumor diameter after the initial surgery is an important prognostic factor in stage III EOC. Hoskins et al. conducted a GOG study and indicated that CCC is a significant prognostic factor in small-volume stage III EOC after cytoreductive surgery based on univariate analysis results [32]. Advanced CCC patients with optimal disease showed a significantly better prognosis than those with suboptimal disease; consequently, the importance of maximum cytoreductive surgery is indicated [27, 33]. A retrospective study of advanced CCC was recently conducted in Japan and showed that the survival rate was low in groups with both a ≥1 cm and <1 cm residual tumor diameter after surgery, and the survival rate in the complete resection group was significantly higher than in the groups with both a ≥1 cm and a <1 cm residual tumor diameter after initial surgery (Fig. 8.3) [34]. For CCC treatment, the postoperative condition without visible lesions, i.e., maximum cytoreduction, should be sought. Some studies have indicated that the success rate of complete resection in CCC does not differ from that in other EOC [35, 36], however, recent studies have shown high success rates and few CCC patients with large residual tumors after surgery [33].

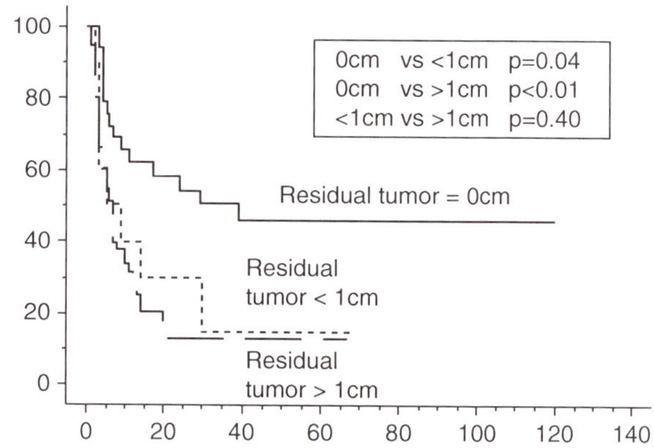

Fig. 8.3 Progression-free survival (PFS) of stage III, IV patients according to the residual tumor (RT) diameter: The patients with no residual tumor had significantly better PFS than those with the tumor diameter less than 1 cm ($p=0.04$) or those with the tumor diameter more than 1 cm ($p<0.01$),r espectively [9]

8.4.2 Lymph-Node Metastasis

Even in pT1 EOC, the incidence of positive lymph-nodes was not low, ranging from 5.1 to 20% [37–39]. It was reported that SAC had a higher incidence of lymph-node involvement than non-SACs [40]. The true incidence of lymph-node metastasis in CCC had not been clear. Takano et al. showed the similar rate of lymph-node metastasis compared with other EOC in a large number of patients with CCC [30]. Lymph-node metastasis was observed in 9.1% in pT1a tumors, 7.1% in pT1c tumors, and 10.8% in pT2 tumors, respectively. Fifteen (8.7%) of 173 patients who had pT1 or pT2 tumors were upstaged as stage IIIc tumors based on lymph-node status. Chen et al. showed that 27.5% of 28,082 EOC patients underwent lymph-node dissection and lymph-node involvement was found in 7.9% of CCC patients, which was significantly lower than 13.6% of SAC patients [5]. In several reports of CCC patients who received a comprehensive surgical staging including lymph-adenectomy, lymph-node status was identified as a strong prognostic factor and it is essential to accurately evaluate the lymph-node status through complete surgical staging procedures. Onda et al. showed that the prognoses for pT1 and pT2 diseases with or without lymph-node metastasis were similar [41]. In contrast, several studies made clear that survival rates with node-positive disease were significantly lower in pT1 and pT2 diseases [38, 42, 43].

Table8.1 Stagedis tribution

Histology	Number of points	I(%)			II (%)	III(%)			IV(%)
		a	b	c		a	b	c	
Serous adenocarcinoma	3085	5.1	1.1	7.6	7.1	3.4	5.5	*53.4*	14.7
Clear cellc arcinoma	494	20.6	1.2	*32.2*	10.5	1.4	3.8	21.9	6.1

FIGO annual report: 1999–2001

8.4.3 *Stage Distribution*

CCC frequently appears at early stages (stage I/II: 59–71%), especially stage IC (Table 8.1) [2, 3]. Approximately 30% of them develop stage III cancer and rarely have a measurable lesion after the initial surgery. In contrast, SAC is found not at early stages but most of them are advanced cancer.

In a review of the study results regarding prognostic factors for EOC, it was found that many studies considered CCC to be a prognostic factor, although some indicated that stage I CCC is not a prognostic factor [44]. The GOG showed that CCC and MAC were significant prognostic factors in 726 patients with stage III-IV EOC [45], and many other studies supported this finding [46]·.

8.5 AdjuvantT reatment

Paclitaxel/Carboplatin using all subtypes of EOC as standard regimen may not be an optimal regimen for CCC because CCC accounts for only 2–5% of cases enrolled in randomized controlled trials.

8.5.1 *Response Rate in Postoperative Chemotherapy* (Table 8.2)

8.5.1.1 ConventionalPl atinum-Based Chemotherapy

CCC patients rarely have a measurable lesion after the initial surgery; there have therefore been no phase II studies of CCC patients. The response rates of conventional platinum-based chemotherapy (carboplatin, platinum and cyclophosphamide, and platinum, cyclophosphamide and doxorubicin) are also poor (11–27%) [47, 48]. In contrast, the progression disease (PD) rate is high in chemotherapy for CCC; CCC is therefore considered to be resistant to platinum-based chemotherapy [49]. In vitro studies in CCC cells have also shownc isplatin-resistance [50, 51].

8.5.1.2 CombinationT herapyo f Paclitaxel and Platinum

The response rates of paclitaxel/platinum chemotherapy, standard regimen for EOC, varied but generally low (18–56%) [48, 52–56]. Pectasides et al. have reported that the response rate of clear cell adenocarcinoma is 45% and significantly lower than that of SAC (81%) [53]. Ho et al. and Utsunomiya et al. have reported response rates of 56 and 53%, respectively [48, 52]. On the other hand, Enomoto et al. conducted a prospective study of paclitaxel/carboplatin and showed response rates of 81 and 18% for SAC and CCC, respectively [55]. In contrast, the PD rate was extremely high, ranging from 40 to 73%. Reporting on a recent preliminary review of the GOG experience with CCC in protocols 97, 111, and 132, Birrer noted in the ASCO 2003 that the response rate in that review (62% for papillary SAC and 38% for CCC; $p=0.07$) did not reach statistical significance, but that the trend wass imilar [56].

8.5.2 *Survival Rate and Time*

8.5.2.1 ConventionalPl atinum-Based Chemotherapy

Of all studies regarding the prognosis of non-CCC (SAC in main), some studies that were published in 1970 or after have suggested that there is no difference in survival by stage between patients with CCC and SAC. In contrast, several recent reports have indicated that CCC is a histologic subtype with poor survival. Approximately, 30% of patients who were diagnosed with Stage I/II EOC were CCC; consequently, it is important to control

Table8.2 Response platinum-basedc hemotherapyf orC CC:r ecentr eports [7]

Authors (year)	Number of points	Response rate (%)	PD rate (%)	Regimen
Sugiyama (2000)	*27*	*11*	*82*	*Conventional platinum-based regimens*
Ho (2004)	*15*	*27*	*73*	*Conventional platinum-based regimens*
Pectasides(2006)	20	45	–	Includingpa clitaxel/platinum
Enomoto(2003)	11	18	73	Paclitaxel/carboplatin
Takano(2006)	22	32	56	Paclitaxel/carboplatin
Ho(2004)	16	56	44	Paclitaxel/platinum
Utsunomiya(2006)	15	53	40	Paclitaxel/platinum
Birrer(2003)		38		Paclitaxel/carboplatin
Takano (2006)	*9*	*43*	*22*	*Irinotecan/cisplatin*

early CCC. Some studies reported that CCC in early stages showed similar survival rate to other EOC [29, 33, 35], but others showed poor outcomes. Jenison et al. [3], O'Brien et al. [57], and we reported that CCC in early stages had a poorer outcome or a tendency toward poor outcome compared early-stage SAC [47]. Behbakht et al. indicted that Stage I CCC had a higher recurrence rate but a similar 5-year survival rate compared with other EOC [35]. Kennedy et al. reported that prognosis of stages I/II CCC was similar to that of SAC but that of Stage IC, CCC was poor in 1989 [2]. However, they reported in 1999 that no significant differences in survival were noted for either limited or advanced cancers in comparison with other histologic types of high-grade EOC [33], and then Kennedy et al. stated that all CCCs be considered high-grade tumors. Our results exhibited that Stage IC CCC with malignant ascites showed a significantly poor prognosis among Stage I CCC [30]. Comprehensively, judging the above results, the recurrence rate of CCC in early stages is higher than that of SAC and the survival rate of CCC is similar or poorer. Many studies reported that CCC in advanced stages (stages III/IV) showed a lower survival rate than other EOC [2, 3, 35, 45, 46, 58]. Some studies reported no difference between them [57], however, the trend was similar. In a comparative study of 1,411 CCC and 13,835 SAC patients who were identified from the Surveillance, Epidemiology, and End Results (SEER) from 1988 to 2001, the 5-year disease-specific survival of CCC was slightly poorer in Stage I/II and significantly poorer in stage III/IV than that of SAC [5]. Kennedy et al. reported that the 5-year survival rate in patients with stages III/IV CCC (17%) was not significantly different from that of other high-grade, stages III/IV EOC (22%) [2]. Recio et al. reported that platinum-based chemotherapy did not appear to improve the survival when compared with nonplatinum-based chemotherapy for CCC [27].

8.5.2.2 CombinationT herapyo f Paclitaxel and Platinum

In studies used as evidence for recommending paclitaxel/carboplatin as the standard treatment for EOC, most of the enrolled patients have had SAC, with only 2.1–4.9% and 2.4–4.4%, respectively, having CCC and MAC [28]. Consequently, these study results do not provide a scientific rationale for recommending paclitaxel/carboplatin as the standard therapy for CCC and MAC. The Gynecologic Intergroup (GCIG) analyzed the results of seven randomized cooperative group trials in 8,704 women with stage III/IV EOC treated with combination therapy of paclitaxel and platinum and confirmed that the subjects included only 221 (2.5%) CCC and 264 (3.0%) MAC patients and that these patients had poorer outcomes than the SAC patients. The above GCIG analysis results do not support the recommendation that combination therapy of paclitaxel and platinum be the standard therapy for CCC and MAC.

Pectasides et al. have reported that the median survivals of CCC and SAC were 25 and 49 months, and the 5-year survival rates were 32 and 39%, respectively, which indicated that CCC had a poorer or similar outcome compared with SAC [55]. Mizuno et al. indicated that there was no difference in the survival rate between CCC and SAC in stage III however, in stages IIIb and IIIc, the 5- and 8-year survival rates of

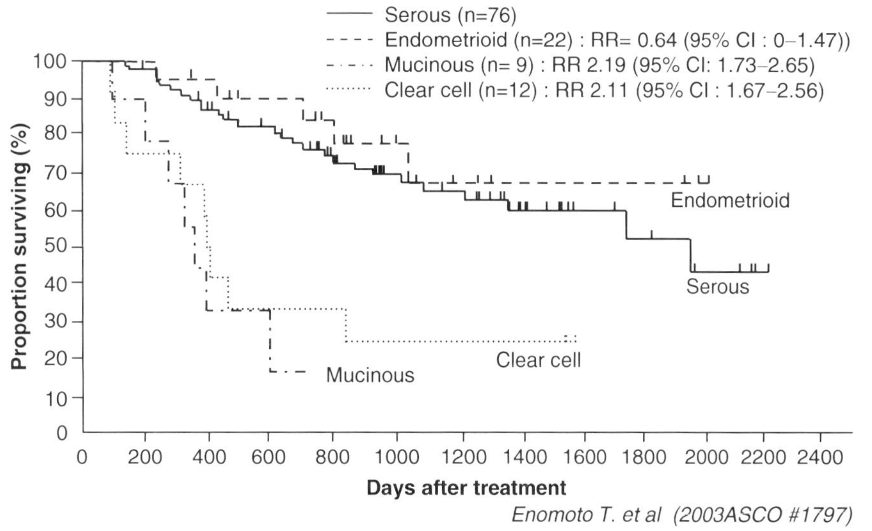

Fig. 8.4 Overalls urvival(OS) in Stage II–IV patients with suboptimal disease (residual disease >1 cm) treated with paclitaxel/carboplatin. The OS of clear cell carcinoma was significantly shorter than that ofs erousa denocarcinoma [55]

CCC were significantly lower than those of SAC [29]. A few studies showed that paclitaxel/platinum chemotherapy was more effective to CCC than conventional platinum-based chemotherapy however, the efficacy for CCC prognosis is still insufficient. Enomoto et al. also conducted a prospective study of TC regimens and showed a significantly shorter survival time of CCC than that of SAC and EAC [55]. In particular, the survival rate of patients with residual tumor after the initial surgery was extremely low (Fig. 8.4). A recent randomized controlled trial comparing tri-weekly and weekly dose-dense TC regimens in Stage II-IV EOC patients confirmed a significant improvement in outcomes of the weekly dose-dense TC regimens (median survival time: 28 months vs. 17 months) [59]. Many subset analyses indicated the superiority of weekly dose-dense TC regimens; however, no difference in clear cell/mucinous histology alone was shown, suggesting the limitation of CCC treatment with paclitaxel/carboplatin. The GCIG analysis of 221 Stage III/IV CCC patients treated with combination therapy of paclitaxel and platinum confirmed that their outcomes were poorer than those of SAC patients.

8.5.2.3 CombinationT herapyw ithI rinotecan

Recurrent tumor after treatment with Paclitaxel/Carboplatin, particularly in paclitaxel/carboplatin-resistant patients, is usually treated with irinotecan mono- and combined therapy in Japan. The standard regimen in monotherapy with irinotecan is 100 mg/m^2 of CPT-11 (days 1, 8 and 15) every 4 weeks, and Matsumoto et al. have shown a 29% response rate in 28 paclitaxel/carboplatin-resistant patients [60]. No results are available, however, for CCC patients alone. The major combination therapy of irinotecan involves irinotecan and cisplatin (CPT-P) regimens [61], and the rationale for this regimen is that there is no cross-tolerance or overlapped toxicity and that there are additive or synergistic effects. Some studies have confirmed a 40–50% response rate in CCC; but all of these have been small-scale studies with approximately ten patients [34, 62–66]. Our retrospective study confirmed a 43% response rate [34]. The Phase II trial of TC and CPT-P regimens in CCC (JGOG3014) confirmed that CPT-P regimens are superior to paclitaxel/carboplatin in patients with residual tumors less than 2 cm, although the survival rates are similar [67]. CPT-P regimens are currently being examined as a research arm in an ongoing international randomized comparative study (GCIG/JGOG 3017). Irinotecan combined with MMC has shown good efficacy to CCC as well as irinotecan/platinum chemotherapy [68–70]. However, these have been small-scale studies, and prospective RCT is required. The sensitivity of SN-38 to CCC was confirmed in an in vitro study by Nishida et al. [71] and the sensitivity of paclitaxel by Ohta et al [72]. Our fundamental study with 5 CCC cell strains confirmed the sensitivity of paclitaxel and SN-38 (irinotecan) in three strains, respectively, and the sensitivity of cisplatin in one strain, while there was no sensitivity of MMC and VP-16 in any of the five strains [73].

8.6 Mechanismso fC hemotherapy Resistance (Table 8.3)

CCC is thought to be resistant to conventional platinum-taxane based chemotherapy. Several mechanisms involved in drug resistance have been suggested, including decreased drug accumulation, increased drug detoxification, and increased DNA repair system [74–76].

8.6.1 ABC Transporter

ABC transporter enhances drug efflux and cause a decrease in the accumulation of the drug. Oishi et al. examined tumor samples from 30 SACs and 20 CCCs for the expression of MDR1, MRP1, MRP2 and MRP3 mRNA using real-time RT-PCR and demonstrated that MRP3 expression in CCC was significantly four times higher than that in SAC [77]. Schaner et al. performed microarray analysis for 55 EOCs and demonstrated that MRP3 was highly expressed in the CCC [78]. *MRP3* is a transporter that may confer resistance to several chemotherapeutic agents including topoisomerase inhibitors, platinums and antimetabolites [79]. We performed genomic and expression array analyses for 30 CCCs and 19 SACs and demonstrated significantly higher ABCF2 DNA and mRNA copy number and protein levels in CCC compared with those in SAC, furthermore, ABCF2 cytoplasmic staining was significantly higher in nonresponders than that in the responders [80]. *ABCF2* gene on 7q35–36 is a member of the ABC transporter superfamily; however, the role of ABCF2 remains unclear.

Table8.3 Chemoresistancer elatedge ne

ABC transporter	
	MRP3 ABCF2
Drugina ctivation	
	ANXA4G LRX
Cellprolife ration	
	CyclinEG FR
Stressre sponse	
	GPX3 SOD2 HIF 1αH IG2
DNAre pair	
	ERCC1 XPB hMLH1 hMSH2
Other	
	HNF1βTW IST

8.6.2 Drug Inactivation

Drug detoxification is also important for drug resistance. Schaner et al. reported that several genes involved in drug resistance such like *annexin IV (ANXA4)* or *glutaredoxin (GLRX)* were highly expressed in the CCC [81]. Schwartz et al. also reported that GLRX and ANXA4 were highly expressed in CCC [19]. ANXA4 has been implicated in drug resistance after exposure of cells to paclitaxel [79], and glutaredoxin, a redox regulating protein, has been implicated in resistance to cisplatin [78].

8.6.3 Low Cell Proliferation

The 60% of CCCs are diagnosed at stage I, and it may mean that growth of CCC is slow. Itamochi et al. demonstrated that CCC has low proliferation activity and proliferation activity was related with chemoresistance and concluded that low proliferation of tumor may be a behavior of CCC that contributes to its resistance to chemotherapy [82, 83]. In addition, they also reported that the expression of galectin-3 in CCC might contribute to its lower cell proliferation and lead to cisplatin resistance [77]. Shimizu et al. reported that in CCC, the Ki67, p53 and cyclin A expression are low [84]. Low proliferating activity is thought to be associated withc hemoresistance.

8.6.4 Stress Response, Glycogenesis and Glycolysis

Schwartz et al. analyzed gene expression in 113 EOCs, using oligonucleotide macroarrays [19]. They demonstrated that CCC was readily distinguished from the SAC and 73 genes expressed 2–29-fold higher in CCC compared with other histological types. Of these genes, *glutathione peroxidase 3* (*GPX3*), *glutaredoxin* (*GLRX*), *superoxide dismutase* (*SOD2*) were included and have all been implicated in oxidative stress response. These antioxidant proteins may render CCC more resistant to chemotherapy [85]. Lee et al. compared the hypoxia-inducible factor 1 alpha (HIF 1alpha) expression in EOC and showed that HIF-1 alpha expression is higher in CCC than in other histological types [86]. In addition, we previously demonstrated that hypoxia-inducible protein 2 (HIG2) expressions is higher in CCC than in SAC [80]. HIF 1alpha and HIG2 proteins are induced in hypoxic condition. *HIF 1alpha* has been reported to be an important predictor of tumor progression for some solid cancer [87, 88]. Togashi et al. showed that HIG2 is a novel potential target for molecular therapy of renal cell cancer [89].

Another possibility of drug resistance is glycogenesis and glycolysis. Morita et al. performed proteomic analysis for 2 CCC cell lines and MAC cell line and demonstrated that selected 12 genes in which elevated in CCC [90]. Of these 12 genes, 5 genes were related with glycolysis. Higashiguchi et al. reported that hepatocyte nuclear factor 1β (HNF1β) expression is higher in CCC than in other histological types [91]. *HNF-1β* has been reported to act antagonistically toward *HNF-1α* which increases expression of sodium-glucose cotransporter 1 [92], glucose 6-phosphate transporter, and glucose 6-phosphatase [93]. Given that glycogen storage was shown in the hepatocytes of *HNF-1α*-null and mutant [93, 94]. Higashiguchi et al. speculated that HNF-1β overexpression might cause clear cytoplasm characteristics. Kiyozuka demonstrated that (1) glycogen concentration in CCC cytoplasm is high and its concentration is positively related with cell doubling time, (2) in glycogen free condition, chemosensitivity of SAC cell line increase, however, that of CCC did not change [95].

8.6.5 Other

TWIST is a highly conserved basic helix-loop-helix transcription factor that regulates the expression of E-cadherin and promotes the epithelial-mesenchymal transition. In addition, TWIST was reported to be involved in the development of acquired resistance to chemotherapeutic agents including paclitaxel [96, 97]. Kajiyama et al. reported that TWIST expression was an independent prognostic factor in CCC [98]. Another important system is DNA repair system. Reed et al. reported that mRNA expression of excision repair cross-complementing rodent repair deficiency, complementation group 1 (ERCC1) and xeroderma pigmentosum group B (XPB) expression were higher in CCC as opposed to other histological types. *ERCC1* and *XPB* are key genes in the nucleotide excision repair pathway, and clinical resistance of platinum-chemotherapy in EOC [99]. Cai et al. showed that high expression of hMLH1 and hMSH2 proteins are related with the development of a subset of CCC and there is a strong correlation between alterations in the expression of hMLH1 and hMSH2 and the status of MSI [100]. Alteration of hMLH1 and hMSH2 are thought to cause the dysfunction of DNA mismatch repair systems and correlatesw ithc hemoresistance [101].

8.7 FutureT herapy

Clinical analysis results showed that outcomes in CCC patients were poorer than those in SAC patients. These results provide strong evidence in support of separate trials targeting the CCC patient population with new therapeutic strategies. CCC has a rare histological type; therefore, international collaborative research is needed. A CCC-specific international clinical trial (GCIG/JGOG3017) is currently ongoing. CCC has a markedly different molecular biology from other EOC, and patients with CCC are more likely to be completely resected than SAC. In addition to chemotherapy after complete resection, effective molecular-targeted drugs inhibiting cancer cell migration and invasion should be investigated.

CCC has a markedly different molecular biology from other EOC, and effective molecular-targeted drugs inhibiting cancer cell migration and invasion should be investigated [28]. Both epidermal growth factor receptor (*EGFR*) and v-erb-b2 erythroblastic leukemia viral oncogene homolog 2 (*HER2*) are cell-surface receptor tyrosine kinases and activate the Akt signaling pathway. Fujimura demonstrated that EGFR expression is high in CCC clinical samples and gefitinib strongly inhibited the growth and invasion of 3 CCC cell lines [102]. Fujimura et al. also reported that *HER2* is frequently over-expressed in CCC clinical samples, and trastuzumab significantly and dose-dependently reduced the growth of CCC cell lines in mice model [103]. Zorn et al. compared the expression profile among CCC, SAC, EAC and renal clear cell carcinoma (RCC) and demonstrated that CCC showed a remarkable similarity across organs (including kidney) [20]. Recently, Motzer et al. demonstrated that sunitinib malate prolonged progression-free survival and response in patients with metastatic RCC compared with interferon alfa [104]. Sunitinib malate is an orally administered small molecular inhibitors of tyrosine kinases, including vascular endothelial growth factor receptor (VEGFR) and platelet-derived growth factor receptor (PDGFR) [105, 106]. Rauh-Hain et al. reported a cases of CCC in whom sunitinib was effective [107]. These molecular targets are promising candidate targets.

References

1. Serov SF, Scully RE, Sobin LH. International histologic classification of tumors. No.9 histologic typing of ovarian tumors. Geneva: World Health Organization; 1973. p. 1–7.
2. Kennedy AW et al. Ovarian clear cell adenocarcinoma. Gynecol Oncol. 1989;32(3):342–9.
3. Jenison EL et al. Clear cell adenocarcinoma of the ovary: a clinical analysis and comparison with serous carcinoma. Gynecol Oncol. 1989;32(1):65–71.
4. McGuire V, Jesser CA, Whittemore AS. Survival among U.S. women with invasive epithelial ovarian cancer. Gynecol Oncol. 2002;84(3):399–403.
5. Chan JK et al. Do clear cell ovarian carcinomas have poorer prognosis compared to other epithelial cell types? A study of 1411 clear cell ovarian cancers. Gynecol Oncol. 2008; 109(3):370–6.
6. Recio FO et al. Lack of improved survival plus increase in thromboembolic complications in patients with clear cell carcinoma of the ovary treated with platinum versus nonplatinum-based chemotherapy. Cancer. 1996;78(10):2157–63.
7. Sugiyama T, Fujiwara K. Clear cell carcinoma of the ovary. ASCO education book. 2007. p. 318–22.
8. Mizuno M et al. Long-term follow-up and prognostic factor analysis in clear cell adenocarcinoma of the ovary. J Surg Oncol.2006;94(2) :138–43.
9. Takano M et al. Clear cell carcinoma of the ovary: a retrospective multicentre experience of 254 patients with complete surgical staging. Br J Cancer. 2006;94(10):1369–74.
10. Ohkawa K et al. Clear cell carcinoma of the ovary: light and electron microscopic studies. Cancer. 1977;40(6): 3019–29.
11. Kobayashi H et al. Risk of developing ovarian cancer among women with ovarian endometrioma: a cohort study in Shizuoka, Japan. Int J Gynecol Cancer. 2007;17(1): 37–43.
12. Komiyama S et al. Prognosis of Japanese patients with ovarian clear cell carcinoma associated with pelvic endometriosis: clinicopathologic evaluation. Gynecol Oncol. 1999;72(3):342–6.
13. Erzen M et al. Endometriosis-associated ovarian carcinoma (EAOC): an entity distinct from other ovarian carcinomas as suggested by a nested case-control study. Gynecol Oncol.2001;83(1) :100–8.
14. Sekizawa A et al. Malignant transformation of endometriosis: application of laser microdissection for analysis of genetic alterations according to pathological changes. Med Electron Microsc. 2004;37(2):97–100.
15. Sato N et al. Loss of heterozygosity on 10q23.3 and mutation of the tumor suppressor gene PTEN in benign endometrial cyst of the ovary: possible sequence progression from benign endometrial cyst to endometrioid carcinoma and clear cell carcinoma of the ovary. Cancer Res. 2000;60(24): 7052–6.
16. Yamamoto S et al. Clear-cell adenofibroma can be a clonal precursor for clear-cell adenocarcinoma of the ovary: a possible alternative ovarian clear-cell carcinogenic pathway. J Pathol. 2008;216(1):103–10.
17. Dent J et al. Cytogenetic alterations in ovarian clear cell carcinoma detected by comparative genomic hybridisation. Br J Cancer. 2003;88(10):1578–83.
18. Suehiro Y et al. Genetic aberrations detected by comparative genomic hybridization in ovarian clear cell adenocarcinomas. Oncology. 2000;59(1):50–6.
19. Okada S et al. Allelotype analysis of common epithelial ovarian cancers with special reference to comparison between clear cell adenocarcinoma with other histological types. Jpn J Cancer Res. 2002;93(7):798–806.
20. Hirasawa A et al. Association of 17q21-q24 gain in ovarian clear cell adenocarcinomas with poor prognosis and identification of PPM1D and APPBP2 as likely amplification targets. Clin Cancer Res. 2003;9(6):1995–2004.
21. Hu J et al. Comparative study of primary and recurrent ovarian serous carcinomas: comparative genomic hybridization analysis with a potential application for prognosis. Gynecol Oncol. 2003;89(3):369–75.
22. Tanner MM et al. Frequent amplification of chromosomal region 20q12-q13 in ovarian cancer. Clin Cancer Res. 2000;6(5):1833–9.
23. Fejzo MS et al. Comprehensive analysis of 20q13 genes in ovarian cancer identifies ADRM1 as amplification target. Genes Chromosom Cancer. 2008;47(10):873–83.
24. Schwartz DR et al. Gene expression in ovarian cancer reflects both morphology and biological behavior, distinguishing clear cell from other poor-prognosis ovarian carcinomas. Cancer Res. 2002;62(16):4722–9.
25. Zorn KK et al. Gene expression profiles of serous, endometrioid, and clear cell subtypes of ovarian and endometrial cancer. Clin Cancer Res. 2005;11(18):6422–30.
26. Milner BJ et al. p53 mutation is a common genetic event in ovarian carcinoma. Cancer Res. 1993;53(9):2128–32.
27. Obata K et al. Frequent PTEN/MMAC mutations in endometrioid but not serous or mucinous epithelial ovarian tumors. Cancer Res. 1998;58(10):2095–7.
28. Eltabbakh GH et al. Clinical and molecular differences between clear cell and papillary serous ovarian carcinoma. J Surg Oncol. 2006;93(5):379–86.
29. Okuda T et al. p53 mutations and overexpression affect prognosis of ovarian endometrioid cancer but not clear cell cancer. Gynecol Oncol. 2003;88(3):318–25.
30. Hashiguchi Y et al. PTEN expression in clear cell adenocarcinoma of the ovary. Gynecol Oncol. 2006;101(1):71–5.
31. Tsuda H et al. Cyclin E amplification and overexpression in clear cell adenocarcinoma of the ovary. Oncology. 2004; 67(3–4):291–9.

32. Hoskins WJ et al. The influence of cytoreductive surgery on recurrence-free interval and survival in small-volume stage III epithelial ovarian cancer: a Gynecologic Oncology Group study. Gynecol Oncol. 1992;47(2):159–66.
33. Kennedy AW et al. Survival probability in ovarian clear cell adenocarcinoma. Gynecol Oncol. 1999;74(1):108–14.
34. Takano M et al. Adjuvant chemotherapy with irinotecan hydrochloride and cisplatin for clear cell carcinoma of the ovary. Oncol Rep. 2006;16(6):1301–6.
35. Behbakht K et al. Clinical characteristics of clear cell carcinoma of the ovary. Gynecol Oncol. 1998;70(2):255–8.
36. Eisenkop SM, Friedman RL, Wang HJ. Complete cytoreductive surgery is feasible and maximizes survival in patients with advanced epithelial ovarian cancer: a prospective study. Gynecol Oncol. 1998;69(2):103–8.
37. Morice P et al. Lymph node involvement in epithelial ovarian cancer: analysis of 276 pelvic and paraaortic lymphadenectomies and surgical implications. J Am Coll Surg. 2003;197(2):198–205.
38. Sakuragi N et al. Prognostic significance of lymph node metastasis and clear cell histology in ovarian carcinoma limited to the pelvis (pT1M0 and pT2M0). Gynecol Oncol. 2000;79(2):251–5.
39. Cass I, Li AJ, Runowicz CD, Fields AL, Goldberg GL, Leuchter RS, et al. Pattern of lymph node metastases in clinically unilateral stage I invasive epithelial ovarian carcinomas. Gynecol Oncol. 2001;80:56–61.
40. Takeshima N et al. Lymph node metastasis in ovarian cancer: difference between serous and non-serous primary tumors. Gynecol Oncol. 2005;99(2):427–31.
41. Onda T et al. Patients with ovarian carcinoma upstaged to stage III after systematic lymphadenctomy have similar survival to Stage I/II patients and superior survival to other Stage III patients. Cancer. 1998;83(8):1555–60.
42. Negishi H, Takeda M, Fujimoto T, Todo Y, Ebina Y, Watari H, et al. Lymphatic mapping and sentinel node identification as related to the primary sites of lymph node metastasis in early stage ovarian cancer. Gynecol Oncol. 2004;94: 161–6.
43. Kanazawa K, Suzuki T, Tokashiki M. The validity and significance of substage IIIC by node involvement in epithelial ovarian cancer: impact of nodal metastasis on patient survival. Gynecol Oncol. 1999;73:237–41.
44. Ahmed FY, Wiltshaw E, AOHern RP, Nicol B, Shepherd J, Blake P, et al. Natural history and prognosis of untreated stage I epithelial ovarian cancer. J Clin Oncol. 1996;14: 2968–75.
45. Omura GA et al. Long-term follow-up and prognostic factor analysis in advanced ovarian carcinoma: the Gynecologic Oncology Group experience. J Clin Oncol. 1991;9(7): 1138–50.
46. Makar AP et al. The prognostic significance of residual disease, FIGO substage, tumor histology, and grade in patients with FIGO stage III ovarian cancer. Gynecol Oncol. 1995; 56(2):175–80.
47. Sugiyama T et al. Clinical characteristics of clear cell carcinoma of the ovary: a distinct histologic type with poor prognosis and resistance to platinum-based chemotherapy. Cancer.2000; 88(11):2584–9.
48. Ho CM et al. Pure-type clear cell carcinoma of the ovary as a distinct histological type and improved survival in patients treated with paclitaxel-platinum-based chemotherapy in pure-type advanced disease. Gynecol Oncol. 2004;94(1): 197–203.
49. Goff BA et al. Clear cell carcinoma of the ovary: a distinct histologic type with poor prognosis and resistance to platinum-based chemotherapy in stage III disease. Gynecol Oncol.1996; 60(3):412–7.
50. Gorai I et al. Establishment and characterization of two human ovarian clear cell adenocarcinoma lines from metastatic lesions with different properties. Gynecol Oncol. 1995;57(1):33–46.
51. Shimizu Y, Umezawa S, Hasumi K. The results of chemosensitivity test for clear cell adenocarcinoma of the ovary. Gan To Kagaku Ryoho. 1996;23(7):945–7.
52. Utsunomiya H et al. Paclitaxel-platinum combination chemotherapy for advanced or recurrent ovarian clear cell adenocarcinoma: a multicenter trial. Int J Gynecol Cancer. 2006;16(1):52–6.
53. Pectasides D et al. Advanced stage clear-cell epithelial ovarian cancer: the Hellenic Cooperative Oncology Group experience. Gynecol Oncol. 2006;102(2):285–91.
54. Pather S, Quinn MA. Clear-cell cancer of the ovary-is it chemosensitive? Int J Gynecol Cancer. 2005;15(3):432–7.
55. Enomoto T, Kuragaki C, Yamasaki M. Is clear cell carcinoma and mucinous carcinoma of the ovary sensitive to combination chemotherapy with paclitaxel and carboplatin? Proc Am Soc Clin Oncol. 2003;22:447(#1797).
56. Fleming G. Gynecologic cancer: advances in management. Annual Meeting Summaries, 2003. p. 133–9.
57. O'Brien MER, Schofield JB, Tan S, Fryatt I, Fisher C, Wiltshaw E. Clear cell epithelial ovarian cancer (mesonephroid): bad prognosis only in early stages. Gynecol Oncol.1993; 49:250–4.
58. McGuire V, Jesser CA, Whittemore AS. Survival among U.S. women with invasive epithelial ovarian cancer. Gynecol Oncol. 2002;84:399–403.
59. Katsumata N, Yasuda M, Takahashi F, et al. Dose-dense paclitaxel once a week in combination with carboplatin every 3 weeks for advanced ovarian cancer: a phase 3, open-label, randomized controlled trial. Lancet. early online publication, 2009.
60. Matsumoto K et al. The safety and efficacy of the weekly dosing of irinotecan for platinum- and taxanes-resistant epithelial ovarian cancer. Gynecol Oncol. 2006;100(2): 412–6.
61. Sugiyama T, Yakushiji M, Nishida T, Ushijima K, Okura N, Kigawa J, et al. Irinotecan (CPT-11) combined with cisplatin in patients with refractory or recurrent ovarian cancer. Cancer Lett. 1998;128:211–8.
62. Adachi S, Ogasawara T, Yamasaki N, Shibahara H, Kanazawa R, Tsuji Y, et al. A pilot study CPT-11 and cisplatin for ovarian clear cell adenocarcinoma. Jpn J Clin Oncol.1999; 29:434–7.
63. Nishida M, Tsunoda H, Ichikawa Y, Yoshikawa H. Complete response to irinotecan hydrochloride and nedaplatin in a patient with advanced ovarian clear cell carcinoma. Int J Clin Oncol. 2004;9:403–5.
64. Takakura S, Saito M, Ueda K, Motegi M, Takao M, Yamada K, et al. Irinotecan hydrochloride (CPT-11) and cisplatin as first-line chemotherapy after initial surgery for ovarian clear cell adenocarcinoma. Int Surg. 2007;92:202–8.

65. Takano M, Sugiyama T, Yaegashi N, Suzuki M, Tsuda H, Sagae S, et al. Progression-free survival and overall survival of patients with clear cell carcinoma of the ovary treated with paclitaxel-carboplatin or irinotecan-cisplatin: retrospective analysis. Int J Clin Oncol. 2007;12:256–60.
66. Kita T, Kikuchi Y, Kudoh K, Takano M, Goto T, Hirata J, et al. Exploratory study of effective chemotherapy to clear cell carcinoma of the ovary. Oncol Rep. 2000;7:327–31.
67. Takakura
68. Nishino K, Aoki Y, Amikura T, et al. Irinotecan hydrochloride (CPT-11) and mitomycin C as the first line chemotherapy for ovarian clear cell adenocarcinoma. Gynecol Oncol. 2005;97:893–7.
69. Shimizu Y, Umezawa S, Hasumi K. A phase II study of combined CPT-11 and mitomycin-C in platinum refractory clear cell and mucinous ovarian carcinoma. Ann Acad Med Singapore.1 998;27:650–6.
70. Tanaka T, Umesaki N, Ogita S. Camptothecin and mitomycin combination chemotherapy on ovarian clear cell carcinoma with multiple systemic metastases. Eur J Gynaecol Oncol.2000;21:377–9.
71. Nishida M. Chemosensitivity of ovarian clear cell carcinoma in vitro (In Japanese). Oncol Chemother. 1992;8:128–36.
72. Ohta I, Gorai I, Miyamoto Y, Yang J, Zheng JH, Kawata N, et al. Cyclophosphamide and 5-fluorouracil act synergistically in ovarian clear cell adenocarcinoma cells. Cancer Lett.2001;162(1):39–48.
73. Itamochi H, Kigawa J, Sultana H, Iba T, Akeshima R, Kamazawa S, et al. Sensitivity to anticancer agents and resistance mechanisms in clear cell carcinoma of the ovary. Jpn J Cancer Res. 2002;93:723.
74. Godwin AK et al. High resistance to cisplatin in human ovarian cancer cell lines is associated with marked increase of glutathione synthesis. Proc Natl Acad Sci USA. 1992; 89(7):3070–4.
75. Kasahara K et al. Metallothionein content correlates with the sensitivity of human small cell lung cancer cell lines to cisplatin. Cancer Res. 1991;51(12):3237–42.
76. Kuwano M et al. Multidrug resistance-associated protein subfamily transporters and drug resistance. Anticancer Drug Des. 1999;14(2):123–31.
77. Ohishi Y et al. ATP-binding cassette superfamily transporter gene expression in human primary ovarian carcinoma. Clin Cancer Res. 2002;8(12):3767–75.
78. Kool M et al. MRP3, an organic anion transporter able to transport anti-cancer drugs. Proc Natl Acad Sci USA. 1999;96(12):6914–9.
79. Han EK et al. Modulation of paclitaxel resistance by annexin IV in human cancer cell lines. Br J Cancer. 2000; 83(1):83–8.
80. Tsuda H et al. Identification of overexpression and amplification of ABCF2 in clear cell ovarian adenocarcinomas by cDNA microarray analyses. Clin Cancer Res. 2005;11(19 Pt1):6880–8.
81. Schaner ME et al. Gene expression patterns in ovarian carcinomas. Mol Biol Cell. 2003;14(11):4376–86.
82. Itamochi H et al. Mechanisms of cisplatin resistance in clear cell carcinoma of the ovary. Oncology. 2002;62(4): 349–53.
83. Itamochi H et al. Low proliferation activity may be associated with chemoresistance in clear cell carcinoma of the ovary. Obstet Gynecol. 2002;100(2):281–7.
84. Shimizu M et al. Clear cell carcinoma has an expression pattern of cell cycle regulatory molecules that is unique among ovarian adenocarcinomas. Cancer. 1999;85(3):669–77.
85. Kong Q, Lillehei KO. Antioxidant inhibitors for cancer therapy. Med Hypotheses. 1998;51(5):405–9.
86. Lee S et al. Over-expression of hypoxia-inducible factor 1 alpha in ovarian clear cell carcinoma. Gynecol Oncol. 2007;106(2):311–7.
87. Kurokawa T et al. Overexpression of hypoxia-inducible-factor 1alpha(HIF-1alpha) in oesophageal squamous cell carcinoma correlates with lymph node metastasis and pathologic stage. Br J Cancer. 2003;89(6):1042–7.
88. Lidgren A et al. The expression of hypoxia-inducible factor 1alpha is a favorable independent prognostic factor in renal cell carcinoma. Clin Cancer Res. 2005;11(3):1129–35.
89. Togashi A et al. Hypoxia-inducible protein 2 (HIG2), a novel diagnostic marker for renal cell carcinoma and potential target for molecular therapy. Cancer Res. 2005;65(11): 4817–26.
90. Morita A et al. Proteomic search for potential diagnostic markers and therapeutic targets for ovarian clear cell adenocarcinoma. Proteomics. 2006;6(21):5880–90.
91. Higashiguchi A et al. Specific expression of hepatocyte nuclear factor-1beta in the ovarian clear cell adenocarcinoma and its application to cytological diagnosis. Cancer Sci.2007; 98(3):387–91.
92. Rhoads DB et al. Circadian periodicity of intestinal Na+/glucose cotransporter 1 mRNA levels is transcriptionally regulated. J Biol Chem. 1998;273(16):9510–6.
93. Lee YH et al. Liver-specific reactivation of the inactivated Hnf-1alpha gene: elimination of liver dysfunction to establish a mouse MODY3 model. Mol Cell Biol. 2003;23(3): 923–32.
94. Hiraiwa H et al. A molecular link between the common phenotypes of type 1 glycogen storage disease and HNF1alpha-null mice. J Biol Chem. 2001;276(11):7963–7.
95. Kiyozuka Y. Glycogen levels in human ovarian clear cell adenocarcinoma in relation to chemosensitivity and cellular growth. Proc Am Soc Clin Oncol. 2002;21:449a.
96. Wang X et al. Identification of a novel function of TWIST, a bHLH protein, in the development of acquired taxol resistance in human cancer cells. Oncogene. 2004;23(2):474–82.
97. Zhang X et al. Anti-apoptotic role of TWIST and its association with Akt pathway in mediating taxol resistance in nasopharyngeal carcinoma cells. Int J Cancer. 2007;120(9): 1891–8.
98. Kajiyama H et al. Twist expression predicts poor clinical outcome of patients with clear cell carcinoma of the ovary. Oncology.2006; 71(5–6):394–401.
99. Reed E et al. Clear cell tumors have higher mRNA levels of ERCC1 and XPB than other histological types of epithelial ovarian cancer. Clin Cancer Res. 2003;9(14):5299–305.
100. Cai KQ et al. Microsatellite instability and alteration of the expression of hMLH1 and hMSH2 in ovarian clear cell carcinoma. Hum Pathol. 2004;35(5):552–9.
101. Claij N, te Riele H. Microsatellite instability in human cancer: a prognostic marker for chemotherapy? Exp Cell Res. 1999;246(1):1–10.
102. Fujimura M, Hidaka T, Saito S. Selective inhibition of the epidermal growth factor receptor by ZD1839 decreases the growth and invasion of ovarian clear cell adenocarcinoma cells. Clin Cancer Res. 2002;8(7):2448–54.

103. Fujimura M et al. HER2 is frequently over-expressed in ovarian clear cell adenocarcinoma: possible novel treatment modality using recombinant monoclonal antibody against HER2, trastuzumab. Jpn J Cancer Res. 2002;93(11):1250–7.
104. Motzer RJ et al. Sunitinib versus interferon alfa in metastatic renal-cell carcinoma. N Engl J Med. 2007;356(2):115–24.
105. Abrams TJ et al. SU11248 inhibits KIT and platelet-derived growth factor receptor beta in preclinical models of human small cell lung cancer. Mol Cancer Ther. 2003;2(5):471–8.
106. Mendel DB et al. In vivo antitumor activity of SU11248, a novel tyrosine kinase inhibitor targeting vascular endothelial growth factor and platelet-derived growth factor receptors: determination of a pharmacokinetic/pharmacodynamic relationship. Clin Cancer Res. 2003;9(1):327–37.
107. Rauh-Hain JA, Penson RT. Potential benefit of Sunitinib in recurrent and refractory ovarian clear cell adenocarcinoma. Int J Gynecol Cancer. 2008;18(5):934–6.

The Continuum of Serous Ovarian Tumors of Low Malignant Potential and Low-Grade Serous Carcinoma of the Ovary

9

David M. Gershenson

9.1 Introduction

Over the past few years, it has become increasingly evident that serous tumors of low malignant potential (LMP) and low-grade serous carcinoma coexist on a continuum. This realization has occurred due to the confluence of information on pathology, molecular biology, and clinical behavior of these two entities. This chapter provides evidence for this intimate relationship and outlines their contemporary clinical management.

9.2 Serous Tumors of Low Malignant Potential

Since serous tumors of LMP were first described approximately 80 years ago, it has only been within the past two decades that our understanding of their biology and clinical behavior has escalated. Ovarian tumors of LMP account for approximately 15% of all epithelial neoplasms. The mean age of patients with this condition is in the early 40s – approximately two decades younger than the average age for women with invasive ovarian cancer. Presenting signs and symptoms associated with ovarian tumors of LMP are similar to those of invasive cancers and include abdominal bloating and abdominal discomfort or distension.

The typical histologic criteria for the diagnosis of serous tumors of LMP include: (1) stratification of the epithelial lining of the papillae; (2) formation of microscopic papillary projections or tufts, often detached, arising from the epithelial lining of the papillae; (3) varying degrees of nuclear atypia; and (4) absence of frank stromal invasion [1]. For women with stage I disease, the standard treatment consists of surgery alone, with a long-term survival rate approaching 100% [2]. Because many patients with serous tumors of LMP are young and desirous of future childbearing, surgical management with fertility-sparing surgery is common, even for patients with advanced stage disease [3–5]. The major controversy surrounding the clinical management of apparent stage I disease is whether comprehensive surgical staging is indicated. Since lymph node involvement is unusual, some have suggested that pelvic and paraaortic lymphadenectomy are not indicated [6]. However, because the omentum and peritoneal surfaces within the pelvis are the most common sites of extra-ovarian disease, omentectomy and peritoneal biopsies are recommended even if the disease appears to be confined to the ovary.

Approximately 30% of patients have associated peritoneal implants. Peritoneal implants are classified as either noninvasive or invasive (Fig. 9.1) [1, 7–10]. Whether these peritoneal implants represent true metastatic disease from the ovarian primary serous tumor of LMP or a common coexistent second primary tumor remains unclear [11, 12]. Although the most reported series include small numbers of patients, the recurrence rates for patients with noninvasive implants vary from 10 to 50%, and 30 to 75% for patients with invasive peritoneal implants. Thus, the type of peritoneal implant is also prognostic. Despite this recurrence risk, no effective postoperative therapy that results in recurrence risk reduction has been identified [8, 9]. Nevertheless, most experts currently recommend postoperative treatment with paclitaxel/carboplatin chemotherapy for

D. M. Gershenson
Department of Gynecologic Oncology, The University of Texas, M.D. Anderson Cancer Center, P.O. Box 301439, Houston, TX 77230-1439, USA
e-mail: dgershen@mdanderson.org

N. Reed et al. (eds.), *Rare and Uncommon Gynecological Cancers*,
DOI: 10.1007/978-3-642-13492-0_9, © Springer-Verlag Berlin Heidelberg 2011

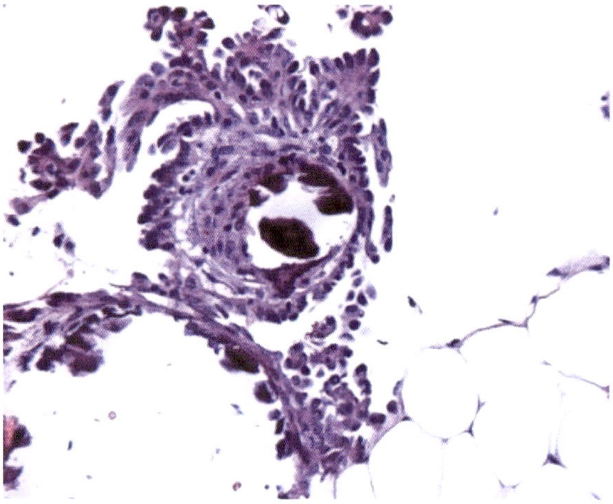

Fig.9.1 Noninvasivep eritoneali mplanti nom entum

those women with serous tumors of LMP and invasive peritoneal implants related to its poor prognosis. The small number of patients in all reported series makes any definitive conclusion regarding the advisability of postoperative chemotherapy extremely difficult, if not impossible.

Thus stage, as defined by the presence or absence of peritoneal implants and the site of the implants, is a prognostic factor in women with serous tumors of LMP. Other factors that have been extensively studied as having prognostic significance include the micropapillary pattern, microinvasion, and lymph node involvement. The micropapillary pattern of serous tumors of LMP, first formally described in 1996, is characterized by a proliferation of micropapillae containing little or no discernible connective tissue cores (Fig. 9.2) [13, 14]. The micropapillae are composed of several cell layers of epithelium that emanate from a central fibrous core, whichishyalinized,edematous,ormyxoid.Occasionally, micropapillae merge with one another, resulting in a cribriform pattern. In these areas, the cells are flattened and display a mesothelial-like appearance. Rather than the columnar cells typical of serous borderline tumors, the most common cell type is a nonciliated cuboidal cell with scant cytoplasm and a high nuclear-to-cytoplasmic (N/C) ratio, followed in frequency by hobnail cells and columnar cells. Although the original reports on the micropapillary pattern essentially advocated that it be considered as an invasive carcinoma [13, 14], the preponderance of subsequent reports support the maintenance of the micropapillary pattern within the classification of serous tumors of LMP [15–17]. Nevertheless, it is true that, compared with the typical pattern of serous tumor of LMP, the micropapillary pattern is associated with a higher frequency of bilateral ovarian involvement, invasive peritoneal implants, and relapse. On the other hand, overall survival is not significantlydif ferent [15–17].

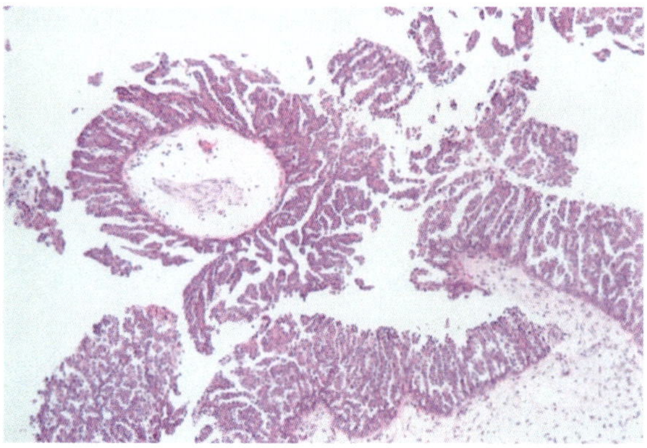

Fig. 9.2 Micropapillary pattern of serous tumor of low malignant potential demonstrating marked epithelial proliferation with long, thin papillae arising from stromal cores

Microinvasion – area(s) of stromal invasion <3 mm – does not apparently have a significant influence on survival [18]. However, microinvasion containing micropapillae may represent a high-risk lesion. Likewise, lymph node involvement also does not appear to affect prognosis, but the presence of discrete nodular aggregates of epithelium may negatively impact survival [19]. Clearly, more studies of both microinvasion and lymph node involvement are warranted to elucidate their true significance.

When women with an original diagnosis of serous tumor of LMP do relapse, approximately 80% do so with invasive low-grade serous carcinoma [8–10, 17, 20]. For the 20% or so who relapse with a serous tumor of LMP, secondary surgery appears to be the most effective therapy [20]. The remainder of this chapter deals with the current state of knowledge regarding the clinicopathological and molecular aspects of low-grade serous carcinoma.

9.3 Low-GradeSer ousC arcinoma

Progress in our understanding of low-grade serous carcinoma of the ovary and peritoneum has been facilitated by an amazing confluence of advances in pathologic classification, clinical behavior information, and molecular biology over the past two decades.

9.3.1 Pathology

As noted previously, low-grade serous carcinoma may arise as a recurrence after an original diagnosis of a serous tumor of LMP. More commonly, low-grade serous carcinoma may arise de novo. Although several studies have indicated that histologic grade is one of the most important prognostic factors in epithelial ovarian cancer, no universal grading system exists. Beginning in the early 1990s, our group at M.D. Anderson Cancer Center developed and refined a simpler, more reproducible, more clinically meaningful two-tier grading system for invasive serous carcinoma – low-grade and high-grade. After more than a decade of clinical use, we published the details of this proposed two-tier grading system and subsequently found it to be highly reproducible [21, 22]. This grading system is based primarily on the degree of nuclear atypia, with mitotic count as a secondary feature (Figs. 9.3 and 9.4) [21]. In fact, grade 1 serous carcinoma according to the grading system of the International Federation of Gynecology and Obstetrics (FIGO) usually coincides with low-grade serous carcinoma, whereas grade 3 serous carcinoma usually coincides with high-grade serous carcinoma. The problem is basically with grade 2 by the FIGO system; while most are classified as high-grade in the two-tier system, a sizable minority is classified as low-grade. A subsequent report from the Gynecologic Oncology Group, in which serous carcinomas of patients enrolled in a phase III chemotherapy study were reclassified using the two-tier system from the FIGO grading system, indicated that the two-tier system was associated with significant advantages over the FIGO system [23]. While both systems were prognostic, in the FIGO system, the outcomes of patients with grades 2 and 3 tumors were indistinguishable. But more than just representing a more clinically meaningful grading system, the two-tier classification has actually facilitated our understanding of both clinical and molecular aspects of this histologic type. Additional evidence to support the fact that serous tumor of LMP and low-grade serous carcinoma exist on a continuum, was also embedded in the initial report of the two-tier grading system; in fact, 60% of the low-grade serous carcinomas also contained areas of serous tumor of LMP within the same ovary [21].

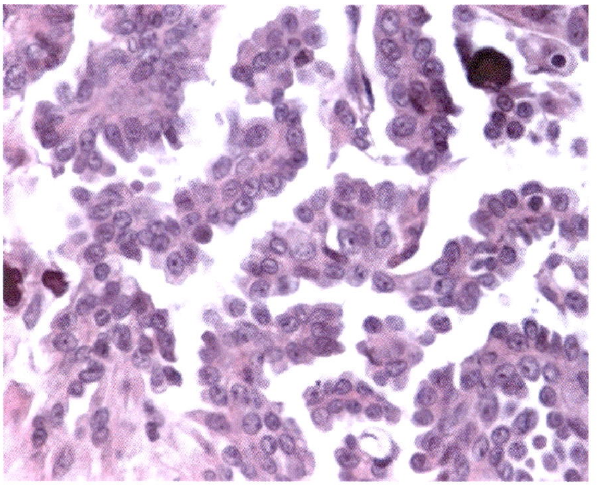

Fig. 9.3 Low-grade serous carcinoma demonstrating uniformity of nucleia ndf ewm itoses

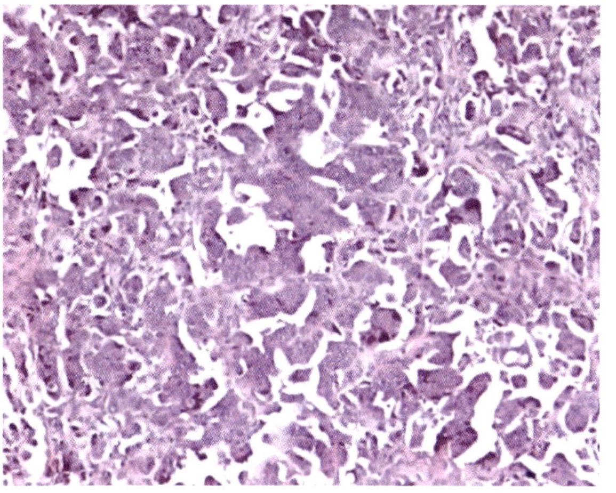

Fig. 9.4 High-grade serous carcinoma displaying marked nuclear pleomorphisma ndm itotica ctivity

Other investigators have also lent support to use of the two-tier grading system for serous carcinoma. Seidman et al. compared the M. D. Anderson and the Washington Hospital Center two-tier grading systems for grading of serous carcinoma and found the former to be more promising [24]. Vang et al., analyzing p53 mutations and in vitro extreme drug resistance assays, found the subclassification of high-grade serous carcinomas into grade 2 and grade 3 irrelevant [25].

9.3.2 Clinical Behavior and Management

The development and implementation of the binary grading system for serous carcinomas has actually facilitated the conduct of studies of the clinical behavior of low-grade serous carcinoma and the molecular biology. In the initial review of our experience with low-grade serous carcinoma of the ovary, we reviewed the clinical behavior of 112 women with stages II–IV disease [26]. The major findings from this study included the following: a relatively young median age (43 years), relative chemoresistance (only 52% were clinically disease-free at the completion of chemotherapy), and prolonged overall survival (median = 82 months). In a multivariate analysis, only persistent disease after primary chemotherapy was associated with shorter overall survival time.

In a subsequent study, Schmeler et al. reviewed our experience with 25 women who underwent neoadjuvant chemotherapy for advanced-stage low-grade serous ovarian carcinomas [27]. Only a single patient had an objective response, although 88% had stable disease. This report lent additional support to the concept that these tumors are relatively chemoresistant. And in our study of women with recurrent low-grade serous carcinomas, of 58 evaluable patients who received a total of 108 separate chemotherapy regimens, there were only four responses, for an overall response rate of 3.7% [28]. Stable disease was observed in 60% of the 108 patient regimens, and median overall survival for this cohort was 87 months. Whether the high rate of stable disease was attributable to tumor biology or influence of chemotherapy remains unclear and warrants further study.

Currently, the clinical management of women with low-grade serous carcinoma remains identical to that of ovarian cancer in general. For patients who develop low-grade serous carcinoma recurrence after an original diagnosis of a serous tumor of LMP, there is some evidence to suggest that secondary cytoreductive surgery may be beneficial in selected patients [20, 29]. If debulking surgery is performed, some type of postoperative systemic therapy is recommended (see below). For patients with stage I low-grade serous carcinoma, there are no robust data to guide therapy. Nevertheless, surgery alone seems appropriate. Of course, the diagnosis of stage I disease should include comprehensive surgical staging. For patients with stages II–IV low-grade serous carcinoma or primary peritoneal low-grade serous carcinoma, standard management includes primary surgery with an objective of maximal cytoreduction followed by systemic therapy (see below) [26]. However, as with high-grade ovarian cancers, selected patients who present with extensive metastatic disease may be candidates for neoadjuvant chemotherapy followed by interval debulking surgery [27].

There is no standard systemic therapy for women with low-grade serous carcinoma of the ovary or peritoneum. Of course, if a clinical trial is available, this would be our primary recommendation. For newly diagnosed patients with stage II–IV disease, primary peritoneal carcinoma, or a recurrent low-grade serous carcinoma following a diagnosis of serous tumor of LMP, we continue to recommend initial therapy with taxane/platinum chemotherapy. For persistent or recurrent disease, options include cytotoxic chemotherapy, hormonal agents, or biologic agents. For platinum-sensitive disease, retreatment with a platinum-based regimen is generally recommended. Options include paclitaxel/carboplatin, gemcitabine/carboplatin, or pegylated liposomal doxorubicin/carboplatin. For platinum-resistant disease, conventional chemotherapy options include pegylated liposomal doxorubicin, topotecan, gemcitabine, oral etoposide, capecitabine, weekly paclitaxel, vinorelbine, or docetaxel. As indicated above, the objective response rate to any of these agents appears to be extremely low [28]. However, the high frequency of stable disease could be potentially a direct result of therapy.

Hormonal therapy for low-grade serous carcinoma has not been well studied. However, our extensive clinical experience indicates that some patients may have objective response or prolonged stable disease to a variety of agents, including tamoxifen, leuprolide acetate, letrozole, or Arimidex. Clearly, further study is warranted to better define the role of these therapies.

Biologic or targeted agents have been used, but there is little information available. Drugs such as bevacizumab, sorafenib, and sunitinib have been administered to a few patients. Bidus et al. reported on three patients with low-grade serous carcinoma who had sustained responses to bevacizumab [30]. We have already entered an era of drug discovery for these rare tumors, with emphasis on the development of targeted agents. A current Gynecologic Oncology Group trial is testing an oral MEK inhibitor, AZD6244, in women with recurrent low-grade serous carcinoma of the ovary or peritoneum. And a series of follow-up trials is being planned.

9.3.3 Molecular Biology

Concomitant with the increase in clinicopathologic information about low-grade serous carcinoma has been the emergence of advances in our understanding of its molecular biology. These studies have included mutational analysis investigations, immunohistochemical staining studies, and genomic profiling studies.

9.3.3.1 Mutational Analyses

The MAP kinase pathway appears to play a prominent role in the pathogenesis of low-grade serous carcinoma. Singer et al. observed KRAS mutations in approximately 50% of serous tumors of LMP and low-grade serous carcinomas and no KRAS mutations in high-grade serous carcinoma [31]. Subsequent studies confirmed those previous observations and further demonstrated that either BRAF or KRAS mutations occurred in 68% of low-grade serous carcinomas and in 61% of serous tumors of LMP but in none of the 72 high-grade serous carcinomas [32]. Other investigators have also observed KRAS or BRAF mutations in low-grade serous carcinomas, albeit at different frequencies [33, 34]. Our own unpublished data indicates that the KRAS/BRAF mutation rate in low-grade serous carcinomas is 21%. CHEK2, a protein kinase involved in cell cycle arrest, is also apparently associated with serous tumors of LMP and low-grade serous carcinoma in its missense variant but not with high-grade serous carcinomas [35]. On the other hand, p53 mutations occur with high frequency in high-grade serous carcinomas but are very rare in serous tumors of LMP or low-grade serous carcinomas [36, 37].

9.3.3.2 Expression Profiling Studies

Genomic profiling studies have indicated that low-grade and high-grade serous carcinomas have distinctly different gene expression profiles but that serous tumors of LMP appear to cluster with the former [38–41]. Jazaeri et al. compared the expression profiles of eight high-grade and four low-grade serous carcinomas [40]. They found 99 separate genes that were differentially expressed; 49 were more highly expressed in low-grade tumors, and the other 50 were more highly expressed in high-grade tumors. Bonome et al. used gene expression profiles to demonstrate that serous tumors of LMP are distinct from high-grade serous carcinomas but similar to low-grade serous carcinomas (Fig. 9.5) [38].

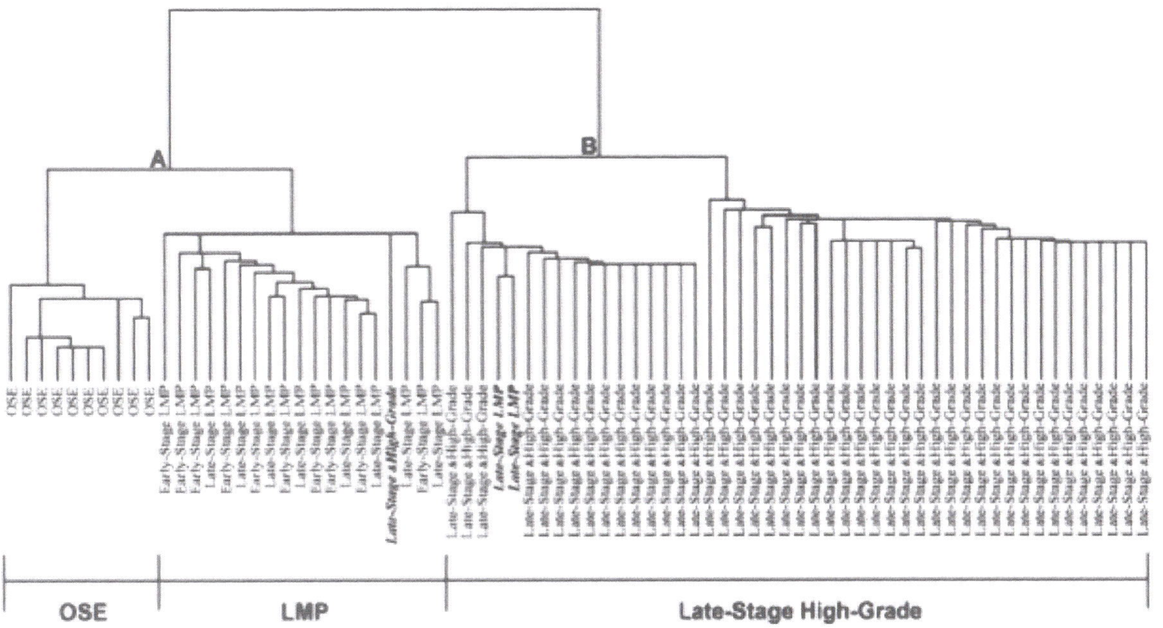

Fig. 9.5 Hierarchical clustering analysis of the 16,178 probe sets passing the filtering criteria for LMP tumors, late-stage high-grade cancers, and ovarian surface epithelium (OSE). Clustering analysis was completed using a 1-correlation metric with centroid linkage. OSE specimens grouped independently from LMP specimens (node A), whereas late-stage high-grade tumors clustered in two distinct groups (node B). Misclassified specimens are bold italicized (from Bonome et al. [38])

Specifically, in LMP tumors and low-grade carcinomas, pathways present in high-grade tumor (i.e., cell cycle progression, cellular proliferation, and chromosomal instability) were absent.

Meinhold-Heerlein et al. used oligonucleotide arrays and comparative genomic hybridization to profile serous tumors of LMP and serous carcinomas of varying grade [41]. They observed a striking similarity between serous tumors of LMP and low-grade serous carcinomas and a significant difference compared with high-grade serous carcinomas in a number of genes, including p21/WAF1, STAT-1, and STAT-3/JAK-1/2-induced gene expression. And Gilks et al. found that serous tumors of LMP and serous carcinomas are distinguished at the molecular level by a relatively small genes et [39].

9.3.3.3 OtherB iomarkers

O'Neill et al. investigated the immunohistochemical expression of a number of proteins in 22 low-grade and 47 high-grade serous carcinomas [36]. They found a significantly higher expression of p53, MIB1, BCL2, HER-2/neu, and c-KIT in high-grade compared with low-grade serous carcinomas. Wong et al. performed a series of immunohistochemical studies in paraffin-embedded specimens from 47 low-grade and 49 high-grade serous carcinomas [42]. Low-grade serous carcinomas expressed significantly higher levels of estrogen receptor, progesterone receptor, and E-cadherin than did high-grade serous carcinomas. On the other hand, high-grade serous carcinomas had increased expression of MMP-9, BCL1, p53, and Ki-67.

9.4 Summary

Over the past decade, molecular and clinicopathologic evidence increasingly suggests that serous tumors of LMP and low-grade serous carcinomas exist on a continuum and have a common pathogenesis. Additionally, the binary grading system for serous carcinoma has facilitated the study of serous carcinoma and led to advances in the molecular biology and clinical management of low-grade serous carcinomas. The establishment of the Rare Tumor Committee within the Gynecologic Oncology Group in 2005 allowed the development of separate clinical trials for women with low-grades erousc arcinomas.

References

1. Russell P, Merkur H. Proliferating ovarian epithelial tumors: a clinico-pathological analysis of 144 cases. Aust N Z J Obstet Gynaecol. 1979;19:45–51.
2. Barnhill DR, Kurman RJ, Brady MF, et al. Preliminary analysis of the behavior of Stage I ovarian serous tumors of low malignant potential: a Gynecologic Oncology Group study. J Clin Oncol. 1995;13:2752–6.
3. Morice P, Camatte S, El Hassan J, et al. Clinical outcomes and fertility after conservative treatment of ovarian borderline tumors. Fertil Steril. 2001;75(1):92–6.
4. Morris RT, Gershenson DM, Silva EG, et al. Outcome and reproductive function after conservative surgery for borderline ovarian tumors. Obstet Gynecol. 2000;95(4):541–7.
5. Rao GG, Skinner EN, Gehrig PA, et al. Fertility-sparing surgery for ovarian low malignant potential tumors. Gynecol Oncol.2005; 98(2):263–6.
6. Rao GG, Skinner E, Gehrig PA, et al. Surgical staging of ovarian low malignant potential tumors. Obstet Gynecol. 2004;104:261–6.
7. Bell DA, Weinstock MA, Scully RE. Peritoneal implants of ovarian serous borderline tumors: histologic features and prognosis. Cancer. 1988;62:2212–22.
8. Gershenson DM, Silva EG, Levy L, et al. Ovarian serous borderline tumors with invasive peritoneal implants. Cancer. 1998;82:1096–103.
9. Gershenson DM, Silva EG, Tortolero-Luna G, et al. Ovarian serous borderline tumors with noninvasive peritoneal implants. Cancer. 1998;83:2157–63.
10. Silva EG, Gershenson DM, Malpica A, et al. The recurrence and the overall survival rates of ovarian serous borderline neoplasms with noninvasive implants is time dependent. Am J Surg Pathol. 2006;30:1367–71.
11. Gu J, Roth LM, Younger C, et al. Molecular evidence for the independent origin of extra-ovarian papillary serous tumors of low malignant potential. J Natl Cancer Inst. 2001;93: 1147–52.
12. Lu KH, Bell DA, Welch WR, et al. Evidence for the multifocal origin of bilateral and advanced human serous borderline ovarian tumors. Cancer Res. 1998;58:2328–30.
13. Burks RT, Sherman ME, Kurman RJ. Micropapillary serous carcinoma of the ovary. A distinctive low-grade carcinoma related to serous borderline tumors. Am J Surg Pathol. 1996;20:1319–30.
14. Seidman JD, Kurman RJ. Subclassification of serous borderline tumors of the ovary into benign and malignant types: a clinicopathologic study of 65 advanced stage cases. Am J Surg Pathol. 1996;20:1331–45.
15. Deavers MT, Gershenson DM, Tortolero-Luna G, et al. Micropapillary and cribriform patterns in ovarian serous tumors of low malignant potential: a study of 99 advanced stage cases. Am J Surg Pathol. 2002;26:1129–41.
16. Eichhorn JH, Bell DA, Young RH, et al. Ovarian serous borderline tumors with micropapillary and cribriform patterns: a

study of 40 cases and comparison with 44 cases without these patterns. Am J Surg Pathol. 1999;23:397–409.

17. Longacre TA, McKenney JK, Tazelaar HD, et al. Ovarian serous tumors of low malignant potential (borderline tumors) outcome-based study of 276 patients with long-term follow-up. Am J Surg Pathol. 2005;29:707–23.
18. McKenney JK, Balzer BL, Longacre TA. Patterns of stromal invasion in ovarian serous tumors of low malignant potential (borderline tumors): a reevaluation of the concept of stromal microinvasion. Am J Surg Pathol. 2006;30:1209–21.
19. McKenney JK, Balzer BL, Longacre TA. Lymph node involvement in ovarian serous tumors of low malignant potential (borderline tumors): pathology, prognosis, and proposed classification. Am J Surg Pathol. 2006;30:614–24.
20. Crispens MA, Bodurka D, Deavers M. Response and survival in patients with progressive or recurrent serous ovarian tumors of low malignant potential. Obstet Gynecol. 2002; 99(1):3–10.
21. Malpica A, Deavers MT, Lu K, et al. Grading ovarian serous carcinoma using a two-tier system. Am J Surg Pathol. 2004; 28(4):496–504.
22. Malpica A, Deavers MT, Tornos C, et al. Interobserver and intraobserver variability of a two-tier system for grading ovarian serous carcinoma. Am J Surg Pathol. 2007;31(8): 1168–74.
23. Bodurka DC, Deavers MT, Tian C, et al. Ancillary study of GOG 158: survival based on reclassification to a two-tier grading system for serous carcinoma of the ovary. Gynecol Oncol.2008;108:S 33.
24. Seidman JD, Horkayne-Szakaly I, Cosin JA, et al. Testing of two binary grading systems for FIGO stage III serous carcinoma of the ovary and peritoneum. Gynecol Oncol. 2006; 103:703–8.
25. Vang R, Shih I-M, Salani R, et al. Subdividing ovarian and peritoneal serous carcinoma into moderately differentiated and poorly differentiated does not have biologic validity based on molecular genetic and in vitro drug resistance data. Am J Surg Pathol. 2008;32(11):1667–74.
26. Gershenson DM, Sun CC, Lu KH, et al. Clinical behavior of stage II–IV low-grade serous carcinoma of the ovary. Obstet Gynecol.2006;108(2):361–8.
27. Schmeler KM, Sun CC, Bodurka DC, et al. Neoadjuvant chemotherapy for low-grade serous carcinoma of the ovary or peritoneum. Gynecol Oncol. 2008;108(3):510–4.
28. Gershenson DM, Sun CC, Bodurka D, et al. Recurrent low-grade serous carcinoma of the ovary is relatively chemoresistant. Gynecol Oncol. 2009;114:48–52.
29. Bristow RE, Gossett DR, Shook DR, et al. Recurrent micropapillary serous ovarian carcinoma: the role of secondary cytoreductive surgery. Cancer. 2002;95:791–800.
30. Bidus MA, Webb JC, Seidman JD, et al. Sustained response to bevacizumab in refractory well-differentiated ovarian neoplasms. Gynecol Oncol. 2006;102:5–7.
31. Singer G, Kurman RJ, Chang HW, et al. Diverse tumorigenic pathways in ovarian serous carcinoma. Am J Pathol. 2002; 160:1223–8.
32. Singer G, Oldt 3rd R, Cohen Y, et al. Mutations in BRAF and KRAS characterize the development of low-grade ovarian serous carcinoma. J Natl Cancer Inst. 2003;95:484–6.
33. Mayr D, Hirschmann A, Lohrs U, et al. KRAS and BRAF mutations in ovarian tumors: a comprehensive study of invasive carcinomas, borderline tumors and extraovarian implants. Gynecol Oncol. 2006;103(3):883–7.
34. Sieben NL, Macropoulos P, Roemen GM, et al. In ovarian neoplasms BRAF, but not KRAS, mutations are restricted to low-grade serous tumours. J Pathol. 2004;202:336–40.
35. Szymanska-Pasternak J, Szymansha A, Medrek K, et al. CHEK2 variants predispose to benign, borderline and low-grade invasive ovarian tumors. Gynecol Oncol. 2006;102: 429–31.
36. O'Neill CJ, Deavers MT, Malpica A, et al. An immunohistochemical comparison between low-grade and high-grade ovarian serous carcinomas: significantly higher expression of p53, MIB1, BCL2, HER-2/neu, and c-KIT in high-grade neoplasms. Am J Surg Pathol. 2005;29:1034–41.
37. Singer G, Stohr R, Cope L, et al. Patterns of p53 mutations separate ovarian serous borderline tumors and low- and high-grade carcinomas and provide support for a new model of ovarian carcinogenesis: a mutational analysis with immunohistochemical correlation. Am J Surg Pathol. 2005;29: 218–24.
38. Bonome T, Lee JY, Park DC, et al. Expression profiling of serous low malignant potential, low-grade, and high-grade tumors of the ovary. Cancer Res. 2005;65:10602–12.
39. Gilks CB, Vanderhyden BC, Zhu S, et al. Distinction between serous tumors of low malignant potential and serous carcinomas based on global mRNA expression profiling. Gynecol Oncol. 2005;96:684–94.
40. Jazaeri AA, Lu K, Schmandt R, et al. Molecular determinants of tumor differentiation in papillary serous ovarian carcinoma. Mol Carcinog. 2003;36:53–9.
41. Meinhold-Heerlein I, Bauerschlag D, Hilpert F, et al. Molecular and prognostic distinction between serous ovarian carcinomas of varying grade and malignant potential. Oncogene.2005; 24:1053–65.
42. Wong KK, Lu KH, Malpica A, et al. Significantly greater expression of ER, PR, and ECAD in advanced-stage low-grade ovarian serous carcinoma as revealed by immunohistochemical analysis. Int J Gynecol Pathol. 2007;26(4): 404–9.

SexC ord-StromalT umors

10

Jubilee Brown and David M. Gershenson

10.1 OvarianS exC ord-StromalT umors

10.1.1 Overview and Epidemiology

The predicted incidence for all new cases of ovarian cancer in the United States is estimated to be 21,550 for 2009, accounting for 14,600 deaths. This accounts for 3% of cancers and 6% of all deaths in the United States [63]. Ninety percent of these malignancies are epithelial in origin, with the remaining 10% comprised of sex cord-stromal tumors, germ cell tumors, soft tissue tumors not specific to the ovary, unclassified tumors, and metastatic tumors [60]. Histologic classification is presented in Figs. 10.1 and 10.2 [60]. However, these data do not specify the exact numbers for stromal tumors of the ovary. Likewise, estimates from the SEER database between 1975 and 1998 suggest that for each five-year interval between ages 15 and 40, the incidence of non-germ cell ovarian malignancy increases from 8 per million to 79 per million women per year [12]. However, these data are also nonspecific for stromal ovarian tumors. In general, it has been estimated that malignant stromal tumors of the ovary account for between 3 and 10% of all ovarian malignancies [46, 62, 70].

Granulosa cell tumors, the most common histologic subtype, represent 90% of stromal ovarian tumors and comprise between 2 and 5% of all ovarian cancers, with an incidence of 0.58–1.6 cases per 100,000 women [7, 122, 132]. Granulosa cell tumors occur as adult and juvenile types; most adult types occur during the reproductive or perimenopausal years, whereas most juvenile types occur during childhood and adolescence. Although juvenile granulosa cell tumors represent only 5% of granulosa cell tumors, they are

I. Common epithelial tumors

II. Sex cord-stromal tumors

- A. Granulosa stromal cell
- B. Androblastomas; Sertoli-Leydig cell tumors
- C. Lipid cell tumors (steroid cell tumors)
- D. Gynandroblastoma
- E. Unclassified

III. Germ cell tumors

- A. Dysgerminoma
- B. Endodermal sinus tumor
- C. Embryonal carcinoma
- D. Polyembryoma
- E. Choriocarcinoma
- F. Teratomas
- G. Mixed forms
- H. Gonadoblastoma

IV. Soft tissue tumors not specific to the ovary

V. Unclassified tumors

VI. Metastatic (secondary) tumors

VII. Tumor-like conditions

Fig. 10.1 Modified World Health Organization comprehensive classification of ovarian tumors. Modified from International Histologic Classification of Tumors, No. 9, Geneva, World HealthO rganization,1 973

J.B rown (✉) and D.M. Gershenson
Department of Gynecologic Oncology, The University of Texas, M.D. Anderson Cancer Center, 1155 Herman Pressler Drive, Unit1362 , Houston, TX 77230-1439, USA
e-mail:jbbro wn@mdanderson.org; dgershen@mdanderson.org

N. Reed et al. (eds.), *Rare and Uncommon Gynecological Cancers*,
DOI: 10.1007/978-3-642-13492-0_10, © Springer-Verlag Berlin Heidelberg 2011

Classification of Stromal Tumors of the Ovary

1. Granulosa stromal cell tumors
   a. Granulosa cell tumors
      i. Juvenile
      ii. Adult
   b. Thecomas / fibromas
      i. Thecoma
         1. Typical
         2. Luteinized
      ii. Fibroma
   c. Cellular fibroma
   d. Fibrosarcoma
   e. Stromal tumor with minor sex cord elements
   f. Sclerosing stromal tumor
   g. Stromal luteoma
   h. Unclassified (fibrothecoma)
2. Sertoli-stromal cell tumors; androblastomas
   a. Well differentiated
      i. Sertoli cell tumor; tubular androblastoma
      ii. Sertoli-Leydig cell tumor
      iii. Leydig cell tumor
   b. Intermediate differentiation
      i. Variant – with heterologous elements
   c. Poorly differentiated (sarcomatoid)
      i. Variant – with heterologous elements
   d. Retiform
   e. Mixed
3. Sex cord tumor with annular tubules (SCTAT)
4. Gynandroblastoma
5. Steroid (lipid) cell tumor
   a. Stromal luteoma
   b. Leydig cell tumor

Unclassified

Fig. 10.2 Classification of stromal tumors of the ovary. Modified from International Histologic Classification of Tumors, No. 9, Geneva,W orldH ealthO rganization,1 973

distinct from their adult counterpart in natural history and pathologic characteristics.

Many of these tumors occur in adolescent and young women and require special consideration with regard to fertility preservation. Although most adolescents and young adults with ovarian malignancies do have ovarian germ cell tumors, 10–15% of childhood ovarian tumors are sex cord-stromal [121], with juvenile granulosa cell tumors most often occurring in childhood and Sertoli-Leydig cell tumors and unclassified sex cord-stromal tumors occurring during puberty [119]. One study identified 38 cases of pediatric ovarian tumors, and 15% were stromal ovarian tumors, all of which were juvenile granulosa cell tumors [50]. Neonatal presentations of juvenile granulosa cell tumorsha vea lsobe enre ported [11, 19, 22, 109].

Conversely, thecomas, fibromas, and fibrothecomas typically occur in postmenopausal women, and only 10% of patients are under the age of 30 years [8, 39]. The mean age at diagnosis is 48 years. These tumors are largely benign, and are not usually considered as malignant ovarian neoplasms; however, of all stromal ovarian tumors, ovarian fibromas are the most common. Together, these tumors account for 1% of all ovarian neoplasms.

Sertoli-Leydig cell tumors may contain only Sertoli cells, only Leydig cells, or both. These rare tumors represent less than 1% of all ovarian tumors. As noted in Fig. 10.2, they are classified in five groups: well differentiated, intermediately differentiated, poorly differentiated, retiform, and mixed. Well-differentiated tumors include Sertoli cell tumors, Leydig cell tumors, and Sertoli-Leydig cell tumors. Sertoli-Leydig cell tumors tend to occur in young adult women with a mean age of 25 years. Well-differentiated tumors tend to occur approximately 10 years later than intermediate or poorly differentiated tumors. Conversely, the retiform type is usually diagnosed at a younger age than intermediate or poorly differentiated types [114, 154]. Pure Sertoli tumors are seen in young women, and Sertoli-Leydig tumors tend to occur in women in their teens and twenties. Thus, fertility preservation is an important consideration in many of these patients, and this is usually appropriate as over 95% of all tumorsa reunila teralw itha norma lute rus [2, 44, 45].

Sex cord tumor with annular tubules (SCTAT) was first described in 1970 by Scully as a tumor associated with Peutz-Jeghers syndrome [123]. Since that time the behavior of this tumor has become better characterized, and it is now known that approximately 15% of these tumors are associated with adenoma malignum of the cervix [129]. These tumors are uncommon in adolescents, but have been reported to present with isosexual precocity [94].

Gynandroblastomas are a separate, rare type of stromal tumor, accounting for less than 1% of all ovarian stromal tumors. These tumors usually occur during the third to fifthde cadesoflife [3, 36, 37].

Steroid (lipid) cell tumors consist of stromal luteomas, Leydig cell tumors, and steroid cell tumors not otherwise specified (NOS). Combined, these three neoplasms represent less than 0.1% of all ovarian tumors. Stromal luteomas represent approximately one-fourth of steroid cell tumors, and may occur during pregnancy but are most common during the postmenopausal years. These are benign lesions. Leydig cell tumors represent 15–20% of all steroid cell tumors of the ovary and usually occur in postmenopausal women. Steroid cell tumors NOS are a distinct category of steroid cell tumor; these are the most common type of steroid cell tumor and can be malignant and aggressive, differing from the other types of steroid cell tumors. These neoplasms usually present at an earlier age, with a mean age of 43 years [55].

Sclerosing stromal tumor of the ovary is an extremely rare benign ovarian neoplasm which occurs primarily in women under 30 years of age and is usuallyunila teral [24].

Stromal tumors of the ovary represent a small portion of ovarian cancers, and an even smaller portion of the overall world cancer burden. However, stromal tumors have a distinct histologic origin, clinical pattern, and treatment paradigm compared with other ovarian cancer histologies and, as such, are treated with different guidelines. For women with these neoplasms, many of whom are in their reproductive years, successful treatment is critical. This chapter presents the current science to inform the optimal management of these patients, emphasizing recent progress in the field of stromal tumors.

10.1.2 Pathology, Molecular Characteristics, and Associated Biomarkers

10.1.2.1 Pathology

Specialized gonadal stromal cells and their precursors can give rise to sex cord-stromal tumors of the ovary, which arise as masses in the pelvis, originating within one or both ovaries. These tumors can occur as an isolated histologic subtype or in combination. The classification is presented in Fig. 10.1 [60]. Specifically, granulosa cells and Sertoli cells arise from sex cord cells, while theca cells, Leydig cells, lipid cells, and fibroblasts arise from stromal cells and their pluripotent mesenchymal precursors.

Granulosa cell tumors occur in two distinct histologic varieties, adult and juvenile. The patient profile, histologic appearance, natural history, and recommended treatment differ between these subtypes. Adult granulosa cell tumors represent 95% of granulosa cell tumors. The gross appearance of both subtypes is similar, most commonly presenting with a tumor with cystic and solid components. Uniformly solid tumors, uniformly cystic tumors, and hemorrhagic cysts can also occur. On microscopic examination, two characteristics distinguish juvenile from adult granulosa cell tumors: the nuclei of juvenile granulosa cell tumors are rounded and hyperchromatic with moderate to abundant eosinophilic or vacuolated cytoplasm, and the theca cell component is luteinized [16] (Figs. 10.3 and 10.4).

Thecomas and fibromas are a category of ovarian stromal tumor representing a spectrum of neoplasms with significant overlap, each of which has clinically benign behavior and is derived from ovarian stromal

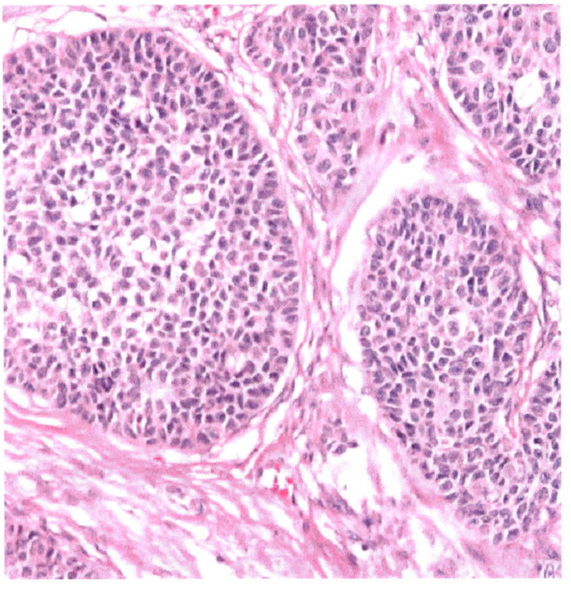

Fig. 10.3 Adult granulosa cell tumor: hematoxylin and eosin, × 100. Call-Exner bodies are seen amid insulae of uniformly stainingc ell

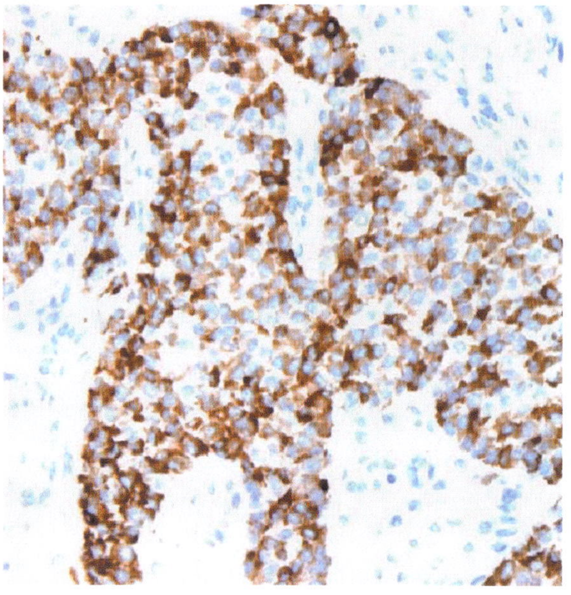

Fig. 10.4 Juvenile granulosa cell tumor immunostained for inhibin A, ×100. Uniform cells are seen amid an edematous, loose stroma. Cytoplasmic staining for inhibin A is present in the majorityofc ells

cells. These tumors share many similar clinical characteristics and often cannot be assigned to either the distinct thecoma or fibroma category based on the clinical or microscopic examination [16]. Histologically, thecomas are composed of lipid-laden stromal cells which may or may not demonstrate luteinization. Their clinical behavior is usually benign and the prognosis is excellent. Occasionally, tumors may exhibit nuclear atypia and mitoses; these may represent low-grade stromal sarcomas or fibrosarcomas and may have a malignant course [145]. Fibromas are usually solid and white, although degenerative cystic cavities are not uncommon. The average size is 6 cm but size increases with the age at diagnosis [33]. Approximately 10% of fibromas will show light microscopic evidence of hypercellularity, as well as pleomorphism and mitoses. Tumors of low malignant potential (cellular fibromas) are designated as those with an increased cellular density, mild nuclear atypia, and less than three mitotic figures per high power field. Fully malignant fibrosarcomas have greater cellular density, marked pleomorphism and more than ten mitoses per high power field. In contrast to the benign fibroma, fibrosarcomas are highly aggressive tumors, which are usually large, unilateral, and highly vascular with rupture, adhesions, hemorrhage, and necrosis often seen at the time of surgery [107].

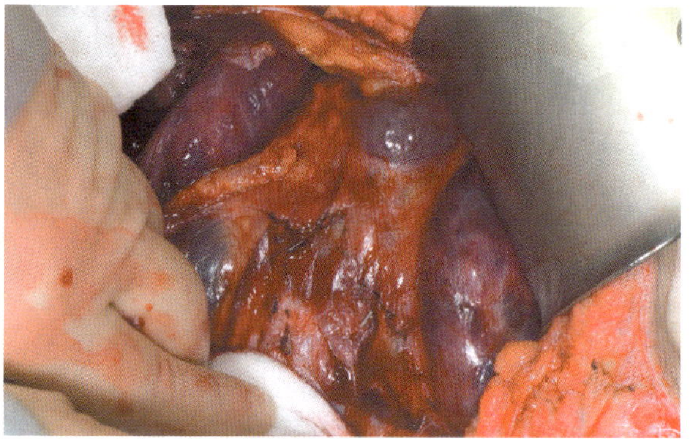

Fig. 10.5 Sertoli-Leydig cell tumor: gross photograph of appearance at time of surgery. Recurrent tumor filled the abdomen and pelvis, investing small bowel, diaphragm, and liver. Tumor appears as *dark maroon*, hemorrhagic, fleshy,a nds olid

Sertoli-stromal cell tumors, also known as androblastomas, represent a group of tumors which differentiate toward testicular structures. These tumors were originally described as arrhenoblastomas in 1931 by Meyer [85], but were renamed Sertoli-Leydig cell tumors in 1958 by Morris and Scully [89]. Gross examination shows Sertoli-Leydig cell tumors to be solid or mixed cystic and solid (Fig. 10.5), with no features pathognomonic for Sertoli-Leydig cell tumors on visual inspection. The size is variable, ranging from microscopic to 25 cm [97, 114]. Well-differentiated tumors tend to be smaller, and poorly differentiated tumors tend to be larger [154]. Microscopic examination shows that well-differentiated tumors, which account for 11% of cases, have a predominantly tubular pattern. The Sertoli cells are cuboidal or columnar with round nuclei, but with no prominent nucleoli. Atypical nuclei are absent or rare and few mitotic figures are seen. The stroma consists of a nest of Leydig cells. The most common variants are intermediate differentiation (54%) and poor differentiation (13%). These subgroups are characterized by a continuum of different patterns and combinations of cell types, with both Sertoli and Leydig components exhibiting various degrees of maturity. A retiform component is present in 15% of tumors, demonstrating tubules and cysts arranged in a pattern that resembles the rete testis (Fig. 10.6). Twenty-two percent of cases contain heterologous elements, such as carcinoid.

SCTAT are characterized by either simple or complex ring-shaped tubules. It is controversial whether these tumors are more closely related to granulosa cell tumors or Sertoli-Leydig cell tumors, as the cellular

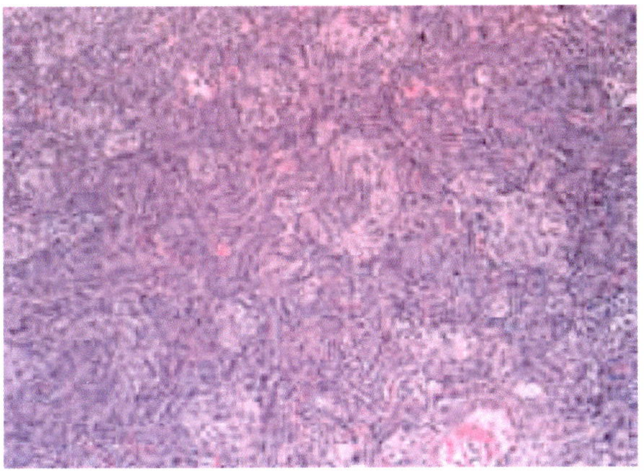

Fig. 10.6 Sertoli-Leydig cell tumor demonstrates both Sertoli and Leydig cells in trabeculae. Hematoxylin and eosin, ×100

elements appear to be somewhat intermediate in nature, but they do seem to represent a distinct entity [16].

Gynandroblastomas are comprised of granulosa cell elements, tubules, and Leydig cells. The specific cell of origin remains debated, but it may arise from undifferentiated mesenchyme [3]. Most of these tumors are solid and large, measuring between 7 and 10 cm in size, with yellow-white cystic areas present. Microscopically, these combine elements of both "male and female directed cells" [91]. These tumors must show unequivocal granulosa/theca cell elements, must be well differentiated, and must demonstrate intimate mixing of all the constituent cell types.

Steroid cell tumors, one of the more rare subtypes of stromal ovarian tumor, were historically designated as lipid cell tumors. However, it was determined that a substantial percentage of these tumors had no fatty component, so the name was changed to steroid cell tumors [152]. As noted, steroid cell tumors consist of stromal luteomas, Leydig cell tumors, and steroid cell tumors NOS. Stromal luteomas are often small; half measure under 5 cm [54]. Microscopically, they consist of large, rounded, or polyhedral cells resembling Leydig cells, luteinized ovarian stromal cells, and adrenocortical cells. Leydig cell tumors are subdivided into tumors of hilar and non-hilar type, and both are benign. Inspection reveals small, unilateral tumors with a median size less than 3 cm [34, 100, 113]. Histologically, they consist solely of Leydig cells, and crystals of Reinke are seen. Steroid cell tumors NOS are larger than the other steroid cell tumors and have an average size of 8.5 cm. They are not infrequently bilateral [55]. Histologically, these lipid cell tumors lack the specific characteristics of stromal luteomas or Leydig cell tumors. Negative prognostic factors included age, size, increased mitosis, pleomorphism, and presence of necrosis [54]. The strongest prognostic factor other than stage is the number of mitotic figures, since over 90% of tumors with over 2 mitoses per 10 high power fields are malignant.

10.1.2.2 MolecularC haracteristics

Molecular and pathologic markers have recently been evaluated as prognostic indicators for adult granulosa cell tumors. A high mitotic count appears to confer a worse prognosis, but the impact of atypia is less clear [69, 80, 86]. Aneuploidy and Ki-67 expression, markers of cellular proliferation, appear to confer a worse prognosis, but these results are somewhat controversial [29, 40, 69, 115]. Other molecular markers associated with poor prognosis in other tumors do not appear to play a role in granulosa cell tumors. These include p53, c-*myc*, p21-*ras*, c-*erbB2*, and *PTEN* [5, 40, 69, 78]. The presence of the *gsp* oncogene may play a role in the development of granulosa cell tumor [141]. Of note, the mitotic index and Ki-67 expression have been shown to be similar between the primary tumor and corresponding metastases in patients with adult granulosac elltumor [134].

Vascular endothelial growth factor is overexpressed in a majority of stromal ovarian tumors, which may account for the vascularity, angiogenesis, and response toa ntiangiogenica gents [118, 136](Fig. 10.7).

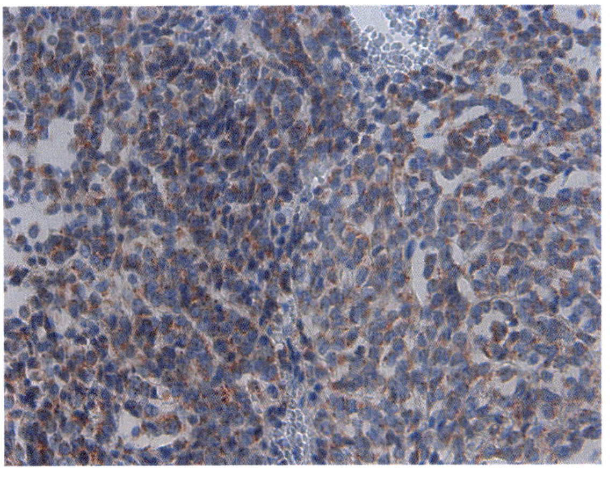

Fig. 10.7 Adult granulosa cell tumor after immunostaining for vascular endothelial growth factor (VEGF) showing overexpression with cytoplasmic staining. Hematoxylin and eosin, ×100

Chromosomal abnormalities have also been recently evaluated in granulosa cell tumors. Detected abnormalities include trisomy 12, monosomy 22, and deletion of chromosome 6, but these studies await confirmation [32, 42, 76, 77, 103, 137]. Monosomy 22, often in conjunction with trisomy 14, has been detected in these tumors, as have deletions in 22q [76] and frequent microsatellite instability [32]. A single recurrent somatic mutation (402 C–G) in the *FOXL2* gene has been identified as occurring in adult granulosa cell tumors [126]. Validation and confirmation as a driver mutation has yet to be published.

Among juvenile granulosa cell tumors, cytogenetic studies have identified trisomy 12 [112] and a deletion in chromosome 6q [153]. Additionally, a high mitotic index may be a negative prognostic factor [18].

Abnormalities in chromosome 12 have been described for thecomas, but these have not been specifically related to prognosis [61]. Trisomy 8 may be identified and may prove useful in differentiating fibrosarcoma from the benign fibroma [139].

10.1.2.3 AssociatedB iomarkers

Preoperative laboratory tests which may be helpful include inhibin A, inhibin B, and, less often, CA-125, in addition to routine preoperative laboratory testing. These levels may act as tumor markers, facilitating preoperative diagnosis but more importantly, serving as a baseline by which to judge efficacy of therapy [25, 26, 111].

Inhibin and calretinin may be helpful immunohistochemical stains to aid in the pathologic diagnosis of sex cord-stromal ovarian tumors [82, 101, 104, 110]. In a panel of 29 stromal ovarian tumors, all were positive for inhibin A, 59% were positive for inhibin B, and all but one were positive for CD99 [26]. Inhibin B may be particularly helpful in identifying recurrent disease [87]. SF-1 is a diagnostically useful immunohistochemical marker that aids in the differential diagnosis of Sertoli cell tumors [156]. Immunostaining can sometimes be used to differentiate among the various stromal ovarian tumors; androgen receptor and vimentin are preferentially expressed in granulosa cell components, whereas CD10 and low molecular weight cytokeratin are seen more in Sertoli components [142]. This may suggest derivation from granulosa versus Sertoli cell lines in the genesis of the tumor, and therefore these markers may overlap in mixed stromal tumors.

Patients with adult granulosa cell tumors should be followed with serum inhibin A and CA-125 levels [10, 13, 64, 74]. Patients with Sertoli-Leydig cell tumors can be followed with serum alpha-fetoprotein, inhibin, and testosterone levels. Mullerian inhibiting substance and inhibin are useful tumor markers in patients with sex cord tumors with annular tubules (SCTAT). Estradiol may be elevated at the time of diagnosis [94]. Gynandroblastoma often produces androgens. Therefore, preoperative testing usually reveals elevated levels of testosterone [3, 23, 95] or urinary 17-ketosteroids [91], and may also reveal elevated levels of androstenedione, dehydroepiandrosterone, and dihydrotestosterone, and estradiol [72, 79, 128]. Serum estrogens or androgens can be followed as tumor markers.

10.1.3 Diagnosis

Definitive diagnosis of a stromal tumor of the ovary is based upon histologic evaluation of the removed tumor specimen. However, the history and physical examination, appropriate imaging, and directed laboratory testing may suggest the diagnosis prior to tumor removal at the time of surgery.

The history may suggest a stromal tumor of the ovary based on the age of the patient in her adolescent or young adult years. The physical examination usually suggests a pelvic mass, with associated signs and symptoms typical for patients with a pelvic mass, including bloating, pelvic pressure or pain, increase in abdominal girth, and gastrointestinal or urinary symptoms. In some patients, particularly those with granulosa cell tumors, evidence of hemoperitoneum can be present, with abdominal pain and tenderness, peritoneal signs, a fluid wave, and even hemodynamic instability.

As noted, since stromal tumors of the ovary arise from steroid-producing cells, these tumors are often hormonally active, producing estrogen, progesterone, and androgens. Therefore, physical manifestations of excess estrogens or androgen production can be the presenting symptoms or signs of a stromal tumor [149]. These cells are involved in the production of steroid hormones, and therefore physical manifestations of excess estrogen or androgen production are not infrequent at the time of diagnosis, leading to hirsutism or virilism, or if adolescents, they may describe isosexual precocious puberty [149]. For patients during the reproductive years, presenting signs and symptoms related to hormonal changes include menorrhagia, irregular menstrual bleeding, and amenorrhea. Postmenopausal patients may note vaginal bleeding, breast enlargement or tenderness, and vaginal cornification [48].

Patients with adult granulosa cell tumors can frequently present with abnormal vaginal bleeding, abdominal distention and/or pain, and occasionally signs of virilism [39, 48, 90, 96], and usually present with a unilateral pelvic mass. When adult granulosa cell tumors are diagnosed during pregnancy, hormonal manifestations are less common, and the tumors are large and often complicated by rupture [135, 151]. One report exists of adult granulosa cell tumors of the ovary in two first-degree relatives, but this is an isolated instance and may not speak to a hereditary component [133].

Patients with a juvenile granulosa cell tumor typically present with a palpable mass on pelvic or rectal examination, and over 95% are unilateral [73, 150]. Of note, an association has been described between juvenile granulosa cell tumors and Ollier disease (enchondromatosis)andMaffuccisyndrome(enchondromatosis and hemangiomatosis). An increased risk for the development of breast cancer has also been reported [120].

Thecomas are often hormonally active and may cause abnormal vaginal bleeding, which is the most common presenting symptom. Additionally, 37–50% of patients with thecomas have endometrial hyperplasia and up to 27% have an associated endometrial carcinoma [8, 39, 131]. Therefore, just as in granulosa cell tumors, patients presenting with abnormal bleeding should always have the endometrium sampled. Thecomas may also be luteinized, which may cause androgenproduc tiona ndviriliz ation [155].

In contrast, fibromas are usually benign, unilateral, and hormonally inactive tumors, and therefore patients may present with pelvic heaviness or pain and a mass. The presence of ascites is not uncommon, and it tends to occur with increasing tumor size; for example, ascites is present in 30% of patients with tumors greater than 6 cm. One percent of patients will develop a hydrothorax,c alledM eigss yndrome [83].

Sertoli-Leydig cell tumors cause virilization in approximately 50% of patients. The differential diagnosis includes adrenal and gonadal hyperplasia and a neoplasm. The presence of a unilateral adnexal mass, however, palpated on examination or visualized on imaging, suggests an ovarian neoplasm as the source of the virilization. The size of the tumor, however, does not predict the ability to cause virilization, however; so a very small neoplasm can be responsible for a significant testosterone elevation and cause virilization [114]. The evaluation of a patient with virilization, or androgen excess, includes a transvaginal pelvic ultrasound to visualize the ovaries. Also, serum dehydroepiandrostenedione sulfate (DHEAS) and testosterone levels should be measured. An elevated DHEAS suggests that the adrenal gland is the source of the androgen excess. Conversely, an elevated testosterone suggests an ovarian source. A CT may visualize an adrenal mass responsible for secretion of DHEAS. Additional studies helpful in the workup of virilization include 17-OH progesterone, elevated in congenital adrenal hyperplasia), and cortisol (elevated in Cushing's disease). Prior to surgical intervention, the offending mass should be detected by imaging or physical examination. It has been suggested that ovarian vein catheter studies can be helpful in detecting the source if the imaging and examination are unrevealing.

Patients with SCTAT usually present with abnormal vaginal bleeding. Abdominal pain and intussusception have been reported but are less common.

Gynandroblastomas present with symptoms and signs related to estrogen and androgen overproduction. Androgen excess is present in 60% of patients with gynandroblastoma. Therefore, virilization is visible, but estrogenic stimulation of specific end organs still occurs, so endometrial hyperplasia is commonly noted [95]. Also, most gynandroblastomas are appreciated on the pelvic examination because of their size.

Patients with steroid cell tumors demonstrate androgenic changes in approximately half of cases [105].

During the diagnostic and/or preoperative evaluation, abnormal uterine bleeding should prompt consideration for an endometrial biopsy. Of course, in women of reproductive age, pregnancy must first be excluded. Since endometrial hyperplasia can be a secondary effect of excess estrogen production by the ovarian stromal tumor, the endometrium must be evaluated. If this is not done in the office preoperatively, it must be done in the operating room upon the diagnosis of the ovarians tromaltumor [140].

10.1.4 Imaging

Imaging tests which may prove useful in the diagnosis of the adnexal mass include transvaginal ultrasound, computerized tomography, and magnetic resonance imaging. Of these, the ultrasound is often the best for distinguishing the details of pelvic anatomy. The findings may also identify hemoperitoneum or ascites. If hemoperitoneum is present, surgery should proceed immediately through a laparotomy, as is discussed later.

Adult granulosa cell tumors have varying appearances on imaging, since they have variable amounts of solid, cystic, hemorrhagic, and necrotic components. They may appear as solid masses, multilocular cystic lesions, or completely cystic tumors [65]. Ultrasound often shows increased vascularity by color flow Dopplerdue tothe tumorc haracteristics [143].

Sertoli-Leydig cell tumors appear as well-defined solid enhancing masses with cysts within the tumor on CT, and appear hypointense with multiple variable-sized cystic areas on MRI. The amount of fibrous stroma determines the low signal intensity on T2-weighted imaging MRI [65].

Radiographically, 79% of thecomas are solid on CT and show delayed accumulation of contrast material [4]. Some have suggested that the diagnosis can be suggested by poor penetration of the mass with acoustic shadowing on ultrasound [148]. Fibromas appear as hypointense on T1-weighted MRI with very low signal intensity on T2-weighted imaging, often with dense calcifications [65].

The specific radiological diagnosis, however, for any stromal ovarian tumor is nonspecific. The utility of this testing in diagnosis and treatment planning cannot beo verstated.

10.1.5 Surgical Therapy and Staging

The appropriate treatment of stromal ovarian tumors is determined by many factors, including patient age, parity, desire for future fertility, extent of disease, and comorbid conditions. The goals of surgical therapy should be to treat the patient by removing the mass, staging appropriately to avoid reoperation, tumor reduction when disseminated disease is present, and preservation of fertility when possible in reproductive aged patients who desire this.

Often, the surgeon does not know the precise histologic classification of the adnexal mass during surgery, even with the pathologic evaluation of frozen tissue sections. General guidelines must then be applied for nonepithelial ovarian tumors during the initial operative management, and the need for adjuvant or additional therapy may be reevaluated based on the final pathology results. With close attention to all details, including histologic type, patient characteristics, and extent of disease, the need for reexploration and more extensive surgery can be minimized. Alternatively, the frozen section diagnosis may be rendered in the intraoperative setting, in which case guidelines for specific stromal ovarian tumors can be followed.

10.1.5.1 GeneralT reatmentG uidelines: Surgical Therapy

When a pelvic mass is first diagnosed, the specific histologic diagnosis is unknown. However, using patient characteristics including age, physical examination, and imaging characteristics, a stromal tumor of the ovary may be suspected. A frank discussion should always be held preoperatively with any woman of childbearing age who has an adnexal mass regarding her wishes for future fertility and her desires for maintaining ovarian and/or uterine function in light of potential operative findings. Although this is often a difficult conversation for the physician to initiate, it is better discussed preoperatively with the patient than intraoperatively with the next of kin when a malignancy is encountered [45].

Minimally invasive surgery (laparoscopy with or without robotic assistance) is appropriate in the occasional patient with a small solid adnexal mass or complex ovarian cyst [21, 84]. However, any patient with a large, solid adnexal mass or evidence of hemodynamic instability should undergo laparotomy through a vertical skin incision to allow for appropriate surgical staging ortumor -reductives urgery,ifne cessary [122].

Upon initial intraoperative inspection, gross characteristics can suggest the diagnosis. A large, unilateral, solid adnexal mass, often yellow and multilobulated in appearance, or hemorrhagic with hemoperitoneum evident, can suggest a granulosa cell tumor or other sex cord-stromal tumor. Upon entering the peritoneal cavity, the surgeon should obtain pelvic washings and evacuate the hemoperitoneum, if present. The site of hemorrhage is most commonly the mass itself, and therefore surgical removal may stop the bleeding. A unilateral mass in a patient of any age should be removed by unilateral salpingo-oophorectomy and sent for immediate histologic evaluation [45, 122].

Cystectomy is not appropriate in this case. The mass should not be ruptured or morcellated, as this results in the disease being classified as a more advanced stage and may adversely affect survival [9, 116]. Intraoperative rupture of granulosa cell tumors during laparoscopic management can result in subsequent peritoneal seeding and convert an early-stage malignancy to one with disseminated disease [116]. Therefore, the tumor should not be morcellated to effect laparoscopic removal. In cases in which laparoscopy is used initially, a bag with an extended incision should be utilized or the procedure should be converted to a laparotomy to avoid morcellating the tumor mass. If a cystectomy is initially performed and the frozen section returns as a stromal ovarian tumor, the remainder of the adnexa should immediately be removed – cystectomy is not appropriate therapy [45, 122]. No support exists in the literature for ovarian cystectomy in premenopausal patients with sex cord-stromal tumors. Articles that summarize "conservative management" of these tumors invariably describe unilateral salpingo-oophorectomy with conservation of the uterus and normal-appearing contralateral ovary in the setting of limited disease. Therefore, unilateral salpingo-oophorectomy is the initial step in the treatment of patients with disease apparently confined to one ovary [45, 122].

Once the diagnosis of a sex cord-stromal tumor is made, the entire abdominopelvic cavity should be explored, with attention paid to all peritoneal surfaces and abdominopelvic organs. A complete staging procedure should be performed, including cytologic evaluation of each hemidiaphragm, infracolic omentectomy, and peritoneal biopsies from each paracolic gutter, the vesicouterine fold, and the pouch of Douglas. Additionally, biopsies of any suspicious areas should be performed. The bowel should be inspected from the ileocecal valve to the ligament of Treitz, with specific evaluation for tumor implants and sites of obstruction. Tumor-reductive surgery should be performed in patients with advanced disease to reduce the tumor burden as much as possible, preferably leaving the patientw ithnoma croscopicdis ease [45, 122].

Historically, pelvic and paraaortic lymphadenectomy were performed as a component of surgical staging. However, lymph node metastasis in stromal ovarian tumors is extremely rare [1, 17]. In one report examining 58 patients with sex cord-stromal ovarian tumors who had lymph nodes sampled during primary surgery, none had positive nodes [17]. These findings suggest that lymphadenectomy may be omitted when staging patients with ovarian SCSTs.

Patients who have completed childbearing should undergo total abdominal hysterectomy and bilateral salpingo-oophorectomy regardless of the stage of disease. However, preservation of fertility is an essential consideration in young patients [45]. In the unusual circumstance that the contralateral ovary and/or uterine serosa are grossly involved by tumor, the surgeon may have no choice but to remove the uterus and both adnexae. If the contralateral ovary and uterine serosa appear normal, conservative management with preservation of the uterus and contralateral adnexa is safe and appropriate, as 95% of sex cord-stromal tumors are unilateral [44, 45, 48, 122]. Staging should still be performed. Fertility-sparing surgery does not obviate the need for staging, and refers to the safe preservation of a normal-appearing contralateral ovary and uterus in the setting of apparent limited disease.

The treatment of patients who have had inadequate staging is a difficult issue. Limited information exists as to the best course of action for these patients. If the patient has documented large amounts of residual disease after a limited initial attempt at tumor reduction, repeat exploration with staging and tumor-reductive surgery would be reasonable. If the patient has had an inadequate exploration, such as through a small Pfannenstiel incision or through a limited laparoscopy, more information needs to be collected prior to making a decision about postsurgical treatment. We have recommended several options, including repeat laparoscopic or open exploration with full surgical staging or, in some circumstances, a physical examination, computed tomography (CT), and measurement of serum inhibin and serum CA-125 levels. If the results of all of these are negative, the decision may be made to observe the patient clinically, with or without hormonal suppression therapy using leuprolide acetate [9]. Lack of lymphadenectomy during staging, however, should not warrant reoperation, as the risk of nodalin volvementa pproachesz ero [17].

With regard to specific tumor types, some limited information and guidelines are available. Adult granulosa cell tumors may present with abnormal uterine bleeding. In this case, a preoperative endometrial biopsy or intraoperative endometrial curettage should be performed, as the excess estrogen produced by many granulosa cell tumors can lead to endometrial hyperplasia or malignancy. Up to 55% of patients have associated endometrial hyperplasia or polyps, independent of age; 4–20% of patients have a synchronous endometrial cancer, a risk identified in patients over 45 years of age [51, 140]. If a uterine malignancy is encountered, the uterus should be removed regardless of patient age.

Juvenile granulosa cell tumors are quite distinct from their adult counterpart, and most are diagnosed as stage IA tumors [73, 150]. Since platinum-based chemotherapy is recommended for any patient with disease over stage IA, it is essential to stage each patient, in order not to miss any occult disease which would mandate treatment.

Conversely, thecomas, fibromas, and fibrothecomas are uniformly benign, so surgical resection alone without staging or adjuvant treatment is the appropriate therapy. Given the age distribution for patients with this tumor, preservation of fertility is not usually an issue. Conservative management may include only removal of the ovary or ovaries, but then the endometrium should be sampled with a dilation and curettage to exclude associated endometrial hyperplasia or carcinoma. If these are identified, or if she is postmenopausal, a total hysterectomy and bilateral salpingo-oophorectomy is appropriate [48].

The management of patients with Sertoli-Leydig cell tumors follows the above guidelines, and fertility preservation is important for many of these patients. In patients of reproductive age, a unilateral salpingo-oophorectomy and staging is usually appropriate, as 95% of lesions are unilateral [44, 45]. However, in patients who have completed their childbearing, a total hysterectomy and bilateral salpingo-oophorectomy with staging procedure is the procedure of choice [48].

Clinically, there appear to be two subgroups of ovarian SCTATs. The first subgroup is associated with Peutz-Jeghers syndrome and is typically multifocal, bilateral, and almost always benign. These tumors are small and rarely palpable on examination. Patients with this tumor should be carefully screened for adenoma malignum of the cervix, as 15% of patients have an occult lesion [129]. Therefore, hysterectomy should be strongly considered in these patients. The second subgroup of ovarian SCTATs is unrelated to Peutz-Jeghers syndrome, and presents with larger tumors which have a significant potential for malignant behavior. The basis of treatment remains surgical resection. These tumors tend to remain lateralized and have a tendency toward lymphatic spread.

Patients with gynandroblastomas should also be staged and subjected to aggressive cytoreduction. In young women in whom reproductive function is important, a unilateral salpingo-oophorectomy and staging procedure are advocated. In postreproductive patients, hysterectomy and bilateral salpingo-oophorectomy are indicated, and in patients with advanced disease, cytoreductive surgery is appropriate.

Stromal luteomas and Leydig cell tumors are benign steroid cell tumors that do not require staging or postoperative therapy. Childbearing potential should be maintained in the occasional young patient with this diagnosis [13]. Conversely, steroid cell tumors NOS can be malignant and aggressive, and therefore, when a steroid cell tumor is diagnosed intraoperatively, it should be staged and aggressively cytoreduced. In the largest series, 43% of patients demonstrated extraovarian disease either at diagnosis or during surveillance. Stage IA tumors in women of reproductive age should be staged, and a conservative therapy is appropriate. Patients not wishing future fertility require hysterectomy and bilateral salpingo-oophorectomy with staging, and patients with advanced disease require cytoreductive surgery [55].

10.1.6 Adjuvant Therapy

Since stromal tumors of the ovary are relatively rare, controlled clinical trials designed to determine which treatment regimens are best for certain histologic subtypes are not feasible. Most published studies combine most or all subtypes of stromal ovarian tumors, and therefore treatment recommendations are based on limited data. Most data have been gathered from patients with adult granulosa cell tumors, but occasionally other tumor types are encountered, and treatment is generalized to these types as well [13, 39, 45].

Adjuvant therapy is not indicated for patients with surgically staged stage I disease [56]. Patients with stage IC disease may benefit from some adjuvant therapy, either using platinum-based chemotherapy or hormonalthe rapyw ithle uprolidea cetate [39].

Patients with more advanced disease are typically treated with combination chemotherapy. The data regarding platinum-based therapy originated in the 1970s and 1980s. Several investigators published anecdotal reports of several complete and partial responses to platinum-containing regimens, including VAC, doxorubicin/cisplatin, CAP, and altretamine/cisplatin [20, 46, 62, 66, 92, 124, 127]. Colombo and colleagues subsequently investigated the combination of bleomycin, vinblastine, and cisplatin in patients with newly diagnosed advanced disease, and found that 9 of 11 patients responded but with severe toxicity [28]. Later trials used etoposide in place of vinblastine, and in 1996 Gershenson and colleagues reported an 83% response rate in nine patients with advanced stromal tumors of the ovary [47]. In 1999, Homesley and colleagues reported GOG 115, with 57 evaluable patients with stage II–IV disease. Sixty-one percent of patients experienced grade four myelotoxicity, and 37% of patients had a negative second-look surgery. Thus, 69% of patients with advanced stage primary and 51% of patients with recurrent disease remained progression-free. The progression-free interval was 24 months. As a result, many patients have been treated with three to four courses of bleomycin, etoposide, and cisplatin (BEP), and this has become a commonly utilized treatment for patients with stromal ovarian tumors [59]. The details of the protocol are listed in Fig. 10.8. Most recently, paclitaxel and carboplatin combination therapy has been reported to be effective in stromal tumors with fewer toxic effects compared with BEP [14, 15]. Of 22 newly diagnosed patients, 11 treated with BEP and 11 treated with a taxane/platinum regimen, nine patients in each group were without evidence of disease at the completion of chemotherapy. No differences were detected in response rate, progression-free survival, or overall survival [15]. Confirmation of equivalent outcomes between these two regimens awaits performance of a larger prospective randomized trial, which is expected to open through the Gynecologic Oncology Group in the near future.

Also, a recent study has suggested that postoperative cisplatin-based chemotherapy may improve survival specifically for the juvenile granulosa cell tumor type [18]. Alternatively, methotrexate, dactinomycin, and cyclophosphamide have been suggested to have benefit in patients with juvenile granulosa cell tumors, butthe ses tudiesa res mall [144].

Over 90% of patients with Sertoli-Leydig cell tumors have stage IA disease. This is largely dependent on grade; in one series, every patient with a well-differentiated tumor was uniformly stage IA, but only 52% of

Protocol for BEP (Bleomycin, etoposide, and cisplatin)

Thirty minutes prior to cisplatin each day, prehydrate with 1 liter normal saline with 20 mEq KCl and 16 mEq magnesium sulfate at 250 ml/hr for 4 hours, and give

- Ondansetron 8 mg in 50 ml NS IVPB, and
- Dexamethasone 20 mg in 50 ml NS IVPB, and
- Diphenhydramine 50 mg in 50 ml NS.

Cisplatin 20 mg/m^2/day in 1 L NS with 50 g mannitol IVPB over 4 hours on days 1–5

Follow cisplatin with 500 ml NS with 10 mEq KCl and 8 mEq magnesium sulfate at 250 ml/hr

Etoposide 100mg/m^2/day in 1 liter D5NS IVPB over 2 hours on days 1–5

Bleomycin 20 units/m^2/day in 250 ml NS IVPB over 24 hours on day 1

Follow with:

- Ondansetron 8 mg in 50 ml NS IVPB q8h, and
- Albuterol nebulizers 2.5 mg q6h for 24 hours, and
- Prochlorperazine 10 mg in 50 ml NS IVPB q6h prn nausea.

Regimen repeated every three weeks.

Fig.10.8 Protocolfor B EP (bleomycin, etoposide, and cisplatin)

patients with poorly differentiated tumors were stage IA [49]. There have been no reported patients with advanced stages or recurrence, and only one death from disease has been reported in a patient with a well-differentiated tumor. However, 10% of intermediate, 60% of poorly differentiated, and 20% of retiform and heterologous subtypes show malignant behavior. Therefore, patients with Sertoli-Leydig cell tumors staged IC disease or greater, with poorly differentiated tumors of any stage, or with heterologous elements should receive adjuvant therapy with either BEP or paclitaxel and carboplatin [13]. Due to the rarity of this histologic subtype, firm recommendations are difficult to make. Radiation and hormone therapy have been described [38, 154], but there is very limited information upon which to base treatment.

Patients with advanced gynandroblastoma have a poor prognosis, and are therefore treated with adjuvant therapy, although the data are very limited [95]. Anecdotal reports of P32 and cyclophosphamide, actinomycin D, and vincristine combination chemotherapy are published.

Patients with steroid cell tumors NOS who have tumors that are pleomorphic, have an increased mitotic count, are large, or are at an advanced stage should be treated with additional postoperative platinum-based chemotherapy [68]. Radiation, melphalan, and hormonal therapies have also been used with variable outcomes [35, 88, 102].

No prospective randomized studies showing the value of radiotherapy in stromal ovarian tumors exist, but several retrospective studies have demonstrated the utility of radiation therapy in select patients with advanced or recurrent disease [75, 117, 122, 146, 147]. In another study, 62 patients were evaluated, of whom eight received radiation therapy for advanced disease that was incompletely resected. Of the eight patients who received radiation therapy, four achieved a complete response, including three with disease-free intervals of at least 4 years [117]. In contrast to these findings, other studies have reported no benefit from adjuvantra diationthe rapy [39, 80, 96].

10.1.7 Treatment for Recurrent Disease

Patients with recurrent disease after a long disease-free interval may be candidates for secondary cytoreductive surgery. This may result in long-term survival, sometimes with multiple tumor-reductive surgeries [14, 99]. In cases of widespread disease or disease refractory to surgery, chemotherapy and hormonal therapy are options for treatment. Given the largest reports, the best chemotherapeutic regimens seem to be platinum-based. Either BEP if not previously used, or a taxane-platinum combination may be the most appropriate chemotherapeutic regimen for recurrent disease, yielding similar response rates of 54 and 72%, respectively [15].

Other chemotherapeutic agents with demonstrated response include carboplatin; BEP; cisplatin, doxorubicin, and cyclophosphamide; etoposide and cisplatin; vincristine, actinomycin D, and cyclophosphamide (VAC); oral etoposide; topotecan; liposomal doxorubicin; paclitaxel; and ifosfamide and etoposide [14, 41, 106]. Paclitaxel and carboplatin remain the most commonly used single agents at first and second relapse.

Many adult and juvenile granulosa cell tumors express steroid receptors, so treatment with gonadotropin-releasing hormone antagonists [41, 52, 81] and progestins [52, 106, 138] has been performed. Several responses to both categories of hormone have been reported. Early in the treatment of recurrent disease, leuprolide acetate frequently results in the regression or stabilization of disease [138]. One case has been reported of a partial response to leuprolide acetate in a patient with recurrent steroid cell tumor of the ovary [105]. Recently reported are four patients with recurrent adult granulosa cell tumors who responded to aromataseinhibitors [71].

The use of radiation for the treatment of recurrent disease has also been reported, with some responses noted in patients with localized or symptomatic disease [75, 117, 122, 146, 147]. However, based on the small numbers of patients, the data are anecdotal, the response rates are short, and the impact on survival remains unknown [75, 99, 122, 124, 146, 147, 170???]. Wolf reported on 14 patients with advanced or recurrent granulosa cell tumors. With a median follow-up time of 13 years, ten patients were treated with whole abdominal/pelvic radiation therapy and four patients received only pelvic radiation therapy. Of these 14 patients, six achieved a complete clinical response and these responders were followed for 5–12 years, and three remained in remission at the end of the study. The other three patients experienced relapse between 4 and 5 years after radiation. In a recent case report, one patient with recurrent juvenile granulosa cell tumor responded to palliative radiotherapy with symptomatic andra diologicimpro vementofdis ease [58].

Antiangiogenic agents have also been investigated in patients with recurrent adult granulosa cell tumor, due to the overexpression of vascular endothelial growth factor and vascularity of these tumors. Promising results have been noted [67, 136].

Factors surrounding recurrence have been reported in several large series [7, 9, 31, 39, 43, 93]. The overall 20-year survival approximates 40%. The stage at presentation is the strongest prognostic factor, with the 5–10-year survival over 90% for stage I, 55% for stage II, and 25% for stage III tumors. Adult-type granulosa cell tumors are characterized by late recurrence, and recurrence over a decade after the initial diagnosis is not unusual. The average time to recurrence is 5–10 years, but recurrence up to 30 years later has been reported [6]. Other prognostic factors include tumor size, rupture, and bilaterality. In patients with stage I disease, recurrences are rare for tumors less than 5 cm, but recur at a rate of 20% for tumors 5–15 cm in size and over 30% for tumors greater than 15 cm [9].

When juvenile granulosa cell tumors recur, they usually do so after a shorter progression-free interval than is seen with adult granulosa cell tumors. Although many approaches to treatment have been used, including surgical cytoreduction, radiation therapy, and multiple chemotherapy regimens including high-dose chemotherapy, few sustained responses are seen in patients with recurrent juvenile granulosa cell tumors. In our experience, responses have been achieved with BEP; paclitaxel and/or carboplatin; topotecan; bleomycin, vincristine, and cisplatin; etoposide and cisplatin; cisplatin, doxorubicin, and cyclophosphamide; high-dose chemotherapy; and gemcitabine [14]. According to a single report, patients with recurrent disease may benefit more from multi-agent chemotherapy than single-agent chemotherapy [18]. Overall, the prognosis for patients with juvenile granulosa cell tumor remains good but is related to stage. The five-year survival for patients with stage IA disease is 99%, but this declines to 60% for patients with advanced disease [18, 73].

Eighteen percent of patients with Sertoli-Leydig cell tumors recur, and of those that recur, two-thirds do so within the first year. Platinum-based chemotherapy is the mainstay of treatment upon recurrence, but anecdotal reports show that outcomes are poor for patients withre currentdis ease [13].

A percentage of SCTATs recur and metastasize, in which case repeat cytoreductive surgery is usually warranted. Chemotherapy remains unproved outside ofa necdotalc ases [108].

Unfortunately, eventual disease-related prognosis is poor if stromal ovarian tumors recur, with 70% mortality despite treatment with chemotherapy, radiation, or both [39].

10.2 UterineT umorsR esembling Ovarian Sex Cord-Stromal Tumors

Uterine tumors resembling ovarian sex cord-stromal tumors (UTROSCT) are rare neoplasms which resemble granulosa or Sertoli cell tumors of the ovary but occur within the uterus. These tumors have been divided into two distinct categories: Group I, which are endometrial stromal tumors with less than 40% differentiation into sex cord-like aggregates, and Group II, which are myometrial tumors composed of sex cord-like components [27]. Group I tumors have also been called endometrial stromal tumors with sex cord-like elements (ESTSCLE) [27, 98]. Group I tumors are usually yellow or white and are fleshy in appearance. Upon microscopic examination, these have focal differentiation with anastomosing trabeculae with plexiform cords one cell in width, small solid cell groups, and tubules of epithelial-like cells in the background of poorly circumscribed mural masses [57]. The tumors may or may not extend to the endometrium. Group II tumors are usually surrounded with myometrium and do not extend to the endometrium. Grossly, they appear as solid, round myometrial tumors which are yellow, gray, or tan and homogeneous. They do not appear whorled as leiomyomata usually do, and mitotic activity is absent. Sex cords are seen but there is minimal stroma [57].

It appears that the presence of the endometrial stromal component determines the clinical behavior of the neoplasm, as patients without an endometrial stromal component (Group II) have a benign course with only occasional recurrence, but approximately 15% of patients with endometrial stromal tumor (Group I) can have malignant behavior with metastasis and recurrence [53, 125]. The *JAZF1-JJAZ1* translocation which is frequently seen in endometrial stromal tumors and may occur in ESTSCLE, however, does not occur in UTROSCTs [130]. Overall, the prognosis of group I tumors depends on type, grade, and stage of the underlying neoplasm, with definite presence of the endometrial stromal component [30], whereas group II tumors are considered to be of low malignant potential [30].

In general, UTROSCTs are managed by hysterectomy, but several cases of Group II tumors have been reported in the literature with conservative management, with resection of the uterine tumor and preservation of the remainder of the uterus, allowing subsequent pregnancy [57]. Patients who undergo conservative management may be followed up with MRI of the pelvis [57].

References

1. Abu-Rustum NR, Restivo A, Ivy J, et al. Retroperitoneal nodal metastasis in primary and recurrent granulosa cell tumors of the ovary. Gynecol Oncol. 2006;103:31–4.
2. Alam K, Maheshwari V, Rashid S. Bilateral Sertoli-Leydig cell tumor of the ovary: a rare case report. Indian J Pathol Microbiol.2009;5 2:97–9.
3. Anderson MC, Rees DA. Gynandroblastoma of the ovary. Br J Obstet Gynaecol. 1975;82:68.
4. Bazot M, Ghossain MA, Buy JN, et al. Fibrothecomas of the ovary: CT and US findings. J Comput Assist Tomogr. 1993;17:754.
5. Bittinger S, Alexiadis M, Fuller PJ. Expression status and mutational analysis of the *PTEN* and *PI3K* subunit genes in ovarian granulosa cell tumors. Int J Gynecol Cancer. 2009;19:339–42.
6. Bjorkholm E. Granulosa cell tumors: a comparison of survival in patients and matched controls. Am J Obstet Gynecol.1980;13 8:329.
7. Bjorkholm E, Silfversward C. Granulosa and theca cell tumors: incidence and occurrence of second primary tumors. Acta Radiol Oncol. 1980;19:161.
8. Bjorkholm E, Silfverswand C. Theca cell tumors: clinical features and prognosis. Acta Radiol. 1980;19:241.
9. Bjorkholm E, Silfversward C. Prognostic factors in granulosa-cell tumors. Gynecol Oncol. 1981;11:261–74.
10. Boggess JF, Soules MR, Goff BA, et al. Serum inhibin and disease status in women with ovarian granulosa cell tumors. Gynecol Oncol. 1997;64:64.
11. Bonnevalle M, Mazingue F, Nelken B, et al. Precocious pseudopuberty in granulosa cell tumor in children less than 1 year old [2 cases]. Chir Pédiatr. 1990;31:32–4.
12. Brown J. Female genital tract cancer. In: Bleyer A, O'Leary M, Barr R, Ries LAG, editors. Cancer epidemiology in older adolescents and young adults 15-29 years of age, including SEER incidence and survival: 1975-2000. NIH Pub No. 06-5767. Bethesda: National Cancer Institute; 2006.
13. Brown J, Gershenson DM. Treatment for rare ovarian malignancies. In: Eifel PJ, Gershenson DM, Kavanagh JJ, Silva EG, editors. M.D. Anderson Cancer Care Series Gynecologic Cancer. New York: Springer; 2006.
14. Brown J, Shvartsman HS, Deavers MT, et al. The activity of taxanes in the treatment of sex cord-stromal ovarian tumors. J Clin Oncol. 2004;22:3517–23.
15. Brown J, Shvartsman HS, Deavers MT, et al. The activity of taxanes compared with bleomycin, etoposide, and cisplatin in the treatment of sex cord-stromal ovarian tumors. Gynecol Oncol. 2005;97:489–96.
16. Brown J, Jhingran A, Deavers M, et al. Stromal tumors of the ovary. In: Raghaven D, Brecher ML, Johnson DH, Meropol NJ, Moots PL, Rose PG, Mayer IA, editors. Textbook of uncommon cancer. West Sussex: Wiley; 2006.
17. Brown J, Sood AK, Deavers MT, et al. Patterns of metastasis in sex cord-stromal tumors of the ovary: can routine staging lymphadenectomy be omitted? Gynecol Oncol. 2009;113:86–90.
18. Calaminus G, Wessalowski R, Harms D, et al. Juvenile granulosa cell tumors of the ovary in children and adolescents: results from 33 patients registered in a prospective cooperative study. Gynecol Oncol. 1997;65:447–52.
19. Cameron FJ, Scheimberg I, Stanhope R. Precocious pseudopuberty due to a granulosa cell tumour in a seven-month-old female. Acta Paediatr. 1997;86:1016–8.
20. Camlibel FT, Caputo TA. Chemotherapy of granulosa cell tumors. Am J Obstet Gynecol. 1983;145:763–5.
21. Canis M, Mage G, et al. A 12 year experience with long term follow-up. Obstet Gynecol. 1994;83:707–12.
22. Capito C, Flechtner I, Thibaud E, et al. Neonatal bilateral ovarian sex cord stromal tumors. Pediatr Blood Cancer. 2009;52:401–3.
23. Chalvardigjian A, Derzko C. Gynandroblastoma: its ultrastructure. Cancer. 1982;50:710.
24. Chang W, Oiseth SJ, Orentlicher R, et al. Bilateral sclerosing stromal tumor of the ovaries in a premenarchal girl. Gynecol Oncol. 2006;101:342–5.
25. Choi K, Lee HJ, Pae JC, et al. Ovarian granulosa cell tumor presenting as Meigs' syndrome with elevated CA125. Korean J Intern Med. 2005;20:105–9.
26. Choi YL, Kim HS, Ahn G. Immunoexpression of inhibin alpha subunit, inhibin/activin beta subunit, and CD99 in ovarian tumors. Arch Pathol Lab Med. 2000;124:563–9.
27. Clement PB, Scully RE. Uterine tumors resembling ovarian sex-cord tumors. A clinicopathologic analysis of fourteen cases. Am J Clin Pathol. 1976;66:512–25.
28. Colombo N, Sessa C, Landoni F, et al. Cisplatin, vinblastine, and bleomycin combination chemotherapy in metastatic granulosa cell tumor of the ovary. Obstet Gynecol. 1986;37:265–8.
29. Costa MJ, Walls J, Ames P, et al. Transformation in recurrent ovarian granulosa cell tumors: Ki67 (MIB-1) and p53 immunohistochemistry demonstrates a possible molecular basis for the poor histologic prediction of clinical behavior. Hum Pathol. 1996;27:274–81.
30. Czernobilinsky B. Uterine tumors resembling ovarian sex cord tumors: an update. Int J Gynecol Pathol. 2008;27:229–35.
31. Dempster J, Geirsson RT, Duncan ID. Survival after ovarian granulosa and theca cell tumors. Scot Med J. 1987;32:38–9.
32. Dhillon VS, Aslam M, Husain SA. The contribution of genetic and epigenetic changes in granulosa cell tumors of ovarian origin. Clin Cancer Res. 2004;10:5537–45.

33. Dockherty MB, Masson JC. Ovarian fibromas: a clinical and pathologic study of two hundred and eighty three cases. Am J Obstet Gynecol. 1944;47:741.
34. Dunnihoo DR, Grieme DL, Woolf RB. Hilar cell tumors of the ovary. Obstet Gynecol. 1966;27:713.
35. Echt GR, Hadd HE. Androgen excretion patterns in a patient with a metastatic hilus tumor of the ovary. Am J Obstet Gynecol. 1968;100:1055.
36. Emig OR, Hertis AT, Rowe FJ. Gynandroblastoma of the ovary. Am J Pathol. 1943;19:633.
37. Emig OR, Hertig AT, Rowe FJ. Gynandroblastoma of the ovary. Review and report of a case. Obstet Gynecol. 1959; 13:135.
38. Emons G, Schally AV. The use of luteinizing hormone releasing hormone agonists and antagonists in gynaecological cancers. Hum Reprod. 1994;9:1364.
39. Evans AT, Gaffey TA, Malkasian GD, et al. Clinicopathological review of 118 granulosa and 82 thecal cell tumors. Obstet Gynecol. 1980;55:231.
40. Evans MP, Webb MJ, Gaffery TA, et al. DNA ploidy of ovarian granulosa cell tumors: lack of correlation between DNA index or proliferative index and outcome in 40 patients. Cancer. 1995;75:2295–8.
41. Fishman A, Kudelka AP, Tresukosol D, et al. Leuprolide acetate for treating refractory or persistent ovarian granulosa cell tumor. J Reprod Med. 1996;41:393–6.
42. Fletcher JA, Gibas Z, Donovan K, et al. Ovarian granulosa-stromal cell tumors are characterized by trisomy 12. Am J Pathol.1991; 138:515–20.
43. Fox H, Agrawal K, Langley FA. A clinicopathologic study of 92 cases of granulosa cell tumor of the ovary with special reference to the factors influencing prognosis. Cancer. 1975;35:231.
44. Gershenson DM. Management of early ovarian cancer: germ cell and sex cord stromal tumors. Gynecol Oncol. 1994;55(3 Pt 2):S62–72.
45. Gershenson DM. Fertility-sparing surgery for malignancies in women. J Natl Cancer Inst Monogr. 2005;34:43–7.
46. Gershenson DM, Copeland LJ, Kavanagh JJ, et al. Treatment of metastatic stromal tumors of the ovary with cisplatin, doxorubicin, and cyclophosphamide. Obstet Gynecol.1987;70 :765–9.
47. Gershenson DM, Morris M, Burke TW, et al. Treatment of poor-prognosis sex cord-stromal tumors of the ovary with the combination of bleomycin, etoposide, and cisplatin. Obstet Gynecol. 1996;87:527–31.
48. Gershenson DM, Hartmann LC, Young RH. Ovarian sex cord-stromal tumors. In: Hoskins WJ, Perez CA, Young RC, editors. Principles and practice of gynecologic oncology. 4th ed. Philadelphia: Lippincott Williams and Wilkins; 2004.
49. Gordon MD, Ireland K. New developments in sex cord-stromal and germ cell tumors of the ovary. Clin Lab Med. 1995;15:595.
50. Gribbon M, Ein SH, Mancer K. Pediatric malignant ovarian tumors: a 43-year review. J Pediatr Surg. 1992;27:480.
51. Gusberg SB, Kardon P. Proliferative endometrial response to theca-granulosa cell tumors. Am J Obstet Gynecol. 1971;111:633.
52. Hardy RD, Bell JG, Nicely CJ, et al. Hormonal treatment of a recurrent granulosa cell tumor of the ovary: case report and review of the literature. Gynecol Oncol. 2005;96:865–9.
53. Hauptmann S, Nadjari B, Kraus J, et al. Uterine tumor resembling ovarian sex-cord tumor – a case report and review of the literature. Virchows Arch. 2001;439: 97–101.
54. Hayes MC, Scully RE. Stromal luteoma of the ovary: a clinicopathologic analysis of 25 cases. Int J Gynecol Pathol. 1987;6:313.
55. Hayes MC, Scully RE. Ovarian steroid-cell tumors (not otherwise specified): a clinicopathological analysis of 63 cases. Am J Surg Pathol. 1987;11:835.
56. Herbst AL. Neoplastic diseases of the ovary. In: Mishell DR, Stenchever MA, Droegemueller W, Herbst AL, editors. Comprehensive gynecology. 3rd ed. New York: Mosby;1997.
57. Hillard JB, Malpica A, Ramirez PT. Conservative management of a uterine tumor resembling an ovarian sex cord-stromal tumor. Gynecol Oncol. 2004;92:347–52.
58. Hirakawa M, Nagai Y, Yagi C, et al. Recurrent juvenile granulosa cell tumor of the ovary managed by palliative radiotherapy. Int J Gynecol Cancer. 2008;18:913–5.
59. Homesley HD, Bundy BN, Hurteau JA, et al. Bleomycin, etoposide, and cisplatin combination chemotherapy of ovarian granulosa cell tumors and other stromal malignancies: a Gynecologic Oncology Group study. Gynecol Oncol. 1999; 72:131–7.
60. World Health Organization (1973) International histologic classification of tumors. No. 9. WHO, Geneva
61. Izutsu T, Kudo T, Miura F, et al. Numerical and structural chromosome abnormalities in an ovarian fibrothecoma. Cancer Genet Cytogenet. 1995;83:84.
62. Jacobs AJ, Deppe G, Cohen CJ. Combination chemotherapy of ovarian granulosa cell tumor with cis-platinum and doxorubicin. Gynecol Oncol. 1982;14:294–7.
63. Jemal A, Siegel R, Ward E, et al. Cancer statistics, 2009. CA Cancer J Clin. 2009;59:225–49.
64. Jobling T, Memers P, Healy DL, et al. A prospective study of inhibin in granulosa cell tumors of the ovary. Gynecol Oncol.1994; 55:285.
65. Jung SE, Rha SE, Lee JM, et al. CT and MRI findings of sex cord-stromal tumor of the ovary. AJR Am J Roentgenol. 2005;185:207–15.
66. Kaye SB, Davies E. Cyclophosphamide, adriamycin, and cisplatinum for the treatment of advanced granulosa cell tumors, using serum estradiol as a tumor marker. Gynecol Oncol.1986; 24:261–4.
67. Kesterson JP, Mhawech-Fauceglia P, Lele S, et al. The use of bevacizumab in refractory ovarian granulosa-cell carcinoma with symptomatic relief of ascites: a case report. Gynecol Oncol. 2008;111:527–9.
68. Khoo SK, Buntine D. Malignant stromal tumor of the ovary with virilizing effects in an XXX female with streak ovaries. Aust N Z J Obstet Gynaecol. 1980;20:123.
69. King LA, Okagaki T, Gallup DG, et al. Mitotic count, nuclear atypia, and immunohistochemical determination of Ki-67, c-myc, p21-ras, c-erbB2, and p53 expression in granulosa cell tumors of the ovary: mitotic count and Ki-67 are indicators of poor prognosis. Gynecol Oncol. 1996;61: 227–32.
70. Koonings PP, Campbell K, Mishell Jr DR, et al. Relative frequency of primary ovarian neoplasms: a 10-year review. Obstet Gynecol. 1989;74:921–6.

71. Korach J, Perri T, Beinar M, et al. Promising effect of aromatase inhibitors on recurrent granulosa cell tumors. Int J Gynecol Cancer. 2009;19:830–3.
72. Laatikainen T, Pelkonen R, Vihko R. Plasma steroids in two subjects with ovarian androgen producing tumors, arrhenoblastoma, gynandroblastoma. J Clin Endocrinol Metab.1972; 34:580.
73. Lack EE, Perez-Atayde AR, Murthy ASK, et al. Granulosa theca cell tumors in premenarchal girls: a clinical and pathological study of ten cases. Cancer. 1981;48:1846.
74. Lappohn RE, Burger HG, Bouma J, et al. Inhibin as a marker for granulosa cell tumors. New Engl J Med. 1989; 321:790.
75. Lee IW, Levin W, Chapman W, et al. Radiotherapy for the treatment of metastatic granulosa cell tumor in the mediastinum: a case report. Gynecol Oncol. 1999;73: 455–60.
76. Lin YS, Eng HL, Jan YJ, et al. Molecular cytogenetics of ovarian granulosa cell tumors by comparative genomic hybridization. Gynecol Oncol. 2005;97:68–73.
77. Lindgren V, Waggoner S, Rotmensch J. Monosomy 22 in two ovarian granulosa cell tumors. Cancer Genet Cytogenet. 1996;89:93–7.
78. Liu FS, Ho ES, Lai CR, et al. Overexpression of p53 is not a feature of ovarian granulosa cell tumors. Gynecol Oncol. 1996;61:50–3.
79. Luca V, Halalau F, Obresui I, et al. Gynandroblastoma of the ovary. Morphol Embryol. 1983;29:117.
80. Malmstrom H, Hogberg T, Risberg B, et al. Granulosa cell tumors of the ovary; prognostic factors and outcome. Gynecol Oncol. 1994;52:50–5.
81. Martikainen H, Penttinen J, Huhtaniemi I, et al. Gonadotropin-releasing hormone agonist analog therapy effective in ovarian granulosa cell malignancy. Gynecol Oncol.1989;35:406.
82. McCluggage WG, Maxwell P, Sloan JM. Immunohistochemical staining of ovarian granulosa cell tumors with monoclonal antibody against inhibin. Hum Pathol. 1997;28: 1034–8.
83. Meigs JV. Fibroma of the ovary with ascites and hydrothorax – Meigs syndrome. Am J Obstet Gynecol. 1954;67:962.
84. Mettler L, Semm K, Shive K. Endoscopic management of adnexal masses. JSLS. 1997;2:103–12.
85. Meyer R. Pathology of some special ovarian tumors and their relation to sex characteristics. Am J Obstet Gynecol. 1931;22:697.
86. Miller BE, Barron BA, Wan JY, et al. Prognostic factors in adult granulosa cell tumor of the ovary. Cancer. 1997;79: 1951–5.
87. Mom CH, Engelen MJA, Willemse PHB, et al. Granulosa cell tumors of the ovary: the clinical value of serum inhibin A and B levels in a large single center cohort. Gynecol Oncol.2007;105:365–72.
88. Montag TW, Murphy RE, Belinson JL. Virilizing malignant lipoid cell tumor producing erythropoietin. Gynecol Oncol.1984;19:98.
89. Morris JM, Scully RE. Endocrine pathology of the ovary. St. Louis: Mosby; 1958.
90. Nakashima N, Young RH, Scully RE. Androgenic granulosa cell tumors of the ovary. Arch Pathol Lab Med. 1984; 108:786.
91. Neubecker RD, Breen JL. Gynandroblastoma. Am J Clin Pathol.1962; 38:60.
92. Neville AJ, Gilchrist KW, Davis TE. The chemotherapy of granulosa cell tumors of the ovary: experience of the Wisconsin Clinical Cancer Center. Med Pediatr Oncol. 1984;12:397–400.
93. Norris HJ, Taylor HB. Prognosis of granulosa-theca cell tumors of the ovary. Cancer. 1968;21:255.
94. Nosov V, Park S, Rao J, et al. Non-Peutz-Jeghers syndrome associated ovarian sex cord tumor with annular tubules: a case report. Fertil Steril. 2009;92:1497.
95. Novak ER. Gynandroblastoma of the ovary: review of 8 cases from the Ovarian Tumor Registry. Obstet Gynecol. 1967;30:709.
96. Ohel G, Kaneti H, Schenker JG. Granulosa cell tumors in Israel: a study of 172 cases. Gynecol Oncol. 1983;15:278.
97. O'Hern TM, Neubecker RD. Arrhenoblastoma. Obstet Gynecol.1962; 19:758.
98. Pang LC. Endometrial stromal sarcoma with sex cord-like differentiation associated with tamoxifen therapy. South Med J. 1998;91:592–4.
99. Pankratz E, Buyes DA, White GW, et al. Granulosa cell tumors: a clinical review of 61 cases. Obstet Gynecol. 1978;52:718.
100. Paraskevas M, Scully RE. Hilus cell tumor of the ovary. Int J Gynecol Pathol. 1989;8:299.
101. Pelkey TJ, Frierson Jr HF, Mills SE, et al. The diagnostic utility of inhibin staining in ovarian neoplasms. Int J Gynecol Pathol. 1998;17:97–105.
102. Peng-Hui W, Hsiang-Tai C, Wen-Ling L. Use of a long-acting gonadotropin-releasing hormone agonist for treatment of steroid cell tumors of the ovary. Fertil Steril. 1998;69:353.
103. Persons DL, Hartmann LC, Herath JF, et al. Fluorescence in situ hybridization analysis of trisomy 12 in ovarian tumors. Am J Clin Pathol. 1994;102:775–9.
104. Portugal R, Oliva E. Calretinin: diagnostic utility in the female genital tract. Adv Anat Pathol. 2009;16:118–24.
105. Powell JL, Dulaney DP, Shiro BC. Androgen-secreting steroid cell tumor of the ovary. South Med J. 2000;93:1201–4.
106. Powell JL, Connor GP, Henderson GS. Management of recurrent juvenile granulosa cell tumor of the ovary. Gynecol Oncol. 2001;81:113–6.
107. Prat J, Scully RE. Cellular fibromas and fibrosarcomas of the ovary. Cancer. 1981;47:2663.
108. Puls LE, Hamous J, Morrow MS, et al. Recurrent ovarian sex cord tumor with annular tubules: tumor marker and chemotherapy experience. Gynecol Oncol. 1994;54:396.
109. Pysher TJ, Hitch DC, Krous HF. Bilateral juvenile granulosa cell tumors in a 4-month-old dysmorphic infant. A clinical, histologic, and ultrastructural study. Am J Surg Pathol.1981; 5:789–94.
110. Rishi M, Howard LN, Brathauer GL, et al. Use of monoclonal antibody against human inhibin as a marker for sex cord-stromal tumors of the ovary. Am J Surg Pathol. 1997;21:583–9.
111. Robertson DM, McNeilage J. Inhibins as biomarkers for reproductive cancers. Semin Reprod Med. 2004;22:219–25.
112. Rodriguez E, Rao P, Reuter V. Cytogenetic analysis of a juvenile granulosa cell tumor. Cancer Genet Cytogenet. 1992;61:207.

113. Roth LM, Sternberg WH. Ovarian stromal tumors containing Leydig-cells. II. Pure Leydig-cell tumor, non-hilar type. Cancer.1973; 32:952.
114. Roth LM, Anderson MC, Govan DT, et al. Sertoli-Leydig cell tumors: a clinicopathologic study of 34 cases. Cancer. 1981;48:187.
115. Roush GR, El-Naggar AK, Abdul-Karim FW. Granulosa cell tumor of ovary: a clinicopathologic and flow cytometric DNA analysis. Gynecol Oncol. 1995;56:430–4.
116. Salani R, Goodrich K, Song C, et al. Three case reports of laparoscopic management of granulosa cell tumor with intraoperative rupture and subsequent upstaging. J Minim Invasive Gynecol. 2008;15:511–3.
117. Savage P, Constenla D, Fisher C, et al. Granulosa cell tumors of the ovary: demographics, survival, and the management of advanced disease. Clin Oncol (R Coll Radiol). 1998;10:242–5.
118. Schmidt M, Kammerer U, Segerer S, et al. Glucose metabolism and angiogenesis in granulosa cell tumors of the ovary: activation of Akt, expression of M2PK, TKTL1 and VEGF. Eur J Obstet Gynecol Reprod Biol. 2008;139:72–8.
119. Schneider DR, Calaminus G, Harms D, et al. Ovarian sex cord-stromal tumors in children and adolescents. J Reprod Med.2005;50:439–46.
120. Schoefield DE, Fletcher JA. Trisomy 12 in pediatric granulosa-stromal cell tumors. Am J Pathol. 1992;141:1265.
121. Schultz KA, Sencer SF, Messinger Y, et al. Pediatric ovarian tumors: a review of 67 cases. Pediatr Blood Cancer. 2005;44:167–73.
122. Schumer ST, Cannistra SA. Granulosa cell tumor of the ovary. J Clin Oncol. 2003;21:1180–9.
123. Scully RE. Sex cord tumor with annular tubules: a distinctive ovarian tumor of the Peutz-Jeghers syndrome. Cancer. 1970;25:1107.
124. Schwartz PE, Smith JP. Treatment of ovarian stromal tumors. Am J Obstet Gynecol. 1976;125:402–11.
125. Seki H, Takagi A, Takada S, et al. A case of recurrent intramural uterine stromal tumor with epithelial differentiation effectively treated with oral low-dose administration of etoposide. Asia Oceania J Obstet Gynaecol. 1994;20:59–65.
126. Shah SP, Kobel M, Senz J, et al. Mutation of FOXL2 in granulosa-cell tumors of the ovary. N Engl J Med. 2009;360: 2719–29.
127. Slayton RE. Management of germ cell and stromal tumors of the ovary. Semin Oncol. 1984;11:299–313.
128. Soules MR, Abraham GE, Bossen EH. The steroid profile of a virilizing ovarian tumor. Obstet Gynecol. 1978;52:73.
129. Srivasta PJ, Keeney GL, Podratz KC. Disseminated cervical adenoma malignum and bilateral ovarian sex cord tumors with annular tubules associated with Peutz-Jeghers syndrome. Gynecol Oncol. 1994;53:256.
130. Staats PN, Garcia JJ, Dias-Santagata D. Uterine tumors resembling ovarian sex cord tumors (UTROSCT) lack the *JAZF1-JJAZ1* translocation frequently seen in endometrial stromal tumors. Am J Surg Pathol. 2009;33:1206–12.
131. Stage AH, Grafton WD. Thecomas and granulosa-theca cell tumors of the ovary: an analysis of 51 tumors. Obstet Gynecol.1977;50 :21.
132. Stenwig JT, Hazekamp JT, Beecham JB. Granulosa cell tumors of the ovary: a clinicopathologic study in 118 cases with long term follow-up. Gynecol Oncol. 1979;7:136.
133. Stevens TA, Brown J, Zander DS, et al. Adult granulosa cell tumors of the ovary in two first-degree relatives. Gynecol Oncol. 2005;98:502–5.
134. Stewart CJR, Brennan BA, Crook ML, et al. Comparison of proliferation indices in primary adult-type granulosa cell tumors of the ovary and their corresponding metastases. Int J Gynecol Pathol. 2009;28:423–31.
135. Tanyi J, Rigo Jr J, Csapo Z, et al. Trisomy 12 in juvenile granulosa cell tumor of the ovary during pregnancy. A report of 2 cases. J Reprod Med. 1999;44:826–32.
136. Tao X, Sood AK, Deavers MT, et al. Anti-angiogenesis therapy with bevacizumab for patients with ovarian granulosa cell tumors. Gynecol Oncol. 2009;114:431–6.
137. Teyssier JR, Adnet JJ, Pigeon F, et al. Chromosomal changes in an ovarian granulosa cell tumor: similarity with carcinoma. Cancer Genet Cytogenet. 1985;14:147.
138. Tresukosol D, Kudelka AP, Edwards CL, et al. Recurrent ovarian granulosa cell tumor: a case report of a dramatic response to Taxol. Int J Gynecol Cancer. 1995; 5:156–9.
139. Tsuji T, Kawauchi S, Utsunomiya T, et al. Fibrosarcoma versus cellular fibroma of the ovary: a comparative study of their proliferative activity and chromosome aberrations using MIB-1 immunostaining, NDA flow cytometry, and fluorescence in situ hybridization. Am J Surg Pathol. 1997;21:52.
140. Unkila-Kallio L, Tiitinen A, Wahlstrom T, et al. Reproductive features in women developing ovarian granulosa cell tumour at a fertile age. Hum Reprod. 2000;15:589–93.
141. Vallar L. Oncogenic role of heterotrimeric G proteins. Cancer Surv. 1996;27:325–38.
142. Vang R, Herrmann M, Tavassoli FA. Comparative immunohistochemical analysis of granulosa and sertoli components in ovarian sex cord-stromal tumors with mixed differentiation: potential implications for derivation of Sertoli differentiation in ovarian tumors. Int J Gynecol Pathol.2004; 23:151–61.
143. Van Holsbeke C, Domali E, Holland TK. Imaging of gynecological disease: clinical and ultrasound characteristics of granulosa cell tumors of the ovary. Ultrasound Obstet Gynecol.2008; 31:450–6.
144. Vassal G, Flamant F, Caillaud JM, et al. Juvenile granulosa cell tumor of the ovary in children: a clinical study of 15 cases. J Clin Oncol. 1988;6:990–5.
145. Waxman M, Vultein JC, Urcuyo R, et al. Ovarian low grade stromal sarcoma with thecomatous features. Cancer. 1979; 44:2206.
146. Wessalowski R, Spaar HJ, Pape H, et al. Successful liver treatment of a juvenile granulosa cell tumor in a 4-year-old child by regional deep hyperthermia, systemic chemotherapy, and irradiation. Gynecol Oncol. 1995; 57:417–22.
147. Wolf JK, Mullen J, Eifel PJ, et al. Radiation treatment of advanced or recurrent granulosa cell tumor of the ovary. Gynecol Oncol. 1999;73:35–41.
148. Yaghoobian J, Pinck RL. Ultrasound findings in thecoma of the ovary. J Clin Ultrasound. 1983;11:91.
149. Young RH, Scully RE. Endocrine tumors of the ovary. Curr Top Pathol. 1992;85:113–64.
150. Young RH, Dickersin GR, Scully RE. Juvenile granulosa cell tumor of the ovary. Am J Surg Pathol. 1984;8:575.

151. Young RH, Dudley AG, Scully RE. Granulosa cell, Sertoli-Leydig cell, and unclassified sex cord stromal tumors associated with pregnancy: a clinicopathologic analysis of thirty six cases. Gynecol Oncol. 1984;18:181.
152. Young RH, Path FRC, Scully RE. Sex cord-stromal, steroid cell, and other ovarian tumors with endocrine, paraendocrine, and paraneoplastic manifestations. In: Kurman RJ, editor. Blaustein's pathology of the female genital tract. New York: Springer; 1994.
153. Zaloudek C, Norris HJ. Granulosa cell tumors of the ovary in children: a clinical and pathologic study of 32 cases. Am J Surg Pathol. 1982;6:503.
154. Zaloudek C, Norris HJ. Sertoli-Leydig tumors of the ovary: a clinicopathologic study of 64 intermediate and poorly differentiated neoplasms. Am J Surg Pathol. 1984;8:405.
155. Zhang J, Young RH, Arseneau J, et al. Ovarian stromal tumors containing lutein or Leydig cells – a clinicopathologic analysis of fifty cases. Int J Gynecol Pathol. 1982;1:270.
156. Zhao C, Barner R, Vinh TN, et al. SF-1 is a diagnostically useful immunohistochemical marker and comparable to other sex cord-stromal tumor markers for the differential diagnosis of ovarian sertoli cell tumor. Int J Gynecol Pathol. 2008;27:507–14.

Squamous Cell Carcinomas Arising From Dermoids

11

M. Corona Gainford and Michael Friedlander

Dermoid cysts or mature cystic teratomas are one of the most common tumors that occur in women during their reproductive life, accounting for almost 20% of all ovarian tumors. They are part of a subclass of ovarian germ cell tumor believed to arise from the primordial germ cells. Such origins give rise to the bizarre gross appearance of these tumors. They are generally unilateral and oophorectomy, the operation of choice, is usually curative.

Malignant transformation is rare and occurs in about 1–2% of cases, typically in postmenopausal women. The tumor may arise from any of the three germ cell layers present in the teratoma and has been observed adjacent to both normal and metaplastic cells. Squamous cell carcinoma (SCC) is the most common type of malignancy that arises and makes up over 80% of cancers that are seen (Figs. 11.1 and 11.2). However, a wide variety of different histological subtypes has been reported and includes carcinosarcomas, melanomas, mucinous cancer, and adenocarcinomas and adenosquamous carcinomas. SCCs arising from dermoids cysts are characteristically seen in an older population with the mean age of patients ranging from 45 to 60 years, but it has been reported in all age groups [1].

SCCs arising from dermoid cysts usually grow slowly and cause minimal symptoms until they are large or there are complications such as torsion or rupture. They are not usually diagnosed preoperatively as there are no particular signs or symptoms associated with malignant transformation. Presenting symptoms may include abdominal pain and distension secondary to a pelvic mass, but with locally advanced disease, the patient may also present with bowel or bladder symptoms.

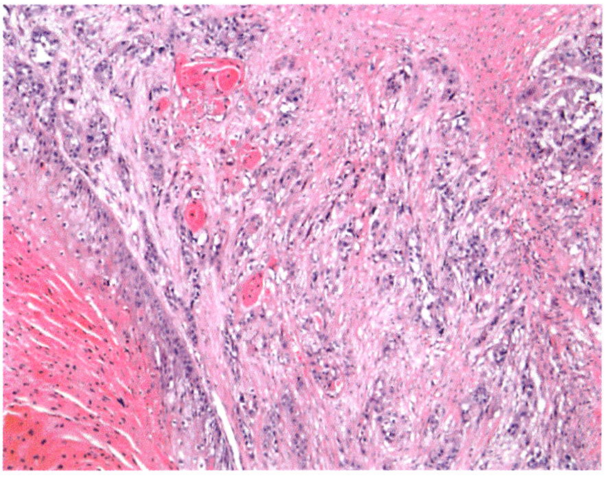

Fig. 11.1 High power: SCC arising in a dermoid. Note the dysplastic squamous lining

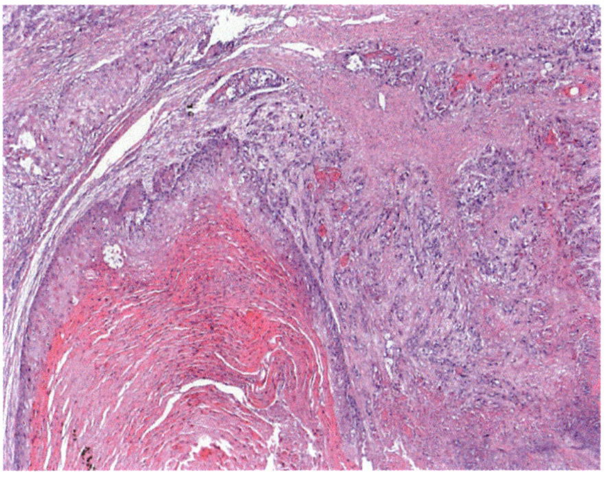

Fig. 11.2 Low power: SCC arising in a dermoid. Note the dysplastic squamous lining

M.C. Gainford
ANZGOG Coordinating Centre, NHMRC Clinical Trials Centre, University of Sydney, Sydney, Australia

M. Friedlander (✉)
Prince of Wales and Royal Womens Hospital, Sydney, Australia
e-mail: michaelfriedlander@unsw.edu.au

N. Reed et al. (eds.), *Rare and Uncommon Gynecological Cancers*,
DOI: 10.1007/978-3-642-13492-0_11, © Springer-Verlag Berlin Heidelberg 2011

Prognosis is dependent on stage with stage I patients having a relatively good prognosis, but the outcome is very poor when the disease has spread beyond the ovary or if the cyst had ruptured. Peterson reported a 75% five-year survival rate in patients with unruptured stage I disease [2]. In a pooled analysis, Kashimura reported a five-year survival rate of 50% in stage I patients vs. 25% in stage II, 12% in stage III, and 0% in stage IV [3]. The most important prognostic indicator of survival has been reported to be confinement of the tumor within the ovarian tunica. Other significant predictors of prognosis include clinical stage, tumor grade, vascular involvement, and the mode of tumor infiltration [4, 5].

Since dermoid cysts are a common ovarian tumor, there is increasing interest in the preoperative risk assessment of these tumors in order to optimize surgical management. Kikkawa reported that age and tumor size were important factors in determining the malignant potential of a dermoid cyst preoperatively among a cohort of 37 patients [6]. The mean age of patients with a benign dermoid cyst was 37.5 years vs. 55.2 years for those with a malignant transformation ($p<0.0001$). The mean tumor size was 88.4 mm vs. 152.3 mm ($p<0.0001$) for benign vs. malignant respectively. Multiple series have investigated the usefulness of serum tumor markers, with variable results [4, 7]. It is generally felt that CA 125 does not have a role as a diagnostic tool. An elevated SCC antigen appears to be the most useful especially when combined with other risk factors [8]. Mori reported that with a serum SCC level less than 2.5 ng/mL and patient's age less than 40 years, the sensitivity for malignant transformation was 77% and specificity was 96%. With regard to radiological studies, MRI appears to be the most useful [9]. Malignant transformation may be demonstrated by the presence of a solid component with contrast enhancement, transmural or transeptal extension, and evidence of adherence to surrounding structures.

Due to its rarity, there is no clear consensus on an optimal management strategy. Surgery including total abdominal hysterectomy, bilateral salpingo-oophorectomy and omentectomy is generally the most widely accepted surgical treatment. If not optimally staged at initial surgery, it is generally recommended that patients undergo a second procedure as complete tumor excision and proper staging are essential to inform prognosis and treatment planning. Laparoscopic removal can be problematic as spillage may occur resulting in inadvertent upstaging [10]. It remains controversial whether this upstaging affects prognosis. Similar to patients with epithelial ovarian cancer, optimal debulking is thought to improve survival in patients with metastatic disease. Tseng reported a statistically significant association between optimal cytoreduction and improved survival among a cohort of 26 patients [11]. Hackethal, in a recently reported meta-analysis reported that omentectomy did not affect overall survival whereas lymphadenectomy improved the chances of survival in patients with advanced stages (59.2 months vs. 40.4 months) [12]. The effectiveness of unilateral oophorectomy and thus fertility-sparing surgery in premenopausal women with early stage disease remains unclear.

The benefits of radiotherapy or chemotherapy have never been prospectively evaluated and remain unclear. The issue of whether pure stage I tumors require further therapy still remains questionable given their relatively good prognosis. For patients with more advanced disease, there are no universally accepted regimens or doses used. Postoperative treatment regimens in the literature include single agent or combination chemotherapy, radiation therapy, or a combination of these approaches. Platinum-based chemotherapy would be a reasonable choice and generally regimens that are active in squamous cell cancer at other sites have been used such as cisplatin-5 FU and carboplatin/cisplatin and paclitaxel. There have been a small number of case reports of prolonged survival in patients with more advanced disease who have been treated with cisplatin-based chemotherapy [13, 14]. Recently, there has been a report of prolonged disease-free survival in a patient with stage III SCC arising in a dermoid who was treated with cisplatin and paclitaxel after debulking surgery [15]. Hackethal in his meta-analysis reported that of patients who received adjuvant chemotherapy with a combination of various cytotoxic drugs (taxanes ($n=5$), anthracyclines ($n=9$), platinum derivatives ($n=60$), vinca alkaloids ($n=29$) and alkylating agents ($n=27$)) showed that only regimens with alkylating drugs were associated with increased survival in tumor stages greater than 1a [12]. These regimens were associated with a mean survival of 57.1 months compared to 25.2 months for regimens without alkylating agents. However, the benefit of chemotherapy was not supported in a multifactorial analysis.

In women at high risk of disease relapse, it has been proposed that postoperative pelvic radiotherapy may be considered on the basis that in patients who did relapse, pelvic disease is common and particularly difficult to manage [1]. However, in his meta-analysis, Hackethal did not find any benefit for postoperative radiotherapy [12].

Secondary debulking surgery has been advocated in some reports where sustained durable remissions have been obtained following relapse [7]. The authors recommend that surgery should be considered as initial management in all women with relapsed disease. It is most likely to be of value in patients with a long disease-free interval and single site of relapse.

As malignant transformation within dermoid cysts is such a rare tumor, a prospective trial to evaluate the optimal treatment strategy is not feasible. We recently proposed an audit of GCIG members to identify the number of cases of SCC arising from dermoids that have been treated by clinicians within GCIG to help clarify the optimal approach to management. Apart from collecting information on age, stage, symptoms at presentation, extent of surgery, adjuvant therapy received, response to treatment, progression, salvage therapy, and survival, the information may help in determining how future patients should be managed.

References

1. Tangjitgamol S, Manusirivithaya S, Sheanakul C, et al. Squamous cell carcinoma arising from dermoid cyst: case reports and review of literature. Int J Gynecol Cancer. 2003; 13:558–63.
2. Peterson WF. Malignant degeneration of benign cystic teratomas of the ovary; a collective review of the literature. Obster Gynecol Surv. 1957;12:793–830.
3. Kashimura M, Shinohara M, Hirakawa T, et al. Clinicopathological study of squamous cell carcinoma of the ovary. Gynecol Oncol. 1989;34:75–9.
4. Kikkawa F, Ishikawa H, Tamakoshi K, et al. Squamous cell carcinoma arising from mature cystic teratoma of the ovary: a clinicopathological analysis. Obstet Gynecol. 1997;89: 1017–22.
5. Hirakawa T, Tsuneyoshi M, Enjoji M. Squamous cell carcinoma arising in mature cystic teratoma of the ovary. Am J Surg Pathol. 1989;13:397–405.
6. Kikkawa F, Nawa A, Tamakoshi K, et al. Diagnosis of squamous cell carcinoma arising from mature cystic teratoma of the ovary. Cancer. 1998;82:2249–55.
7. Hurwitz JL, Fenton A, McCluggage WG, et al. Squamous cell carcinoma arising in a dermoid cyst of the ovary: a case series. BJOG. 2007;114:1283–7.
8. Mori Y, Nishii H, Takabe K, et al. Pre-operative diagnosis of malignant transformation arising from mature cystic teratoma of the ovary. Gynecol Oncol. 2003;90:338–41.
9. Kido A, Togashi K, Konishi I, et al. Dermoid cysts of the ovary with malignant transformation: MR appearance. Am J Roentgenol.1999; 172:445–9.
10. Mayer C, Miller D, Ehlen TG. Peritoneal implantation of squamous cell carcinoma following rupture of a dermoid cyst during laparoscopic removal. Gynecol Oncol. 2002;84: 180–3.
11. Tseng CJ, Ghou HH, Huang KG, et al. Squamous cell carcinoma arising in mature cystic teratoma of the ovary. Gynecol Oncol.1996; 63:364–70.
12. Hackethal A, Brueggmann D, Bohlmann M, et al. Squamous cell carcinoma in mature cystic teratoma of the ovary: systematic review and analysis of published data. Lancet Oncol. 2008;9:1173–80.
13. Arioz DT, Tokyol C, Sahin FK, et al. Squamous cell carcinoma arising in a mature cystic teratoma of the ovary in young patients with elevated carbohydrate antigen 19-9. Eur J Gynae Oncol. 2008;29:282–4.
14. Ding DC, Chu TY, Hsu YH, et al. Multimodality therapy of squamous cell carcinoma arising in mature cystic teratoma of the ovary. A case report. Eur J Obstet Gynecol Reprod Biol.2008; 137:250–1.
15. Powell JL, Stinson JA, Connor P, et al. Squamous cell carcinoma in a dermoid cyst of the ovary. Gynae Oncol. 2003;89: 526–8.

Ovarian Carcinosarcomas

12

Nicholas Reed

Ovarian carcinosarcomas (CSs) are usually considered to be aggressive tumours. There may be pure ovarian sarcomas or more often, mixed tumours with both carcinomatous and sarcomatous elements although molecular studies will usually show a monoclonal origin. This gives rise to the historical name of Malignant Mixed Mullerian tumour or Malignant Mesenchymal tumours (MMMT). However as with uterine CSs, the terminology that is now preferred reflects the fact that these are probably epithelial tumours that are poorly differentiated and this is supported by molecular marker studies. Occasional pure sarcomas may be seen. The importance of central pathological review cannot be underlined enough. In this article, the term carcinosarcoma (CS) will be preferentially deployed. Prior radiation exposure may be causative [45] as reported by Wei et al.

12.1 Incidence and Epidemiology

Since they are often mixed tumours their clinical behaviour will resemble that of epithelial ovarian cancer. Generally they have been considered uncommon and in most series [1–22] they account for 1–2% of ovarian cancer series, but in the Edinburgh experience [18] they accounted for 4% of a consecutive series of patients. This reflects the lack of consensus about how much sarcomatous component is required to label a mixed tumour as a CS. Views range from any sarcomatous component and up to 50%. Clearly some consensus is needed but many would take the view that at least 10% should be sarcomatous. Others might even argue that it does not really matter if they are simply bad type epithelial ovarian cancers with a sarcomatous component! It is more usual that when metastases develop, they are carcinomatous rather than sarcomatous, which supports the view that they are probably epithelial cancers. The clinical presentation, pattern of spread and prognosis are most commonly similar to those of epithelial ovarian cancers. The peak age of incidence for these patients is most frequently in their sixties. The presenting symptoms will be as diverse and as difficult to diagnose as those of ovarian carcinomas. In many situations the diagnosis will only be made after definitive surgery when full histological assessment is obtained. In some series, up to 5% of patients with suspected ovarian carcinoma will turn out to have sarcomatous elements. This has been a concern about relying upon fine needle aspiration of an omental biopsy or pelvic mass or even CT-guided biopsy which may not give a sufficiently representative sample. This may be important for quality control within clinical trials and for prognostic information, although in reality it probably does not affect the treatment planning.

These tumours usually account for 1–2% of ovarian tumours; thus, they are relatively uncommon. Median age of presentation is usually around 60 years. Some series have reported shorter periods of antecedent symptoms: in Prendiville's series [14] it was only 3 months; contrast this with many epithelial cancers! Generally these tumours are staged in the same way as epithelial ovarian carcinomas. It is to be noted that their relative rarity and lack of randomised comparative trial data limit the reviewer in discussing optimal management. There are many descriptive reports but no surgical or adjuvant studies involving RCTs.

N. Reed
Beatson Oncology Centre, Gartnavel General Hospital, 1053 Great Western Road, Glasgow G 120Y N, UK
e-mail: nick.reed@ggc.scot.nhs.uk

N. Reed et al. (eds.), *Rare and Uncommon Gynecological Cancers*,
DOI: 10.1007/978-3-642-13492-0_12,

12.2 Pathology

CSs are probably best viewed as epithelial tumours which contain a sarcomatous component. As mentioned previously, there is no international consensus on what proportion of tumour must be sarcomatous to label the tumour as a CS, although in practice it is often suggested at least 10% should be sarcomatous. They are sub-classified as "heterologous" or "homologous" according to the presence or absence of a stromal component containing mesenchymal tissue not normally found at the primary tumour site [9, 12, 22–24, 48]. This parallels the situation in uterine sarcomas. Previously, it was believed that heterologous CSs carried a worse prognosis than homologous, but recent evidence suggests that this histological feature does not significantly alter prognosis and is not independent of stage. It may well be that heterologous cancers are diagnosed at a later stage with apparent worse prognosis. The term metaplastic carcinoma is increasingly being adopted in uterine CSs and is likely to be accepted in ovarian CS.

Other subtypes aside from CSs include the following:

- Leiomyosarcoma
- Angiosarcoma
- Fibrosarcoma
- Rhabdomyosarcoma

More rarely, chondrosarcoma and osteosarcoma of the ovary have been described but careful exclusion of another primary should be considered. They may also be components of heterologous CSs. Finally, sarcomas arising within a teratoma are reported. Specialist pathology review with a panel of immunocytochemical markers is essential is making a definitive diagnosis.

12.3 Investigationsand I nitial Management

Since these tumours are often initially thought to be epithelial cancers, the initial work-up and investigation are as for any suspected ovarian tumour. CA125 should be measured and is useful for serial measurement and response evaluation, even if it may not be diagnostic. It is also required to calculate the risk of malignancy index (RMI) which may be used to select where patients are sent for operation. The preferred imaging technique reflects local availability and expertise. This is most commonly ultrasound of the pelvis followed by CT scanning or MR imaging. At present there is conflicting evidence about the value of PET CT in ovarian cancers and no strong evidence base for CSs; however, where readily available it can offer additive staging information. In some situations a staging laparoscopy may be a valuable adjunct to making a diagnosis and staging the tumour and its potential resectability. However, unless there is evidence of disease extensively involving the liver or lungs or supracolic omental disease, the standard recommendation would be to proceed to laparotomy to achieve optimal debulking, taking into account the patient's fitness for anaesthesia.

12.4 SurgicalManag ement

Surgical management should be approached as for epithelial carcinomas; however, often the definitive diagnosis will only be confirmed after pathological review. The calculation of the RMI may be useful in selecting whether the patient is referred to a specialist gynaecological oncology team. The approach must be to achieve maximal debulking surgery with no residual disease as the aim. Hence total abdominal hysterectomy, bilateral oophorectomy, omentectomy, and peritoneal washings should be the absolute minimum and depending upon local practice and expertise, blind biopsies from diaphragmatic surfaces and paracolic gutters and selective lymphadenectomy should be performed. The series from Sood confirms the superior survival when optimal debulking is achieved [21]. Specialist surgical units are more likely to carry out procedures that will lead to optimal cytoreduction. Duska et al. [25] showed similar findings and additionally demonstrated the effects of platinum and paclitaxel based therapy in optimally debulked patients. In summary, the goal should always be to aim for optimal surgical cytoreduction [42–44, 49, 51, 52].

In the event of the patient being unfit for surgery or having extensive disease, it is now probably reasonable to recommend neoadjuvant chemotherapy. This has been demonstrated to be non-inferior in epithelial ovarian cancers and it is probably reasonable to extrapolate that in ovarian sarcomas, induction chemotherapy will have a role to play and may render some tumours resectable after three or four induction doses of chemotherapy. Interestingly within the recent EORTC 55971 protocol, between 2 and 3% diagnosed with carcinoma based on initial diagnostic material were ultimately diagnosed with an ovarian sarcoma [26]. This is thought to reflect sampling error with small biopsies of cytological assessment. Further discussion on which agents should be used will follow.

The pathology should be reviewed by a gynaecological pathologist who will carry out immunocytochemical analyses in addition to standard histology. Following the diagnosis and histological assessment the patient should be referred to the Tumour Board for multidisciplinary discussion. It is likely that virtually all cases will be offered some form of chemotherapy because even a tumour that is apparently stage I should be considered as high grade or G3 equivalent and in epithelial ovarian cancers, all patients in this subgroup would be recommended to receive adjuvant treatment [27, 28].

12.5 Post-OperativeMa nagement

The lack of randomised clinical trials means there is no level 1 evidence. Comparisons are made with uterine sarcomas but it is difficult to be certain whether this is a realistic and fair comparison. Certainly many of the older papers cited have drawn from this experience. A major challenge is knowing how to interpret the reports from the older literature given the huge technical advances in diagnostic techniques of the past 20 years. We should not ignore this resource but interpret the information with a degree of caution. The debate is over whether to use epithelial ovarian type schedules or incorporate an anthracycline as these are active agents in sarcomas. Anthracyclines do have moderate activity in epithelial ovarian cancers.

The reasons that adjuvant treatments are recommended are the high risk of relapse and lethality of this tumour in the early reports. An earlier review by Hanjani which collected over 200 cases reported 78% mortality at 1 year [2]. The early series from Prendiville in Manchester UK [14] reported 20 patients over a 10-year period. Nearly half were dead within 1 year with a median survival of 14 months. Harris from the Christie in Manchester, reporting nearly a decade later showed that little progress had been made. The GOG had reported on single agent cisplatin with around a 20% response rate but rather short duration remissions. This was a series collected over a number of years and we would today consider the dose and scheduling less than optimal. However this was an important step towards defining standard treatments [29]. Most reports up till this time showed median survival to be around 8–9 months. An Australian group reviewed 20 cases from the late 1980s and 1990s and reported median survival 8 months but was increased to 23 months in those who received platinum-based chemotherapy (Inthasorn) [30](T able 12.1).

The modern era starts with platinum-based regimens; these range from platinum and a taxane to platinum and ifosfamide. Sit et al. in 2000 using platinum-based chemotherapy reported 19 months' median survival with patients receiving cisplatin and ifosfamide but 23 months' median survival for those receiving carboplatin and paclitaxel [31]. Sood et al. demonstrated the benefit of optimal debulking and its improved prognosis compared to those not optimally

Table12.1 Studiesfro mt heol dere ra

Author	Regimen	RR(%)	PFS(months)	OS(months)
Brown [18]	Mixed 22% no Rx	25	6.4	8.2
Harris [17]	Platinumba sed Non Platinum based	42 33		8.3
Sood [21]	Carboplatin/Pac	80		15 6
Thigpen [29]	Cisplatin	20		
Rutledge [46]	Cisplatin/Ifosfamide/Mesna	88	10	17
Inthasorn [30]	Platinumba sed Mixed			23 8

Table 12.2 Studies from the modern era

Author	Regimen	RR (%)	PFS (months)	OS (months)
Sit [31]	Carboplatin/Paclitaxel Cisplatin/Ifosfamide	NA		33 23
Duska [25]	Carboplatin/Paclitaxel	72		27
Leiser [32]	Platinum/taxane	63		43
Cicin [37]	Platinum based NonPlatinum			26 9.7
Ozoroglu [33]	Carboplatin/Paclitaxel Cisplatin/Ifosfamide	100 60		
Mok [50]	Cis/Ifosfamide	20 (5 years)		46

resectable and also showed the benefit of adding paclitaxel to carboplatin [21]. Most experts would now accept that carboplatin and paclitaxel should be the treatment of choice or these agents be incorporated in the regimen. Subsequent discussions suggest that adding other agents may be useful, such as anthracyclines and ifosfamide (Table 12.2).

Thus the older literature is very cautious if not negative about the value of adjuvant therapies especially in cases more advanced than stage I. However, this may simply reflect the lack of literature and late recognition of ovarian CSs; and if we believe these bear similarities to epithelial ovarian cancers, it is illogical not to treat them in a similar fashion. It also reflects a negativistic attitude prevalent historically about the outcome of ovarian sarcomas. The older literature reports on the disappointing outcome of advanced cases as discussed above. This tends to reflect the pre-platinum era and a less aggressive surgical approach. Contemporary management is far more aggressive with better anaesthesia and back-up, more gynaecological oncologists, multidisciplinary management and better chemotherapy. However, disease biology with more aggressive disease and advanced stage at presentation may account for less than optimal debulking surgery in many cases and the resultant poorer prognosis.

A review of the evolution of chemotherapy schedules will show some overlap with development of regimens for epithelial cancers but also some different directions using sarcoma type regimens. These generally catalogue schedules with poor outcomes. However, historical data has included non-platinum regimens, which include anthracyclines, ifosfamide, vinca alkaloids and actinomycin C and cyclophosphamide. These have been used as single agents such as doxorubicin or ifosfamide, but combinations of cisplatin, ifosfamide and CAP (cisplatin, adriamycin, cyclophosphamide) have been deployed with modest activity. Single agent doxorubicin is reported to have around 25% activity. Most of these early series report short duration responses and we have moved on to better combinations; thus this review concentrates more on the newer approaches. More recent data have shown better outcomes even if they do not match the best for epithelial ovarian cancer. Therefore all cases should be considered for additional chemotherapy assuming the patient is of good performance status and has recovered from surgical procedure.

12.6 Modern Approach to Management

Early series all seem to show survival beyond 2 years to be rare and only associated with stage 1 disease. The more recent series incorporating platinum with or without taxanes is better. However, it is difficult to be certain whether the improvements reflect a more aggressive surgical approach or the introduction of taxanes and platinum! The importance of stage and optimal debulking is confirmed again in Duska's series [25].

Even apparent stage I tumours will have at least an equivalent risk to that of relapse as a G3 epithelial ovarian tumour where chemotherapy will always be offered [27, 28]. It is generally accepted that the agents used for the treatment of ovarian sarcomas will reflect those used in ovarian carcinomas but there are various schools of thought that feel that other drugs should be included or substituted. The standard treatment for epithelial ovarian cancer is carboplatin and paclitaxel and there is a modest literature on the use of these drugs in ovarian sarcoma from the last 5 years. Some authors have argued the case for single agent carboplatin but in those series where it has been used, response rates and survival are inferior to those for platinum combinations. Brown et al. even argue that the low response rates to platinum-based therapies, usually in the range of 25–33% are far inferior to those in epithelial ovarian cancers from the same era [18]. Similarly the median survival was usually in the range of 8–12 months. Harris also using platinum-based therapies reported 42% response rates but still with median survival less than 9 months although a few long term responders [17]. They report a significant number of early deaths on treatment but those who completed therapy had better prospects. However, more recent series do show much better response rates and improved survival.

Given the extensive use of carboplatin and paclitaxel in epithelial ovarian cancers, it is not surprising that a number of recent studies have reported on this combination. Response rates varying from 20 to 80% have been reported but generally the series have had very small numbers and have included a mixture of pure and mixed CSs. Duska reported 72% RR [25] and Sood 80% RR with platinum and taxane combinations but substantially lower when platinum was not used [21]. Sood also demonstrated the importance of achieving optimal debulking surgery [21]. Leiser reported 63% response rate with 40% achieving a complete response [32]. Here we begin to see better overall survival with median survival achieving 43 months. Importantly, 57% were able to undergo optimal cytoreduction. However despite these high response rates, the progression-free survival and overall survival are poorer than in EOC. A recent Turkish paper by Ozguroglu reported on 25 mixed sarcomas from ovary and uterus [33]; a 100% response rate was seen with carboplatin and paclitaxel and 66% with platinum and ifosfamide. Higher response rates were seen when the predominant component was carcinomatous rather than sarcomatous (87.5 vs. 66%). The series reporting platinum and paclitaxel does appear to achieve better responses than the one using platinum ifosfamide, but it is impossible to make absolute comparisons without randomised trials. Recent studies using carboplatin or cisplatin and paclitaxel are starting to set the new standardofc are [31, 32, 34–37].

The MD Anderson group explored CIM, cisplatin, ifosfamide and mesna and reported eight of nine patients responding, with seven out of eight patients achieving CR and one PR but PFS was only 10 months and overall survival 17 months [38]. It was associated with moderate toxicity. Given the modest activity of single agent anthracyclines, adding epirubicin to TC has been tried. The Scandinavian group have attempted to improve first line treatment by adding in epirubicin using the TEC regimen, taxol, epirubicin and carboplatin [34]. The number of patients treated has been small but there is an impression that this is an active regimen although whether it is superior to the standard remains open to debate. The author has treated over 25 patients using this TEC regimen, and found it to be very well tolerated and worthy of consideration for treatment; the data are currently being analysed. One of the difficulties here is that the rarity of the tumour makes it very difficult to do clinical trials and show any benefit from one particular schedule over another. The schedule of TIP (taxol, ifosfamide and cisplatin) is also worthy of consideration; it has been shown to be effective in relapsed cervix cancer and germ cell tumours [39]. It is toxic but when used by experienced teams it is safe. A small series of carboplatin, ifosfamide and paclitaxel was reported at ASCO in 2005 by Kosmas et al. [40]. Sadly we will never be able to mount a study of TIP vs. TEC and anyway these approaches will probably be considered obsolete given the new agents discussed in the next paragraph. Mano et al. have reviewed the management of ovarian sarcomas in a recent article [41]. A report from Hsieh et al [53] has shown that liposomal doxorubicin may be effective.

12.7 TheFut ure

New options include the use of biological or targeted agents and there is some interest in this. To date there have not been any significant series reporting on this but there are phase 1 and 2 studies evaluating some of the tyrosine kinase inhibitors and anti-angiogenesis agents in these tumours. Once again a better understanding of the biology of the disease will hopefully lead to better targeting by newer agents. A recent proposal to the GCIG has proposed a combination of carboplatin and liposomal doxorubicin with a targeted agent such as sorafenib and this is currently being worked up into a definitive protocol, but examples like this are indicative of future approaches. We have still to learn whether to use these new compounds synchronously, sequentially or as single agents! It is probably reasonable to say that the future approach will be more scientific and based on molecular markers in addition to traditional surgical, radiological and histopathological expertise.

12.8 Conclusions

These are rare cancers and should be managed by expert teams. Optimal surgical debulking is important and recent data shows improved survival with platinum-based regimens compared to historical series. Platinum and paclitaxel may be superior to platinum and ifosfamide and is certainly less toxic. The author strongly believes that carboplatin and paclitaxel should be used but that the addition of epirubicin as in the "TEC" regimen is deliverable and may possibly be beneficial. Ifosfamide may be incorporated in first line management but is more likely to be kept for relapse. For recurrent disease, ifosfamide-based regimens are worthy of exploring but may add to toxicity. Clinical trials with international collaboration and new agents, conventional,mo lecularorc ombined,a rene eded.

References

1. Dehner L, Norris H, Taylor H. Carcinosarcomas and mesodermal tumors of ovary. Cancer. 1971;27:207–16.
2. Hanjani P, Peterson RO, Lipton SE, Nolte SA. Malignant mixed mesodermal tumors and carcinosarcoma of the ovary: report of eight cases and review of literature. Obstet Gynecol Surv.198 3;38:345–537.
3. Morrow CP, d'Ablaing G, Brady LW, Blessing JA, Hreshchyshyn MM. A clinical and pathologic study of 30 cases of malignant mixed mullerian epithelial and mesenchymal ovarian tumors: a Gynecologic Oncology Group study. Gynecol Oncol. 1984;18(3):278–92.
4. Morrow CP, Bundy BN, Hoffman J, Sutton G, Homesley H. Adriamycin chemotherapy for malignant mixed mesodermal tumor of the ovary: a Gynecologic Oncology Group study. Am J Clin Oncol. 1986;9:24–6.
5. Anderson B, Turner DA, Benda J. Ovarian sarcoma. Gynecol Oncol.1987;26:183 –92.
6. Geisinger KR, Dabbas DJ, Marshall RB. Malignant mixed mullerian tumors. An ultrastructural and immunohistochemical analysis with histogenetic considerations. Cancer. 1987;59:1781–90.
7. Terada KY, Johnson TL, Hopkins M, Roberts JA. Clinicopathologic features of ovarian mixed mesodermal tumors and carcinosarcomas. Gynecol Oncol. 1989;32: 228–32.
8. Plaxe SC, Dottino PR, Goodman HM, Deligdisch L, Idelson M, Cohen CJ. Clinical features of advanced ovarian mixed mesodermal tumors and treatment with doxorubicin and cisplatin-based chemotherapy. Gynecol Oncol. 1990;37: 244–9.
9. Clarke TJ. Histogenesis of ovarian malignant mixed mesodermal tumours. J Clin Pathol. 1990;43:287–90.
10. Pfeiffer P, Hardt-Madsen M, Rex S, Holund B, Bertelsen K. Malignant mixed mullerian tumors of the ovary. Report of 13 cases. Acta Obstet Gynecol Scand. 1991;70:79–83.
11. Barakat RR, Rubin SC, Wong G, Saigo PE, Markman M, Hoskins WJ. Mixed mesodermal tumor of the ovary: analysis of prognostic factors in 31 cases. Obstet Gynecol. 1992; 80:660–4.
12. de Brito PA, Silverberg SG, Orenstein JM. Carcinosarcoma (malignant mixed mullerian (mesodermal) tumor) of the female genital tract: immunohistochemical and ultrastructural analysis of 28 cases. Hum Pathol. 1993;24:132–42.
13. Sutton GP, Blessing JA, Homesley HD, Malfetano JH. A phase II trial of ifosfamide and mesna in patients with advanced or recurrent mixed mesodermal tumors of the ovary previously treated with platinum-based chemotherapy: a Gynecologic Oncology Group study. Gynecol Oncol. 1994;53:24–6.
14. Prendiville J, Murphy D, Rennison J, Buckley H, Crowther D. Carcinosarcoma of the ovary treated over a 10 year period at the Christie Hospital. Int J Gynecol Cancer. 1994;4:200–5.
15. Chang J, Sharpe JC, A'Hern RP, Fisher C, Blake P, Shepherd J, et al. Carcinosarcoma of the ovary: incidence, prognosis, treatment and survival of patients. Ann Oncol. 1995;6:755–8.
16. Le T, Krepart GV, Lotocki RJ, Heywood MS. Malignant mixed mesodermal ovarian tumor treatment and prognosis: a 20-year experience. Gynecol Oncol. 1997;65:237–40.
17. Harris MA, Delap LM, Sengupta PS, Wilkinson PM, Welch RS, Swindell R, et al. Carcinosarcoma of the ovary. Br J Cancer.2003; 88:654–7.
18. Brown E, Stewart M, Rye T, Al-Nafussi A, Williams AR, Bradburn M, et al. Carcinosarcoma of the ovary: 19 years of prospective data from a single center. Cancer. 2004;100: 2148–53.
19. DiSilvestro PA, Gajewski WH, Ludwig ME, Kourea H, Sung J, Granai CO. Malignant mixed mesodermal tumors of the ovary. Obstet Gynecol. 1995;86:780–2.
20. Geisler JP, Wiemann MC, Miller GA, Zhou Z, Geisler HE. Estrogen and progesterone receptors in malignant mixed mesodermal tumors of the ovary. J Surg Oncol. 1995;59:45–7.
21. Sood AK, Sorosky JI, Gelder MS, Buller RE, Anderson B, Wilkinson EJ, et al. Primary ovarian sarcoma: analysis of prognostic variables and the role of surgical cytoreduction. Cancer.1998; 82(9):1731–7.
22. Kounelis S, Jones MW, Papadaki H, Bakker A, Swalsky P, Finkelstein SD. Carcinosarcomas (malignant mixed mullerian tumors) of the female genital tract: comparative molecular analysis of epithelial and mesenchymal components. Hum Pathol. 1998;29:82–7.
23. Hellström A-C, Tegerstedt G, Silfverswärd C, Pettersson F. Malignant Mixed Müllerian tumors of the ovary: histopathologic and clinical review of 36 cases. Int J Gynecol Cancer. 1999;9:312–6.
24. Jin Z, Ogata S, Tamura G, Katayama Y, Fukase M, Yajima M, et al. Carcinosarcomas (malignant mullerian mixed

tumors) of the uterus and ovary: a genetic study with special reference to histogenesis. Int J Gynecol Pathol. 2003;22: 368–73.
25. Duska LR, Garrett A, Eltabbakh GH, Oliva E, Penson R, Fuller AF. Paclitaxel and platinum chemotherapy for malignant mixed mullerian tumors of the ovary. Gynecol Oncol. 2002;85:459–63.
26. Vergote I, Trop CG, Amant F, Kristensen G, Sardi JE, Ehlen T, Johnson N, Verheijen R, van der Burg MEL, Lacave AJ, Benedetti-Panici PL, Kenter GG, Casado A, Mendiola C, Coens C, Verleye L, Stuart G, Pecorelli S, Reed NS. EORTC-GCG/NCIC-CTG randomised trial primary debulking surgery with neoadjuvant chemotherapy or in stage IIIC and IV ovarian, fallopian tube and primary peritoneal cancer. Int J Gynecol Cancer. 2008.
27. Trimbos JB, Vergote I, Bolis G, Vermorken JB, Mangioni C, Madronal C, et al. Pecorelli S; EORTC-ACTION collaborators impact of adjuvant chemotherapy and surgical staging in early-stage ovarian carcinoma: European Organisation for Research and Treatment of Cancer-Adjuvant ChemoTherapy in Ovarian Neoplasm trial. J Natl Cancer Inst. 2003;95(2): 113–25.
28. Trimbos JB, Parmar M, Vergote I, Guthrie D, Bolis G, Colombo N, et al. International collaborative ovarian neoplasm trial 1 and adjuvant chemotherapy in ovarian neoplasm trial: two parallel randomized phase III trials of adjuvant chemotherapy in patients with early-stage ovarian carcinoma. International Collaborative Ovarian Neoplasm 1; European Organisation for Research and Treatment of Cancer Collaborators-Adjuvant ChemoTherapy in Ovarian Neoplasm. J Natl Cancer Inst. 2003;95(2):105–12.
29. Thigpen JT, Blessing JA, DeGeest K, Look KY, Homesley HD, Gynecologic Oncology Group. Cisplatin as initial chemotherapy in ovarian carcinosarcomas: a Gynecologic Oncology Group study. Gynecol Oncol. 2004;93:336–9.
30. Inthasorn P, Beale P, Dalrymple C, Carter J. Malignant mixed mullerian tumour of the ovary: prognostic factor and response of adjuvant platinum based chemotherapy. Aust N Z J Obstet Gynaecol. 2003;43:61–4.
31. Sit AS, Price FV, Kelley JL, Comerci JT, Kunschner AJ, Kanbour-Shakir A, et al. Chemotherapy for malignant mixed mullerian tumors of the ovary. Gynecol Oncol. 2000;79: 196–200.
32. Leiser AL, Chi DS, Ishill NM, Tew WP. Carcinosarcoma of the ovary treated with platinum and taxane: the memorial Sloan-Kettering Cancer Center experience. Gynecol Oncol. 2007;105:657–61.
33. Ozguroglu M, Bilici A, Ilvan S, Turna H, Atalay B, Mandel N, et al. Determining predominating histologic component in malignant mixed mullerian tumors: is it worth it? Int J Gynecol Cancer. 2008;18:809–12.
34. Bicher A, Levenback C, Silva EG, Burke TW, Morris M, Gershenson DM. Ovarian malignant mixed mullerian tumors treated with platinum-based chemotherapy. Obstet Gynecol. 1995;85:735–9.
35. Eltabbakh GH, Yadav R. Good response of malignant mixed mullerian tumor of the ovary to paclitaxel and cisplatin chemotherapy. Eur J Gynaecol Oncol. 1999;20(5–6):355–6.
36. Santacruz MR, Gehrig PA, Skinner EN, Boggess JF, Fowler WC, Van Le L. Comparison of paclitaxel and carboplatin with ifosfamide and cisplatin for the treatment of ovarian carcinosarcoma [abstract 5116]. Proc Am Soc Clin Oncol. 2004;22:478s.
37. Cicin I, Saip P, Eralp Y, Selam M, Topuz S, Ozluk Y, et al. Ovarian carcinosarcomas: clinicopathological prognostic factors and evaluation of chemotherapy regimens containing platinum. Gynecol Oncol. 2008;108(1):136–40.
38. Crotzer DR, Wolf JK, Jenkins AD, Gershenson DM, Levenback C. A pilot study of cisplatin, ifosfamide and mesna in the treatment of malignant mixed mesodermal tumors of the ovary. Gynecol Oncol. 2007;105:399–403.
39. Lissoni AA, Colombo N, Pellegrino A, Parma G, Zola P, Katsaros D, et al. A phase II, randomized trial of neo-adjuvant chemotherapy comparing a three-drug combination of paclitaxel, ifosfamide, and cisplatin (TIP) versus paclitaxel and cisplatin (TP) followed by radical surgery in patients with locally advanced squamous cell cervical carcinoma: the Snap-02 Italian Collaborative Study. Ann Oncol. 2009;20(4):660–5.
40. Kosmas C, Mylonakis N, Malamos N, et al. Paclitaxel (T)-ifosfamide (I)-carboplatin (Cb) (TICb) combination in advanced gynecologic malignant mixed mullerian tumors (MMMT) [abstract 5125]. Proc Am Soc Clin Oncol. 2005;23:485s.
41. Mano MS, Rosa DD, Azambuja E, Ismael G, Braga S, D'Hondt V, et al. Current management of ovarian carcinosarcoma. Int J Gynecol Cancer. 2007;17:316–24.
42. Barnholtz-Sloan JS, Morris R, Malone JM, Munkarah AR. Survival of women diagnosed with malignant, mixed mullerian tumors of the ovary (OMMMT). Gynecol Oncol. 2004;93:506–12.
43. Zorzou MP, Markaki S, Rodolakis A, et al. Clinicopathological features of ovarian carcinosarcomas: a single institution experience. Gynecol Oncol. 2005;96:136–42.
44. Morrow C, d'Ablaing G, Brady L, Blessing J, Hreschyshyn M. A clinical and pathologic study of 30 cases of malignant mixed mullerian epithelial and mesenchymal ovarian tumors: a Gynecologic Oncology Group study. Gynecol Oncol. 1984;18:278–92.
45. Wei LH, Huang CY, Cheng SP, Chen CA, Hsieh CY. Carcinosarcoma of ovary associated with previous radiotherapy. Int J Gynecol Cancer. 2001;11:81–4.
46. Rutledge TL, Gold MA, McMeekin DS, Huh WK, Powell MA, Lewin SN, et al. Carcinosarcoma of the ovary – a case series. Gynecol Oncol. 2006;100:128–32.
47. Jonson AL, Bliss RL, Truskinovsky A, et al. Clinical features and outcomes of uterine and ovarian carcinosarcoma. Gynecol Oncol. 2006;100:561–4.
48. Ariyoshi K, Kawauchi S, Kaku T, Nakano H, Tsuneyoshi M. Prognostic factors in ovarian carcinosarcoma: a clinicopathological and immunohistochemical analysis of 23 cases. Histopathology.2000; 37:427–36.
49. Muntz HG, Jones MA, Goff BA, Fuller Jr AF, Nikrui N, Rice LW, et al. Malignant mixed mullerian tumors of the ovary: experience with surgical cytoreduction and combination chemotherapy. Cancer. 1995;76:1209–13.
50. Mok JE, Kim YM, Jung MH, Kim KR, Kim DY, Kim JH, et al. Malignant mixed mullerian tumors of the ovary: experience with cytoreductive surgery and platinum-based combination chemotherapy. Int J Gynecol Cancer. 2006;16(1):101–5.
51. Silasi D-A, Illuzzi JL, Kelly MG, Rutherford TJ, Mor G, Azodi M, et al. Carcinosarcoma of the ovary. Int J Gynecol Cancer.2008; 18:22–9.

52. Muller H, Nakchbandi V. Cytoreductive surgery plus intraperitoneal hyperthermic perfusion is an effective treatment for metastasized malignant mixed mesodermal tumours (MMMT) – report of six cases. Eur J Surg Oncol. 2004;30: 573–7.
53. Hsieh CL, Chang TC, Lai CH, Jung SM, Chou HH. Excellent progression-free survival with liposomal doxorubicin for a patient with recurrent ovarian malignant mixed mullerian tumor: case report and literature review. Gynecol Oncol. 2004;94:854–7.

13 Small Cell and Neuroendocrine Cancers of the Ovary

Nicholas Reed

13.1 Introduction

Small cell and neuroendocrine (NE) carcinomas of the ovary are uncommon, constituting about 1% of ovarian cancers. They were really recognised as a separate entity only in 1979 [1], with several further reports in the 1980s [2–4]. These tumours are often very highly aggressive and carry a poor prognosis and unless they are diagnosed at a very early stage, they usually are associated with a high level of lethality. There are four recognised types and the differential diagnosis may be challenging. Furthermore, these tumours may be associated with the ectopic secretion of neuropeptides which may give distinctive clinical syndromes including hypercalcaemia, hypoglycaemia, hyponatraemia with SIADH (syndrome of inappropriate ADH secretion) and myaesthenic syndromes. Carcinoid tumours and struma ovarii are covered more fully in a separate chapter, given their usually very different and more indolent clinical behaviour.

The more aggressive tumours have a small round cell pattern and may cause challenges in establishing a firm histological diagnosis. New immunocytochemical techniques have helped to reduce the diagnostic dilemmas and pitfalls. Nevertheless occasional patients may be seen in whom there remains continuing uncertainty over the final diagnosis so that expert pathological opinion is required. Up to four types of primary tumour are described, but most frequently seen are small cell cancers. Metastatic disease should also be excluded.

Small cell carcinoma of ovary of pulmonary type (SCCOPT)
Small cell carcinoma of ovary of hypercalcaemic type (SCCOHT)
Non-small cell neuroendocrine carcinoma (large cell variant) (NSCNEC)
Classical primary carcinoid (well differentiated neuroendocrine cancer)
Classical carcinoid metastatic from primary gastrointestinal site

13.2 Pathology

The terminology of these tumours has recently tended to follow that of pulmonary small cell cancers rather than the proposed terms from WHO and ENETS [5–8] for other NE cancers. This can seemingly lead to some confusion over terminology. These rare tumours can be classified as pulmonary and non-pulmonary in type and, confusingly, as having a classical (or typical) small cell morphology or a large cell variant. This is a further reason for specialist pathological review. The non-pulmonary type occurs in younger women and is often associated with hypercalcaemia, whereas the pulmonary type is associated with women of perimenopausal age.

In this section we will start with Small Cell Cancer of Ovary of Pulmonary Type (SCCOPT). These ovarian small cell tumours are usually pure, in contrast to cervical tumours which may have a mixed pattern. They strongly resemble pulmonary small cell (oat cell) lung cancers. It is necessary to carry out detailed imaging to exclude a small primary lung cancer and nowadays, ^{18}-FDG PET CT imaging may be an additional useful tool given the aggressive metabolic pattern. One of the principal difficulties in evaluating small cell ovarian tumours is distinguishing them either from metastatic

N. Reed
Beatson Oncology Centre, Gartnavel General Hospital,
1053 Great Western Road, Glasgow, G12 0YN Scotland, UK
e-mail: nick.reed@ggc.scot.nhs.uk

N. Reed et al. (eds.), *Rare and Uncommon Gynecological Cancers*,
DOI: 10.1007/978-3-642-13492-0_13,

small cell disease arising elsewhere or from other small round cell tumours which may have a subtly similar appearance. There are some differences in the immunocytochemical profile but also the method of presentation and age may be relevant. Carcinoids and poorly differentiated sex cord tumours with small cell component may also cause a diagnostic challenge but review by an experienced pathologist should help make the distinction. This diagnosis should always be considered in a younger woman presenting with advanced disease.

Non-pulmonary small cell carcinomas of the ovary may often be associated with hypercalcaemia and are known as Small Cell Cancer Ovary of Hypercalcaemic Type (SCCOHT), which is present in about two thirds of cases and, in spite of the aggressive treatment, may well recur quickly and have a very poor prognosis. Their histological pattern is of poorly differentiated small cells with densely hyperchromatic nuclei and scanty cytoplasm. Confusion with juvenile granulosa cell tumours can occur. Attempts to stain for PTH (parathyroid hormone) are usually unsuccessful but PTHRP (parathyroid hormone related peptide) has been shown in some cases.

Also described but less commonly seen are large/intermediate cell variants which are often called NSCNEC. The largest series was reported by Veras and colleagues [9] in 2007 and included a discussion of previous series. Interestingly these were often associated with simultaneous ovarian tumours including dermoid cysts, teratomas, mucinous borderline tumours and endometrioid cancers. These tumours tended to be solid, cystic and unilateral.

Classical carcinoids (well differentiated neuroendocrine tumours [NET]) are also seen in the ovary but are usually metastatic, and their management is discussed more fully in a separate chapter [10, 11]. More often classical carcinoids present with a diffuse pattern of spread with peritoneal and mesenteric involvement and a primary in appendix, terminal small bowel or ascending colon is likely; but infrequently there may be no other signs of disease and may represent a true primary NET. When they are metastatic to the liver, these patients may often have symptoms of the carcinoid syndrome, but primary ovarian carcinoids may also develop cardiac disease without liver metastases due to the ovarian vein sometimes directly emptying into the inferior vena cava with direct flow into right cardiac chambers. Carcinoid heart disease may be more prevalent in this group, and may arise years after the initial diagnosis. These metastatic tumours should be referred to specialist teams experienced in managing NETs and managed along standard lines [12]. There are good data to support a radical surgical approach in selected patients but this should be done in association with an experienced gastrointestinal or hepatobiliary surgeon. A recent paper from Strosberg discusses the clinical issues of primary vs. metastatic ovarian carcinoids. This is discussed in more detail in as eparatec hapter [11].

13.3 ClinicalPr esentation

There are no specific patterns of presentation although often, the clinical history is short as the tumours tend to grow rapidly. The SCCOHT tend to come from younger age groups and tend to be non-smokers. It is believed that these are more likely to be non-pulmonary small cell cancers. The pulmonary type is more likely to occur in slightly older women around the time of menopause with peak incidence at 50–60 years. A rapidly growing pelvic mass with no other specific symptoms is the likely pattern of presentation. Often there is nothing else to suggest an unusual diagnosis. In younger women, tumour markers for germ cell tumours should be assayed (for example AFP, beta-HCG, LDH, CEA and NSE). Initial imaging of the pelvis will help to make a preliminary diagnosis; a complex solid or semi-solid mass will rule out a borderline tumour but will lead to the usual investigative techniques. Many of these tumours only involve one ovary, and may not be suspected preoperatively. Early cases should be investigated and managed in the usual manner with appropriate staging procedures including laparotomy as for epithelial ovarian cancers; and on occasions, the diagnosis may only be made as an unexpected finding at time of examining the histology. However, a full and thorough staging should be carried out, and in cases of extensive disease in a younger woman with an atypical pattern, small cell carcinoma shouldbe c onsidered [1–6, 9, 13–18].

Thus, a major issue is whether the surgical approach should be as for a suspected epithelial tumour or a more conservative procedure. Frozen section may be considered to assist in this process. Fertility-sparing surgery should always be discussed with the younger woman but until a final histological diagnosis is made, surgical plans have to be tentative. Harrison et al. argue that since most were unilateral, at least in the younger womanc onservings urgeryma ybe of fered [19].

In older women, standard surgical practices should be followed for diagnosis and treatment; a total hysterectomy, bilateral salpingo-oophorectomy, omentectomy and inspection of abdominal cavity with peritoneal washings is the minimum. Whether lymphadenectomy is done will partly depend on whether the procedure is undertaken by a gynaecological oncologist or general gynaecologist together with the surgical findings; however, there is no literature either to support or refute the process of lymphadenectomy. However if the surgeon finds grossly enlarged glands and feels that they can be safely removed at time of surgery, it seems reasonable to proceed. If fertility-sparing surgery is accepted, the patient must be advised about the potential need for a delayed completion procedure although again, there is no specific literature to support this.

While a proportion will be clinically stage 1 (about 20–25% from the published literature), the majority will be diagnosed with advanced metastatic disease. The mode of spread may be similar to common epithelial tumours, but they may have liver metastases at presentation, so a percutaneous liver biopsy may be the quickest way to establish a diagnosis. The finding of hypercalcaemia, particularly with normal bone scan or other imaging, most commonly reflects the ectopic secretion of neuropeptides such as PTHRP and is associated with the distinctive SCCOHT [20]. Other presentations may include hyponatraemia and SIADH, and rarely myaesthenic syndromes. About 70% of the SCCOHT are associated with high serum calcium. A more recent and comprehensive review of small cell cancers of the female genital tract was published in the beginningof200 7 [21].

13.4 Post-OperativeMa nagement

The clinical literature is scanty apart from case reports although there are papers from pathologists who report series of cases sent in for tertiary review, but these are often associated with relatively little clinical information on surgical management and post-surgical management. Careful review by an experienced pathologist specialising in gynaecological oncology pathology is advised as immunocytochemical profile may give important clues (see Chap. 3 where McCluggage and Millan discuss pathology). All cases should be discussed at tumour boards and, if appropriate, referred to regional/national referral centres [22, 23]. This is yet another example where international collaboration and data collection in national registers is needed to help us establish better practices for these rare cancers.

Chemotherapy will usually be advised as an adjuvant even when there is no macroscopic disease and should be recommended in all other advanced cases [17–20, 24–32, 34]. The experience from the older literature is pretty dismal with few cases surviving beyond 12–24 months [17, 18, 24–27, 31]. The conventional approach is to combine platinum with etoposide, as in small cell lung cancer. There is no evidence base to favour cisplatin over carboplatin but the convenience of carboplatin may make it the drug of choice. Hoskins et al. have also added in paclitaxel to carboplatin and etoposide in their patients with small cell cancer of the cervix and this option should also be considered [32]. The numbers are too small to allow confident claims about the superiority but certainly it can be considered. One might also speculate that carboplatin and paclitaxel may be effective in view of its activityins mallc elllungc ancers [29, 33]

13.5 RecentL iterature

A recent review article by Harrison et al. sought case reports from members of the GCIG (Gynaecological Cancer Inter Group) and acquired 17 cases [19]. There is a degree of heterogeneity about the cases collected but it does offer a more contemporary overview and commentary. Not surprisingly, it showed that the best prognosis was associated with early stage disease and an aggressive management including surgery, radiation and chemotherapy. This is clearly controversial and counter-intuitive as adding radiation therapy does not seem logical.

For advanced disease or where optimal debulking surgery cannot be achieved, primary chemotherapy is the treatment of choice. The same combination of a platinum and etoposide will be recommended, usually prescribing up to six cycles. Interval imaging after three cycles is performed to assess response but with continuation to six cycles unless there is progression. There are anecdotal reports of carboplatin and paclitaxel which is used in non-small cell lung cancer and epithelial ovarian cancers regularly, and the author has treated three patients with the dose-dense and dose-intense weekly carboplatin and paclitaxel schedule. All achieved a remission but one relapsed early and died, a second developed isolated brain metastases but remains in remission after further chemotherapy and cranial radiation and the third is still in remission. The importance here may be the weekly dose-dense and dose-intense scheduling rather than the individual drugs.

Unfortunately, many of the patients have a short-lasting response and early relapse either with intra-abdominal disease or even cerebral metastases will occur. Consideration of prophylactic cranial irradiation should be given for those who enter complete remission. For patients who develop early relapse, further chemotherapy may be considered if they are of good performance status. The CAVE regime (cyclophosphamide, adriamycin, vincristine and etoposide) may be considered. Consideration of other non-evidence based schedules including weekly carboplatin and paclitaxel or topotecan may also be active in small cell tumours; otherwise experimental schedules should also be discussed or patients are referred into phase one studies. To date there is no reported experience with any of the newer targeted agents but at the time of writing there is at least one phase one study investigation of bevacizumab (Avastin).

The role of external beam radiation (EBRT) seems paradoxical. It has a very limited role in epithelial ovarian cancers but in Harrison's series those who received adjuvant EBRT had a lower rate of failure [19]. Most important seems to be the presence or absence of residual disease post-surgery. Most of the patients were treated over long time periods with heterogeneous regimens and schedules, and so it is difficult to produce firm evidence-based guidelines. In one of the earliest series, whole abdominal radiotherapy was given but this was in the pre-platinum era and given the additional morbidity one has to question whether this is a useful addition [2]. Nevertheless the conclusion is that platinum-based chemotherapy with or without pelvic radiation should be discussed in all cases. Whilst counter-intuitive it is often recommended in these unusual cases and has to be decided on a case by case basis.

Carcinoid tumours (well differentiated NET) may also involve the ovary and are most frequently metastatic but occasionally no other disease is located and are considered true primary carcinoids. They tend to behave like classical carcinoid tumours and may metastasize and cause carcinoid syndrome when the liver is involved but paradoxically, primary ovarian carcinoids can cause right-sided heart disease in the absence of metastatic disease due to the flow of the ovarian vein directly into the inferior vena cava. The clinical behaviour and the histological appearance should distinguishthe mfroms mallc ellc ancers [11].

References

1. Scully RE. Tumors of the ovary and maldeveloped gonads. Atlas of Tumor Pathology second series, fascicle 16. Washington: Armed Forces Institute of Pathology; 1979.
2. Dickersin GR, Kline IW, Scully RE. Small cell carcinoma of the ovary with hypercalcemia: a report of 11 cases. Cancer. 1982;49:188–97.
3. Abler V, Kjørstad KE, Nesland JM. Small cell carcinoma of the ovary. A report of 6 cases. Int J Gynecol Pathol. 1988;7: 315–29.
4. Aguirre P, Thor AD, Scully RE. Ovarian small cell carcinoma. Histogenetic considerations based on immunohistochemical and other findings. Am J Clin Pathol. 1989;92: 140–9.
5. McCluggage WG, Oliva E, Connolly LE, et al. An immunohistochemical analysis of ovarian small cell carcinoma of hypercalcemic type. Int J Gynecol Pathol. 2004;23:330–6.
6. Clement PB. Selected miscellaneous ovarian lesions: small cell carcinomas, mesothelial lesions, mesenchymal and mixed neoplastic lesions. Mod Pathol. 2005;18 Suppl 2:S113–9.
7. Klöppel G, Perren A, Heitz PU. The gastroenteropancreatic neuroendocrine cell system and its tumors: the WHO classification. Ann N Y Acad Sci. 2004;1014:13–27.
8. Rindi G, Capella C, Solcia E. Introduction to a revised clinicopathological classification of neuroendocrine tumors of the gastroenteropancreatic tract. Q J Nucl Med. 2000; 44(1):13–21.
9. Veras EV, Deavers MT, Silva EG, Malpica A. Ovarian non-small cell neuroendocrine carcinoma. A clinico-pathological and immunohistochemical study of 11 cases. Am J Surg Pathol.2007; 31:774–82.
10. Renshaw AA, Haja J, Lozano RL, Wilbur DC. Distinguishing carcinoid from small cell carcinoma of the lung: correlating cytologic features and performance in the College of American pathologists Non-Gynecologic Cytology programme. Arch Pathol Lab Med. 2005;129(5):614–8.
11. Strosberg J, Nasir A, Cragun J, Gardner N, Kvols L. Metastatic carcinoid tumor to the ovary. A clinicopathologic analysis of seventeen cases. Gynecol Oncol. 2007;106: 65–8.
12. Ramage JK, Davies AH, Ardill J, Bax N, Caplin M, Grossman A, Hawkins R, McNicol AM, Reed N, Sutton R, Thakker R, Aylwin S, Breen D, Britton K, Buchanan K, Corrie P, Gillams A, Lewington V, McCance D, Meeran K, Watkinson A; UKNET work for Neuroendocrine Tumours. Guidelines for the management of gastroenteropancreatic

neuroendocrine (including carcinoid) tumours. Gut. 2005;54 Suppl4:i v1–16.
13. Eichhorn JH, Young RH, Scully RE. Primary ovarian small cell carcinoma of pulmonary type. A clinicopathologic, immunohistologic, and flow cytometric analysis of 11 cases. Am J Surg Pathol. 1992;16:926–38.
14. Peccatori F, Bonazzi C, Lucchini V, Bratina G, Mangioni Z. Primary ovarian small cell carcinoma: four more cases. Gynecol Oncol. 1993;49:95–9.
15. Scully RE. Small cell carcinoma of the hypercalcemic type. Int J Gynecol Pathol. 1993;12:148–52.
16. Young RH, Oliva E, Scully RE. Small cell carcinoma of the ovary, hypercalcemic type. A clinico-pathological analysis of 150 cases. Am J Surg Pathol. 1994;18:1102–16.
17. Reed WC. Small cell carcinoma of the ovary with hypercalcemia: a report of a case of survival without recurrence 5 years after surgery and chemotherapy. Gynecol Oncol. 1995;56:452–5.
18. Hamilton S, Beattie GJ, Williams AR. Small cell carcinoma of the ovary: a report of 3 cases and review of the literature. J Obstet Gynaecol. 2004;2:169–72.
19. Harrison ML, Hoskins P, du Bois A, Quinn M, Rustin GJS, Ledermann JA, et al. Small cell of the ovary, hypercalcemic type – analysis of combined experience and recommendation for management. A GCIG study. Gynecol Oncol. 2006;100:233–8.
20. Chen L, Dinh TA, Haque A. Small cell carcinoma of the ovary with hypercalcemia and ectopic parathyroid hormone production. Arch Pathol Lab Med. 2005;129(4):531–3.
21. Rana S, Warren BK, Yamada SD. Stage IIIC small cell carcinoma of the ovary: surgical with conservative surgery and chemotherapy. Obstet Gynecol. 2004;103:1120–3.
22. Plaxe SC. Chasing zebras: the study and treatment of rare diseases. Gynecol Oncol. 2006;100:227–8.
23. Levels of Evidence and Grades of Recommendation. http://www.cebm.net/Accessed2010
24. Crowder S, Tuller E. Small cell carcinoma of the female genital tract. Semin Oncol. 2007;34(1):57–63.
25. Benrubi GI, Pitel P, Lammert N. Small cell carcinoma of the ovary with hypercalcemia responsive to sequencing chemotherapy. South Med J. 1993;86:247–8.
26. Sholler GL, Luks F, Mangray S, Meech SJ. Advanced small cell carcinoma of the ovary in a pediatric patient with long-term survival and review of the literature. J Pediatr Hematol Oncol.2005; 27(3):169–72.
27. Senekjian EK, Weiser PA, Talerman A, Herbst AL. Vinblastine, cisplatin, cyclophosphamide, bleomycin, doxorubicin, and etoposide in the treatment of small cell carcinoma of the ovary. Cancer. 1989;64:1183–7.
28. Mebis J, De Baekelandt M, Tjalma WAA, Vermorken JB. Primary ovarian small cell carcinoma of pulmonary type; a case report and review of literature. Eur J Gynecol Oncol. 2004;25:239–41.
29. Neubauer MA, Rubins J, Scwattz J, Ilegbodu D, Asmar L. Phase 2 study of weekly paclitaxel and carboplatin in patients with extensive small cell lung cancer with ECOG status of 2 or over age 70. Proc Am soc Clin Oncol. 2003;22:673.
30. Suzuki N, Kameyama K, Hirao T, Susumu N, Mukai M, Aoli D. A case of pulmonary type of small cell carcinoma of the ovary. J Obstet Gynaecol Res. 2007;2:203–6.
31. Powell JL, McAfee RD, McCoy RC, Shiro BS. Uterine and ovary conservation in advanced small cell carcinoma of the ovary. Obstet Gynecol. 1998;91:846–8.
32. Hoskins PJ, Swenerton KD, Pike JA, Lim P, Aquino-Parsons C, Wong F, et al. Small-cell carcinoma of the cervix: fourteen years of experience at a single institution using a combined-modality regimen of involved-field irradiation and platinum-based combination chemotherapy. J Clin Oncol. 2003;21:3495–501.
33. Cheng S, Evans WK, Stys-Norman D, Shepherd FA, Lung Cancer Disease Site Group of Cancer Care Ontario's Program in Evidence-based Care. Chemotherapy for relapsed small cell lung cancer: a systematic review and practice guideline. J Thorac Oncol. 2007;2(4):348–54.
34. Taraszewski R, Rosman PM, Knight CA, et al. Small cell carcinoma of the ovary. Gynecol Oncol. 1991;41:149–51.

14 Primary Ovarian Carcinoids and Neuro-Endocrine Tumours Including StrumaOvar ii

Nicholas Reed

Ovarian carcinoids were first described in 1939 by Stewart et al. [1]. Most commonly ovarian carcinoids will be metastatic rather than primary [2–14, 41]. Of the primary ovarian carcinoids, the insular pattern is the most commonly seen. Carcinoids arising within or associated with an ovarian teratoma are also relatively common but vary with the pathological subtype. Today, it is preferable to adopt the new nomenclature adopted by WHO classification of Neuroendocrine Tumours (NETs) as deployed in other sites, although it is conceded, the old terminology will be used and remains familiar to many clinicians [15, 16]. As well as insular carcinoids, trabecular carcinoids (with trabecular or ribbon pattern) are described and strumal tumours capable of thyroid differentiation. Distinguishing advanced primary from metastatic carcinoid is not always easy but primary tumours tend to involve one ovary whereas metastatic disease usually involves both ovaries. It is suggested that primary insular tumours may commonly be associated with a mature teratoma both in the ipsilateral and sometimes in the contralateral ovary [4, 5, 7, 8, 14, 17]. Finally, goblet cell carcinoids are described, which most probably are adenocarcinomas, with some degree of neuroendocrine differentiation although collision tumours are occasionally described. The new WHO classification refers to these as mixed endocrine–exocrine cancers (MEEC), a term which is probably more useful [18]. This topic of mucinous tumours in the ovary is masterfully reviewed by Young [19, 20].

Ovarian carcinoids (Neuro-endocrine cancers)
Primary type
Insular ± associated mature cystic teratoma
Trabecular ± associated mature cystic teratoma
Strumal carcinoid ± associated mature cystic teratoma
Mucinous carcinoid (goblet cell) ± associated mature cystic teratoma
Mixed endocrine–exocrine type (two or more pure types combined)
Metastatic carcinoids (NETs)

14.1 Primaryl nsularC arcinoids of the Ovary

The most common variant is the insular carcinoma with a histological pattern similar to classical small bowel midgut carcinoids or NETs. They are divided into pure insular and insular with associated mature cystic teratoma. Most of the series show that they commonly arise in association with mature cystic teratomas [4, 5, 7, 8, 14, 17].

14.2 PrimaryT rabecularC arcinoids of the Ovary

These are less common in most series (except for Soga's series where they were of equal incidence) and usually affect post-menopausal women [5, 7, 17, 21, 22]. These appear to arise more commonly within a mature teratoma although there are rare reports of true primary trabecular carcinoids. These may be asymptomatic or present as a pelvic mass. These are said to be less aggressive and rarely metastasise.

N.R eed
Beatson Oncology Centre, Gartnavel General Hospital,
1053G reatW esternR oad, Glasgow G120Y N, Scotland, UK
e-mail:nic k.reed@ggc.scot.nhs.uk

N. Reed et al. (eds.), *Rare and Uncommon Gynecological Cancers*,
DOI: 10.1007/978-3-642-13492-0_14, © Springer-Verlag Berlin Heidelberg 2011

14.3 PrimaryM ucinous Ovarian Carcinoids

Much debate will take place as to whether these are neuroendocrine or mucinous adenocarcinomas or hybrid tumours. They may be mistaken for Krukenberg tumours. There are strong similarities to Goblet cell cancers of appendix and a review of the appendix should be considered. This is discussed in a superb review by Young, who covered the topic most thoroughly [19, 20]. These mixed tumours often behave more akin to adenocarcinomas of the gastro-intestinal tract. There is considerable debate as to how best to manage them. Toumpanakis reviewed the topic recently [23].

14.4 StrumalC arcinoids

Strumal carcinoids or malignant struma ovarii are of endodermal origin with evidence of thyroid or C-cell differentiation. They arise within teratomas. Mature cystic teratomas are common accounting for up to 20% of ovarian tumours and about 15% may contain thyroid tissue. Struma ovarii is a variant which contains in excess of 50% thyroid tissue. They account for about 3% of ovarian teratomas. The incidence of malignant change is difficult to estimate and is certainly uncommon. It is said that the incidence of malignant change may be between 0.1 and 0.3%. Metastases are reported as being very rare, probably less than 5%. Rare metastatic cancers from the thyroid gland are also described and may cause diagnostic difficulties. Logani reported a case of thyroid carcinoma with ovarian metastases so, this must be excluded in all cases but is clearly a very rare clinical situation [24]. A recent report of four cases and a literature review by Roth et al. [25] has expanded our knowledge and the same group have produced a thoughtful review which has challenged some of the precepts of strumal carcinoids and presents an alternative view of their behaviour [26].

The incidence seems to peak post-menopausally with commonest ages of diagnosis being in the fifth and sixth decades of life. They are rarely diagnosed pre-operatively and are usually incidental findings. They are usually unilateral and more commonly arise in the left ovary. The main differential diagnosis will be metastate differentiated thyroid cancers and care should be taken to exclude thyroid primary [37–39].

14.5 Metastases

Typically, they are bilateral and multi-nodular, but are not usually associated with teratomas. Not only is their prognosis much worse, historically they usually caused death within 4 years. Modern surgical practises, together with the introduction of somatostatin analogues have dramatically changed this and many patients with primary ovarian carcinoids will live for longer periods. Metastatic NETs should be referred to specialist teams looking after NETs as the staging and medical management are very different {UKNET and ENETs guidelines} [27, 28]. There may be a strong case for attempting radical debulking surgery including small bowel and mesenteric resection, but patients with advanced disease may need medical preparation with somatostatin analogues or other treatments to get them fit for surgery.

14.6 Pathology

Initially, these tumours were recognised by the presence of cytoplasmic neurosecretory granules and the argentophilic staining; however, modern immunochemistry has aided the diagnosis. Staining for Chromogranin A is now possible and other markers including CD56 and synaptophysin. It is important to seek the advice and opinion of a pathologist with a special interest in Neuro-endocrine cancers [8, 9]. The reader is advised to refer to the chapter by McCluggage and Millan in this book (chapter 3).

14.7 CarcinoidSyndr ome

This occurs in about one third of ovarian carcinoids, although it is a misconception that classical small bowel carcinoids are commonly associated with carcinoid syndrome, as only 35–40% of these will have carcinoid syndrome! What is different is that ovarian carcinoids may be associated with carcinoid heart disease without liver metastases as the ovarian venous system bypasses the hepatic circulation by emptying into the vena cava. Aggressive cardio-vascular management is indicated in these rare situations. This will be discussed later in this chapter. Two recent Japnese reports have identified different disease patterns [36, 42]

14.8 Imaging

Conventional imaging with CT scan will be needed and additional MR scanning was required. The most sensitive imaging technique is usually radionuclide scintigraphy with ^{111}In-Octreoscan. PET-CT if available may in time supplant this but is not universally available. Octreoscan imaging gives both diagnostic and therapeutic information. A negative scan usually correlates with a poorly differentiated tumour and implies somatostatin receptor (SSTR) negativity. Low response rates to somatostatin (SMS) analogues are thus expected and chemotherapy or novel approaches are required. On the other hand, a positive scan suggests a high response rate to SMS. Serial Octreoscan imaging is also useful to assess response and correlates with tumour markers (see below). While not always universally available, ^{67}Ga-Dotatate has improved the quality of imaging and may even be combined with FDG PET which is more likely to pick up less well differentiatedtumours .

14.9 BiochemicalandT umourMar kers

Urine 5HIAA (5-hydroxyindoleacetic acid) has been the classical tumour marker but is messy, fiddly and questionably accurate in its collection. A urine 5HIAA level in excess of 50 μmol/L is usually taken as excessive and abnormal but various dietary products may stimulate its release so a special diet so should be instituted if screening for carcinoids/NETs. Many would now argue that the "Gut Hormone Profile" is better and more accurate and Chromogranin A (CgA) levels measured serially will give good prognostic information [27, 28]. The profile will vary according to the local laboratory but most commonly chromogranins A and B, pancreastatin, neurotensin, VIP, gastrin, pancreatic polypeptide and glucagon are measured. CgA is the most constant and consistent although the other neuropeptides may be variably secreted. It is suggested that neuropeptide secretion correlates with tumour differentiation and in many "non-functioning tumours" only CgA is abnormal. Specialist advice should be sought from the local laboratory as the assays of these neuropeptides are sensitive and need special preparation and transport to the laboratory. Serial measurements are important and correspond to response and progression in most cases, however not all tumours are functional; it is more common for hindgut carcinoids to be non-secretory. Carcinoid heart disease has long been recognised as a distinct problem, principally affecting the right side of the heart but conventionally is associated with systemic disease and extensive liver metastases. However, ovarian carcinoids are unusual and may be associated with cardiac disease without liver metastases as the ovarian vein may drain directly into the inferior vena cava [29, 30]. N-terminal pro-brain natriuretic peptide (BNP) in suspected cardiac disease has recently been shown to be useful in predicting those who will develop cardiac disease needing intervention [31].

14.10 ManagementandC linicalC ourse

Davis et al. in their 1995 paper [17] gave an excellent overview of management in the previous era. Prior to this, much of the literature consisted of small reports, although Robboy et al. collected a series pathological reviews in the 1970s and 1080s [12]. The past 15 years has seen a revolution with modern immunocytochemistry assisting diagnosis, good imaging with CT, nuclear medicine imaging initially with Octreoscan and now PET-CT, together with reliable and accurate tumour markers. However, many would argue that the impact of the somatostatin analogues (Octreotide and Lanreotide) has been even more dramatic. It is thus very challenging to draw on this older experience and applying it to modern management.

In spite of this, a review of some of the historical data is still valuable. Although, first seemingly reported in 1939 with two case reports by Stewart [1], the next 50 years mainly saw anecdotal reports or small series. In 1975 Robboy et al. reviewed 48 cases of primary ovarian insular carcinoids in addition to the 22 in the literature [12]. Localised disease is associated with a good prognosis but 16 of 48 (33%) had carcinoid syndrome. Many of these were retrospectively diagnosed as being confused with the menopause. With careful questioning the flush is really quite different and often provoked by alcohol, specific dietary products and sometimes exercise. However 62% had diarrhoea and other manifestations include wheezing, hypertension and pedal oedema. Unusually, there is a high incidence of cardiac involvement in primary ovarian carcinoids. This may be explained by the drainage of the ovarian vein directly into the vena cava thus bypassing the hepatic circulation.

Davis in 1999 presented a further 17 cases and reviewed the literature [17]. Eleven of their seventeen patients (62%) had stage 1 disease and seven of these had an associated mature teratoma. Five of their 17 had symptoms of carcinoid syndrome. One stage 1, patient went on to develop cardiac disease without other manifestations and required cardiac valve replacement with good outcome. They identified 316 cases in the literature of which 157 had enough detail to discuss care and outcome. Only 21 (13%) had carcinoid syndrome and the vast majority of these (90%) had insular variant. Their discussion includes the treatment of recurrent and metastatic disease in a small number of patients. Stage of disease was the best prognostic predictor with all stage 1 patients alive at 10 years.

A further paper by Timmins et al. in 1999 reported one additional case and re-reviewed the literature [8]. They made some comparisons with ovarian carcinomas of low malignant potential from their pattern of spread, although some would argue this is spurious: the only common link being their relatively slow progression. The main emphasis of their paper is to propose a more radical surgical debulking approach which is in keeping with modern surgical views of management of small bowel carcinoids and NETs. Swedish data do suggest longer survival in patients who were managed more aggressively, although there are no randomisedtria lda tatos upport [32].

Soga reviewed 11,842 NETs cases and reported that the highest 5-year survival rate in the carcinoid group was noted in the ovary (93.6%), the same author also reported specifically on 329 ovarian carcinoids from the Niigata cancer registry [5–7]. Two groups were analysed, i.e. those with and those without associated mature cystic teratomas. The former group consisted of 189 cases (57.4%) and the latter of 140 (42.6%). There were significant differences between the pure carcinoids and those arising with teratomas. The latter were larger, more frequently had metastases and more likely to be associated with carcinoid syndrome. Furthermore, they looked at differences between insular and trabecular tumours. Most previous series suggested insular more common but in this series they were almost equal, (22% vs. 24%). There were significant behavioural differences between the insular and trabecular tumours with 39% of insular tumour patients developing carcinoid syndrome while only 7.8% occurred with trabecular cancers. Five year survival was 93.7% vs. 84% respectively. Their higher incidence of trabecular carcinoids may explain their better prognosis.

The special issue of cardiac disease in non-metastatic ovarian carcinoids is discussed by Botero et al. [29], and we now have potential markers to identify high risk patients [30]. These are rare developments and are explained by the venous drainage directly into the vena cava by passing the liver and causing right heart valvular disease, sometimes occurring many years after the primary diagnosis. Referral to specialist cardiac units is strongly advised as modern cardio-vascular surgery has rendered valvular repair or replacement much safer. Rare reports include tumours arising in the broad ligaments [40].

14.11 Treatmento fR elapsedDi sease

There are good renews of carcinoid tumors [34, 35]. Management of relapsed disease is usually influenced by presence of symptoms including carcinoid syndrome and rate of change of CgA or progression on imaging. A well and asymptomatic patient may not require any immediate intervention. However, initial management of carcinoid syndrome requires Somatostatin (SMS) analogue therapy [27, 28]. Some very recent data from the PROMID study has hinted that early treatment of low volume metastatic disease may delay time to progression [33]. There is probably little to choose between octreotide and lanreotide even though the latter may have theoretical advantages due to different receptor profile. However, in the author's opinion there is no convincing difference and swapping from one to the other may occasionally lead to secondary response. A new analogue pasireotide is expected commercially within the next 2 years and a new chimeric SMS-DOPA antagonist is under development. It is often up to local preference to select which product to be used. The management would normally be overseen by a specialist interested in NETs. Symptomatic responses occur in up to 80% while only 50–60% may show biochemical response and objective imaging response may occur in as few as 10%. Responses last in excess of a year usually and sometimes for several years. On progression, increasing the dose or frequency of administration of SMS analogues may gain some additional benefit.

The next step is usually more controversial as multiple options are available and the choice will depend on local experience, expertise and prejudice! It will include the following options: hepatic artery embolisation (especially when liver metastases are predominant), interferons, radionuclide therapy, conventional chemotherapy and targeted novel agents. A fuller discussion of the management of relapsed disease is beyond the remit of this article. For more detailed information about management the reader is referred toothe rs ourcesofinforma tion [27, 28, 34, 35].

Goblet cell or MEEC are also challenging and prove more difficult to control. Toumpanakis reviewed the experience at the Royal Free Hospital London. They should probably be best managed as for colorectal cancers with pyrimidine based regimes using 5 Fluorouracil orc apecitabinea ndoxa liplatin [23].

14.12 Treatmento fOva rian Strumal Carcinoids

There is considerable debate in the literature not only about the primary surgical management but also about the need for any adjuvant investigations and treatment. Most series advise that if a strumal carcinoid is diagnosed unexpectedly in a post-menopausal woman, or in one who has completed her family, then a hysterectomy and bilateral salpingo-oophorectomy is advised. Conservative surgery may be considered in a younger woman with no extra-capsular spread and no associated mature cystic teratoma. However, some have advised that completion surgery should be carried out when family is completed. In cases with obvious spread more aggressive surgery must be advised [25, 26, 36–39, 40– 42].

For malignant struma ovarii, post-operative care should involve referral for discussion of total thyroidectomy and management as for differentiated thyroid carcinoma. Thyroidectomy is an essential pre-requisite to radio-iodine imaging, and ablation otherwise any administered radio-iodine will be taken up preferentially by the thyroid and not by any strumal tissue. This will involve whole body imaging with radio-iodine to search for any other functioning tissue and to destroy any residual thyroid tissue which in turn allows thyroglobulin to be used as a tumour marker. It is argued that this may be an excessive treatment but those series reporting this as a standard of care do report the best outcomes. Thyroid hormone replacement in doses which fully suppress the TSH is needed. Serial measurement of thyroglobulin has replaced whole body radio-iodine scintigraphy. Thyroglobulin levels should be undetectable and any rising levels or the development of new thyroglobulin antibodies is a case for investigation of possible relapse. To date there is no reported value of PET-CT scanning.

References

1. Stewart MJ, Willis RA, Saram GSW. Argentaffine carcinoma (carcinoid tumour) arising in ovarian teratomas – a report of two cases. J Pathol Bacteriol. 1939;49:207–12.
2. Modlin IM, Sandor A. An analysis of 8305 cases of carcinoid tumours. Cancer. 1997;79:813–29.
3. Modlin IM, Lye KD, Kidd M. A 5-decade analysis of 13,715 carcinoid tumors. Cancer. 2003;97(4):934–59.
4. Robboy SJ, Norris HJ, Scully RE, Robboy SJ, Norris HJ, Scully RE. Insular carcinoid primary in the ovary. A clinicopathologic analysis of 48 cases. Cancer. 1975;36(2):404–18.
5. Soga J, Osaka M, Yakuwa Y. Carcinoids of the ovary: an analysis of 329 reported cases. J Exp Clin Cancer Res. 2000;19:271–80.
6. Soga J. Carcinoids and their variant endocrinomas. An analysis of 11842 reported cases. J Exp Clin Cancer Res. 2003;22(4):517–30.
7. Soga J, Osaka M, Yakuwa Y. Carcinoids of the ovary: an analysis of 329 reported cases. J Exp Clin Cancer Res. 2000;19(3):271–80.
8. Timmins PF, Kuo DY, Anderson PS, Fields AL, Whitney KD, Goldberg GL. Ovarian carcinoid: management of primary and recurrent tumours. Gynecol Oncol. 2000;76:112–4.
9. Wolfe SA. Metastatic carcinoid tumor of the ovary. Am J Obstet Gynecol. 1955;70(3):563–71.
10. Lincoln JC. Malignant argentaffinoma with metastases to the ovaries. Br J Surg. 1966;53(12):1071–3.
11. Shuster M, Mendoza-Divino E, Joselson H. Carcinoid tumor metastasizing to the ovaries. Obstet Gynecol. 1970;36(4): 515–9.
12. Robboy SJ, Scully RE, Norris HJ. Carcinoid metastatic to the ovary. A clinicopathologic analysis of 35 cases. Cancer. 1974;33(3):798–811.
13. Strosberg J, Nasir A, Cragun J, Gardner N, Kvols L. Metastatic carcinoid tumor to the ovary: a clinicopathologic analysis of seventeen cases. Gynecol Oncol. 2007;107:65–8.
14. Talerman A. Carcinoid tumors of the ovary. J Cancer Res Clin Oncol. 1984;107(2):125–35.

15. Rindi G, Capella C, Solcia E. Introduction to a revised clinicopathological classification of neuroendocrine tumors of the gastroenteropancreatic tract. Q J Nucl Med. 2000;44(1): 13–21.
16. Klöppel G, Perren A, Heitz PU. The gastroenteropancreatic neuroendocrine cell system and its tumors: the WHO classification. Ann N Y Acad Sci. 2004;1014:13–27.
17. Davis KP, Hartmann LK, Keeney GL, Shapiro H. Primary ovarian carcinoid tumors. Gynecol Oncol. 1996;61(2): 259–65.
18. Baker PM, Oliva E, Young RH, Talerman A, Scully RE. Ovarian mucinous carcinoids including some with a carcinomatous component. A report of 17 cases. Am J Surg Pathol. 2001;25(5):557–68.
19. Young RH. From krukenberg to today: the ever present problems posed by metastatic tumors in the ovary part I. Historical perspective, general principles, mucinous tumors including the krukenberg tumor. Adv Anat Pathol. 2006;13:205–27.
20. Young RH. From krukenberg to today: the ever present problems posed by metastatic tumors in the ovary part II. Historical perspective, general principles, mucinous tumors including the krukenberg tumor. Adv Anat Pathol. 2007;14:149–77.
21. Azzena A, Zannol M, Bertezzelo M, Zen T, Chiarelli S. Epidermoid cyst and primary trabecular carcinoid of the ovary: case report. Eur J Gynaecol Oncol. 2002;23:317–9.
22. De la Torre J, García A, Castellví J, López M, Gil A. Primary ovarian trabecular carcinoid tumour: a case report with an immunohistochemical study and a review of the literature. Arch Gynecol Obstet. 2004;270(4):274–7.
23. Toumpanakis C, Standish RA, Baishnab E, Winslet MC, Caplin ME. Goblet cell carcinoids (adenocarcinoid) of the appendix. Dis Colon Rectum. 2007;50(3):315–22.
24. Logani S, Baloch ZW, Snyder PJ, Weinstein R, LiVolsi VA. Cystic ovarian metastasis from papillary thyroid carcinoma: a case report. Thyroid. 2001;11(11):1073–5.
25. Roth LM, Miller AW, Talerman A. Typical thyroid carcinoma arising in struma ovarii: a report of 4 cases and review of literature. Int J Gynecol pathol. 2008;27(4):496–506.
26. Roth LM, Talerman A. The enigma of struma ovarii. Pathology.2007;39(1):139–46.
27. Ramage JK, Davies AH, Ardill J, Bax N, Caplin M, Grossman A, et al. Guidelines for the management of gastroenteropancreatic neuroendocrine (including carcinoid) tumours. Gut. 2005;54 Suppl 4:v1–16.
28. Rindi G, de Herder W, O'Toole D, Wiedenmann B. Consensus Guidelines for the management of patients with digestive neuroendocrine tumors: the second event and some final considerations. Neuroendocrinology. 2008;87:5–7.
29. Botero M, Fuchs R, Paulus DA, Lind DS. Carcinoid heart disease: a case report and literature review. J Clin Anesth. 2002;14:57–63.
30. Wilkowske MA, Hartmann LC, Mulany C, Behrenbeck T, Kvols LK. Progressive carcinoid heart disease after resection of primary ovarian carcinoid. Cancer. 1994;73:1889–91.
31. Bhattacharyya S, Toumpanakis C, Caplin ME, Davar J. Usefulness of N-terminal pro-brain natriuretic peptide as a biomarker of the presence of carcinoid heart disease. Am J Cardiol.2008; 102:938–42.
32. Akerstrom G, Hellman P. Surgery on neuroendocrine tumours. Best Prac Res Clin Endocrinol Metab. 2007;21(1): 87–109.
33. Rinke A, Muller HH, Schade-Brittinger C, et al. PROMID study group. Placebo controlled double-blind prospective randomised study on the effect of octreotide LAR in the control of tumor growth in patients with metastatic neuro-endocrine midgut tumors: a report from the PROMID Study group. J Clin Oncol. 2009;27(28):4656–63.
34. Jafri NH, Theodore H, Nicklin JL, Copeland LJ. A carcinoid tumour of the broad ligament. Obstet Gynecol. 1998; 92:708.
35. Maggard MA, O'Connell JB, Ko CY. Updated population-based review of carcinoid tumors. Ann Surg. 2004;240(1): 117-22.
36. Caplin ME, Buscombe JR, Hilson AJ, Jones AL, Watkinson AF, Burroughs AK. Carcinoid tumour. Lancet. 1998; 352(9130):799-805.R eview.
37. Kulke MH, Mayer RJ. Carcinoid tumors. N Engl J Med. 1999;340(11):858-68.R eview.
38. Yaegashi N, Tsuiki A, Shimizu T, Kobayashi N, Sato S, Namiki T, Motoyama T, Katayama Y, Yajima A. Ovarian carcinoid with severe constipation due to peptide YY production. Gynecol Oncol. 1995;56(2):302-6.
39. Matsuda K, Maehama T, Kanazawa K. Strumal carcinoid tumor of the ovary: a case exhibiting severe constipation associated with PYY. Gynecol Oncol. 2002; 87(1):143-5.
40. Griffiths AN, Jain B, Vine SJ. Papillary thyroid carcinoma of struma ovarii. J Obstet Gynaecol. 2004;24(1):92-3.
41. Soto Moreno A, Venegas EM, Rodriguez JR, Sánchez F, Robles MJ, Martinez MA, Gonzalez D, Navarro E, Astorga R. Thyroid carcinoma on an ovarian teratoma: a case report and review of the literature. Gynecol Endocrinol. 2002;16(3): 207-11.
42. Hemli JM, Barakate MS, Appleberg M, Delbridge LW. Papillary carcinoma of the thyroid arising in struma ovary: report of a case and review of management guidelines. GynecolE ndocrinol.2001; 15(3):243-7.

Part III

Uterine Rare Cancers

ReedU terineC arcinosarcomas

15

Nicholas Reed

15.1 Introduction

Uterine sarcomas present a challenging group of tumours to manage. They represent a diverse group of tumours and it is argued whether they are true sarcomas. There is now increasing evidence that the carcinosarcomas (CS) – which have been known under a variety of names in the past – are most probably poorly differentiated epithelial carcinomas [1–11]. This switch to propose calling them CS has come from the WHO as well as the International Society of Gynaecological Pathologists. There is a proposal to adopt yet another term, metaplastic carcinomas which may be more helpful in understanding their status [1]. Their molecular profile suggests monoclonality from an epithelial pathway. Nevertheless, historically these tumours have been lumped together and are usually treated by Gynaecological Cancer Specialist teams rather than Soft Tissue Sarcoma Specialists. Historically there were usually three main types of uterine sarcoma – malignant mixed mullerian tumour or MMMT (now known as carcinosarcoma (CS), endometrial stromal sarcomas (ESS), and leiomyosarcomas (LMS)) and a small proportion of unclassifiable high grade tumours with sarcomatous elements. There is a move towards a simpler classification of high grade vs. low grade tumours which takes cognizance of CS not being true sarcomas. Increasingly, CS are recognised and treated as being more akin to poorly differentiated endometrial carcinomas which is supported by their clinical behaviour. Furthermore, there is an increasing recognition on immunocytochemistry and molecular markers that the distinction between LMS and ESS may be more blurred than we previously recognised. This chapter will focus on CS as they most likely are different!

Traditionalc lassification	Modern classification
MMMT(carcinosarcomas)	
Endometrial stromal sarcomas	High grade
Leiomyosarcomas	Lowgr ade
High grade undifferentiated sarcomas	

15.2 Presentation

These are relatively uncommon cancers accounting for between 3 and 8% of all uterine malignancies. However, CS now seems to account for over 50% of uterine sarcoma; historically around 40% of tumours were LMS, 40% CS (MMMT), 15% endometrial stromal sarcomas and about 5% unclassifiable. Recent data suggests a rising incidence of CS in comparison to LMS so about 50–60% of sarcomas are CS in more recent experience. One source suggests about 17 cases per million populations [3–5]. While they are now considered as distinct tumours, it is often helpful to make comparisons between the different sarcoma subtypes which help us to understand their clinical and behavioural patterns. Furthermore, most early series did not distinguishthe s ubtypes [1, 2, 6–12] Table 15.1.

These tumours tend to present with post-menopausal bleeding (PMB) and arise in the same age group as endometrial carcinomas. It is important to remember, there may be background causation from prior exposure to radiation therapy or the use of tamoxifen, and a good thorough clinical history should always be

N.R eed
Beatson Oncology Centre, Gartnavel General Hospital,
1053G reatW esternR oad, Glasgow G120Y N, Scotland, UK
e-mail:nic k.reed@ggc.scot.nhs.uk

N. Reed et al. (eds.), *Rare and Uncommon Gynecological Cancers*,
DOI: 10.1007/978-3-642-13492-0_15,

Table15. 1 Pathologyc lassifications

Oldc lassification	New classification
Carcinosarcomas (MMMT)	Metaplastic carcinomas
Endometrial stromal sarcomas	Low grade Highgr ade
Leiomyosarcomas	
Undifferentiated or unclassifiable	Highgr ade

obtained [13, 14]. There are also big differences in the ages at which these patients present. Leiomyosarcomas often occur in women of peri-menopausal age but CS and endometrial stromal sarcomas tend to be associated with women beyond the menopause. The peak incidence is reported as 62–67 years compared to 48–54 years for leiomyosarcomas. CS also shares many characteristic with type II endometrial cancers [15]. This would be consistent with the view that CS is simply bad-type endometrial epithelial tumours. Epidemiological studies have suggested the same risk factors for development as EEC again supporting the view that they are carcinoma and not sarcomas.

They may have a history of breast cancer and tamoxifen exposure. There is also an increased risk of developing CS when patients had received prior pelvic radiation. This may be remote and up to 30 years previously, although the mean latent period will often be between 8 and 15 years, typically these develop on the edge (penumbra) of the radiation fields. Given the increasing use of (chemo-) radiation for cervix cancers it will be necessary to monitor this closely over the next 20–30 years. This confirms the importance of establishing a detailed history. The story of tamoxifen exposure is interesting and initially was thought to be associated mainly with endometrioid endometrial carcinomas, usually polypoid lesions with endometrial hyperplasia and only occasional evolution to cancers, but there are now a number of small reports of CS [13, 14]. Early reports suggested the usual pattern of presentation was within a polyp and often showed pre-malignant changes, imaging with transvaginal ultrasound often shows multiple polyps as well as endometrial thickening. However the author has over 60 in his data base, and their behaviour is variable.

Systemic symptoms such as weight loss, loss of appetite and pain generally portend a more advanced stage at diagnosis. Until recently, there was no separate staging system but most experts have adapted the FIGO staging system for endometrial cancer. In 2008, FIGO proposed to adopt a new system for the uterine sarcomas,w hichis be ingintroduc edin2009 [16].

15.3 Stagingl nvestigations

Most will present with PMB, and the investigations will be as for PMB of any cause. There is often little to suggest that the tumour is a sarcoma rather than carcinoma. Increasingly patients are referred to one stop clinics for rapid diagnosis. A full history and examination are performed, and the next steps are likely to be a transvaginal ultrasound (TVS) to assess uterine thickness and a pipelle endometrial biopsy. Prior tamoxifen exposure may cause endometrial thickening due to hyperplasia and polyps and often gives a characteristic appearance. Alternatively, a hysteroscopy and curettage can be performed for diagnosis. Many tumours will arise in polyps so removal of this may be needed. Some tumours do arise as isolated polyps and are true stage 1A and seem to have a better prognosis; it may be fortunate if they present with PMB and are diagnosed at such an early stage.

The next step will be more detailed imaging to assess extent of myometrial thickness and any nodal extension. The incidence of lymph node metastases is higher in CS than endometrioid endometrial cancer (EEC), many series report 15–30% as opposed to around 13–20% in endometrial carcinomas [17, 18]. MR scanning is generally viewed as best technique for local pelvic imaging whereas CT scanning will image the upper abdomen and chest better. Imaging should include the upper abdomen and chest to assess metastatic spread. ^{18}FDG-PET CT imaging has the potential to supplement or even replace both of these but is neither universally available nor universally approved in this setting. Functional imaging developments include dynamic contrast enhancement (DCE) and BOLD MR imaging, and Ultra Small Particles of Iron Oxide (USPIO) with MR but again they have yet to make widespread impact. Another technique which falls into same category is the use of sentinel lymph node biopsy. To date no tumour markers have yet been shown to be of value.

Screening programmes are not used in uterine sarcomas but in a patient with previous breast cancer and tamoxifen usage, it would be prudent to advice about the importance of reporting PMB and investigating at the earliest opportunity. Given the increasing incidence of obesity, we will see more endometrial cancers and future health policies may consider obese women as candidates for screening. Primary care physicians should be alert to the possibility of diagnosing uterine malignancy in higher risk groups. Occasional patients may be diagnosed with small incidentally found lesions at the time of hysterectomy for other reasons but this is more likely with LMS.

15.4 Pathology

The pathology of these tumours has caused much debate over the years. Recent evidence has started to allow this debate to be more scientific as we better understand these tumours and their biology. One definition in use is that these are carcinomas with metaplastic sarcomatous components hence the monoclonality of origin and indeed the metastases are almost universally carcinomatous [1, 2, 5–12, 17–25]. Although the phenotype is a mixture of carcinoma and sarcoma this is now generally regarded as an epithelial tumour, rather than a biclonal malignancy, with mutations in TP53 being a common early event. As a reflection of their similarity to uterine carcinoma they are highly responsive to platinum compounds and taxanes irrespective of the site of origin and as such are not generally treated as sarcomas. These are tumours that show high grade nuclear changes and biphasic pattern, hence the name. Differential diagnosis especially on small endometrial biopsies can be challenging! Anaplastic sarcomas probably cause the most difficulties in interpretation. The epithelial component may be of any of the recognised variants of EEC, e.g. serous, endometrioid, mucinous, squamous, clear cell, undifferentiated or mixtures, although endometrioid is most commonly identified. Traditionally, the stromal component could contain smooth muscle components, stromal sarcoma or fibrosarcoma giving rise to the term "homologous", while if the tumour contained rhabdomyosarcoma, chondrosarcoma, osteosarcoma or liposarcoma elements it is known as a "heterologous" carcinosarcoma. The practical significance is at best unknown and probably of little real value. There is an impression that heterologous may be more aggressive, and in the GOG series they had slightly higher rates of lymph node metastases (21 vs. 15%). This distinction is now beginning to fall out of use as it gives little practical benefit although may be interesting to demonstrate at clinico-pathological conferences!

There are important differences in the ways in which these tumours grow and metastasise with CS tending to have a higher incidence of lymphatic spread and lymph node metastases, whereas LMS are more likely to have early haematogenous spread and the first metastases may well be in the lungs or the liver [17, 18, 20, 21]. Some recent small series have reported high levels of nodal disease in LMS but this does seem substantiated in the larger series and may reflect some degree of case selection. The reader is advised to refer to the separate section on LMS. This therefore has important implications for the investigations, staging and surgical management of these patients. This article focuses predominantly on the clinical management of the diagnosed patient, and when the diagnosis of a sarcoma is suspected from the initial investigations, it would be assumed that full radiological staging with CT and/or MRI of the chest, abdomen and pelvis will be carried out. At present there would appear to be no justification for routine PET-CT or other functional imaging techniques which are worthy of further clinical research. There are no tumour markers of proven value.

There are rare reports of pure adult rhabdomyosarcomas, chondrosarcomas, angiosarcomas and liposarcomas. They are considered to be beyond the scope of the first edition of this book. The reader is advised to refer to a review chapter such as the one by Hendrickson et al. [2].

15.5 SurgicalManag ement

The surgical management should involve referral to a specialist Gynaecological Oncology Surgeon if a carcinosarcoma is suspected on initial investigations. This will allow careful staging procedures to be carried out and the surgery should involve a minimum of total abdominal hysterectomy, bilateral salpingo-oophorectomy, careful and thorough inspection of the abdominal and pelvic contents, sampling of fluid for cytological assessment of the washings and perhaps – a little more contentiously – pelvic and/or para-aortic lymph node dissection (PLND). In CS the lymph node metastases incidence may vary from 15 to 30% and therefore a staging lymphadenectomy should be considered in suitable fit patients (contrast this with the low incidence in

LMS) [17, 18, 23–25]. There will be cases where the diagnosis was not recognised pre-operatively and a simple hysterectomy and BSO is carried out without PLND. A dilemma arises as to whether to recommend re-operation and perform nodal dissection or to offer adjuvant pelvic radiation. This topic will be debated at tumour boards regularly and there is probably no right answer. It may be determined by the patient's fitness, choice, and local prejudice and availability of services.

Following surgery the pathology should be examined by a specialist pathologist interested in gynaecological cancer and the patient's management should be discussed at the local Multi-Disciplinary Team meeting (MDT) or tumour board. Specialist immunocytochemistry may be a valuable aid in the differential diagnosis of these tumours and the use of relatively simple techniques such as oestrogen and progestagen receptor (ER and PR) staining should also be carried out as this may provide therapeutic as well as prognostic guidance. For those working in smaller centres, consideration should be given to discussing these patients with colleagues from the larger regional services who will see these tumours more frequently. It is not suggested that all cases should be referred to these central units but networking with commonly agreed protocols is recommended. Ideally these should be recorded on a local or regional data bases and eventually aspire to national and international registries.

15.6 PostoperativeA djuvantT herapies

Adjuvant therapies to be discussed will include radiation, chemotherapy or both. There may be situations as above where further discussion of the need for pelvic lymph node dissection takes place if the original surgery did not include this.

15.6.1 To Irradiate or Not?

For many years there has been a debate about the role of adjuvant post operative radiotherapy in CS. The historical literature from the 1960s and 1970s from non-randomised trials would appear to show there was a survival advantage for adjuvant post-operative radiation when compared to those patients who were treated with surgery alone or radiation alone [26–30]. There have been other more recent studies which have given inconsistent and discordant results [31–35]. These have generally come from retrospective reviews in larger cancer centres and have variably shown some improvement in local control of limited benefit but rarely with any survival advantage; however one has to question case selection and referral patterns to these specialist units. In the 1980s the EORTC Gynaecological Cancer Co-operative Group decided to address this question by mounting a randomised clinical trial comparing adjuvant pelvic irradiation with no immediate treatment [36]. In the 1990s the GOG set up a trial comparing whole abdominal irradiation (WAI) vs. chemotherapy with cisplatin, ifosfamide and mesna (CIM). These are the only two randomised large trials that have been carried out and their results should really inform us and advise us how to proceed with futuretre atments [36, 37].

The EORTC study contained 224 patients with stage 1 and occult stage 2 sarcomas of the uterus, with the majority being divided between leiomyosarcomas – 103 cases and CS – 99 cases. They underwent total hysterectomy and bilateral salpingo-oophorectomy and it was advised that lymphadenectomy be included but it was optional and a local decision. They were randomised to receive External Beam Radiotherapy (EBRT) to the pelvis or no immediate treatment. This study showed no survival advantage when patients were given adjuvant EBRT [36]. However, perhaps not surprisingly the patients with CS, given adjuvant radiation showed a reduction in the incidence of local relapse, paralleling the situation in high risk endometrial cancer. For CS local control was 61 vs. 47%, while PFS was 6.2 years vs. 4.9 years and OS 8.5 years vs. 6.8 years (see Tables 15.2 and 15.3). On the basis of

Table 15.2 EORTC55874l ocalc ontrol

Carcinosarcoma local relapse		Leiomyosarcoma local relapse	
EBRT	Obs	EBRT	Obs
39%	53%	56%	47%

Table 15.3 EORTC55874s urvival

Survivalye ars	CS	LMS
PFS	6.2	4.9
OS	8.5	6.7

this, it is difficult to justify recommending routine immediate use of adjuvant pelvic irradiation in this group of patients. Insufficient numbers underwent PLND to allow a meaningful analysis of the effect.

The GOG 150 study was carried out over a broadly similar time-span and took over 10 years to complete its accrual [37]. Patients were randomised either to receive WAI followed by a pelvic boost or chemotherapy with cisplatin, ifosfamide and mesna (CIM). The entry criteria included stage 3 patients who had been optimally staged. While it shows a small survival advantage to the patients treated with chemotherapy, it must be conceded that neither group of patients fared particularly well and not surprisingly the patients with radiation treatment had lower local failure rates but with higher rates of distant metastases, whereas the converse was seen in the chemotherapy patients. Are there any lessons to be learnt from this? We know that adjuvant radiotherapy will improve local control but used alone seems to lead to higher failure rates suggesting some change in the biological behaviour. Therefore while we should consider systemic treatment as part of the package of care, can we justify any place for pelvic radiation?

Is it possible to extrapolate from the situation in endometrial carcinomas where the same debate is focusing on the role of chemotherapy and radiation in the high risk cancers and an increasing body of opinion that believes these high risk cases should receive chemotherapy with radiation, particularly if no PLND or positive nodes; these reports and reviews include the following from NSGO and PORTEC trial groups and Cochrane meta-analyses [38–41]. Many arguments were put forward to allow CS to be included in the current PORTEC 3 trial in which high risk endometrial cancers are randomised post-operatively to either EBRT or concomitant chemo-radiotherapy followed by four cycles of carboplatin and paclitaxel [80].

So, how can we resolve these circular arguments? At present, most experts still advocate PLND for uterine CS, where the patient is fit. If nodes are negative EBRT can be omitted, but adjuvant EBRT with or without chemotherapy tends to be offered if nodes are positive. Amant has proposed a study to investigate whether comprehensive surgical staging is sufficient or can be improved by adding chemotherapy [42]. The proposed hypothesis is that optimal comprehensive staging may lead to omission of any systemic therapy. His protocol concept randomises optimally staged CS to no adjuvant therapy or 4–6 cycles of chemotherapy, but because of the relative rarity of the condition and lack of sexy new drugs it is impossible to fund such a study.

However, it still does not really justify the use of routine EBRT in these patients! So what about systemic adjuvant treatments? The obvious clinical trial would be chemotherapy vs. chemoradiation. Given the relatively low incidence of these tumours, would it be possible to mount a further clinical trial, which could be completed in a reasonable time in which we compare chemoradiation against chemotherapy alone? Or, alternatively, should we be considering chemotherapy alone vs. no treatment, particularly if the patient has undergone pelvic lymph node resection as proposed by Amant. The justification for PLND in uterine sarcomas still remains controversial in itself but if done avoids routine use of EBRT, but what should we do if nodes are only sampled or not done? At present the level one evidence suggests no survival benefit so EBRT should be kept for relapse.

15.6.2 Adjuvant Hormonal Therapy

As with endometrial carcinomas, there is no proven benefit for the use of adjuvant therapies with hormones if there has been complete surgical resection. It may be valuable to test ER and PR status on the original sample for future reference but it has no immediate therapeutic gain and should be kept in hand for relapse. Tamoxifen alone or combined tamoxifen and a progestagenma ybe us edinthe re lapseds etting [43, 44].

15.6.3 Adjuvant Chemotherapy

In this article so far the role of adjuvant chemotherapy has been covered only briefly. The GOG has carried out a number of adjuvant studies in the 1980s with doxorubicin [45] or ifosfamide [46] and although there was a tendency to reduction in risk recurrence, the survival benefit was absent. In the 1990s ifosfamide with or without cisplatin failed to achieve a survival benefit [46, 47]. In 1997 Tierney, on behalf of the MRC, looked at adjuvant chemotherapy in all soft tissue sarcomas [48]. There were 264 uterine sarcomas amounting to 17% of the total within the meta-analysis but again there was no convincing evidence to support the routine use of adjuvant chemotherapy in sarcomas. At this point in time, it is probably correct to state that adjuvant chemotherapy remains of unproven benefit.

Other approaches that have been reported include the combination of adjuvant chemotherapy and radiation. A phase-2 study from Pautier of France in a mixture of uterine sarcomas, looked at three cycles of cisplatin/doxorubicin/ifosfamide followed by external radiotherapy and appeared to show a significant benefit compared to historical controlled radiation alone, 76 vs. 43% progression-free survival and 100 vs. 76% 5-year overall survival [49]. Manolitsas looked at the sandwiched treatment of chemotherapy, radiation and chemotherapy on a background of aggressive surgery and showed 90% of patient's disease free with a combined approach compared to 47% in a group who had no combined modality [50]. However, these are small non-randomised phase-2 studies and it is difficult to be certain of the real benefit when applied to real world unselected patients. The EORTC GCG proposed a concept of investigating radical surgery followed by randomisation to chemotherapy or no treatment with the option of giving adjuvant radiotherapy if the nodes were positive. However, history has shown that these studies, however well designed, take longer to complete than originally planned!

The role of chemotherapy is of unproven value as yet, however there is the danger of lumping CS together with other sarcomas of uterus. If we accept that CS are really epithelial cancers, and if we accept the newly emerging data on chemotherapy as an adjunct in high risk endometrial cancers [51], then strong consideration must be given to using adjuvant schedules in the same way as we do for high risk carcinomas. The traditional standard treatment has been the combination of an anthracycline and platinum, i.e. cisplatin and doxorubicin (or possibly carboplatin and epirubicin) but less toxic options are needed. New data from Hoskins has shown that for relapsed disease, carboplatin and paclitaxel is an effective alternative [52]. It is anticipated that increasingly community gynaecologists and oncologists will adopt this.

15.7 Recommendationso fC are

Following surgery, patient management should be discussed at MDT/tumour board meeting. EBRT will not be advised unless there is residual disease in pelvis or positive nodes. In cases where the nodes are not done, there is a conflict with the changing practise in high risk carcinomas where EBRT is increasingly being adopted but survival does not seem to be improved with EBRT alone. For cervical extension, vault brachytherapy is usually recommended. Given the data in NSGO 9505 trial [40], where estimated difference in PFS was 72–79% and for OS 74–82% in high risk endometrial cancers, adjuvant chemotherapy should at least be discussed. There is an urgent need to develop trials but a locally agreed policy to use chemotherapy which can be audited is encouraged as a second best setting. Later in the paper, the choices of agents in relapsed/advanced disease are discussed, but platinums and anthracyclines are the only proven agents. A recent report from Hoskins [52] in Vancouver has shown carboplatin and paclitaxel to be effective. None of these agents or combinations is "licensed" and unlikely to ever achieve such status in uterine sarcomas. Cisplatin and doxorubicin remains the gold standard, but carboplatin and epirubicin may be substituted with some reduction in toxicity and gain in convenience. The GOG investigated ifosfamide and cisplatin in a phase-2 and this is another option but with reservations over its toxicity. More recently Homesley reported ifosfamide and paclitaxel superior to ifosfamide alone. The author would welcome the adoption of carboplatin and paclitaxel as a standard alternative by the health funding bodies given its safety profile and far greater conveniencew ithle sstoxic ity [48, 53].

15.8 RecurrentandA dvancedDi sease

This section will deal with patients who have recurrent or metastatic disease but will also include those patients who present with locally advanced unresectable cancer. The latter make up a small proportion but remain very challenging in terms of management. It is again vital to stress the significant differences between the different tumour sub-types when it comes to using systemic treatment. Some agents that are active in CS for example are virtually inactive in LMS and vice versa. As a generalisation, the stromal sarcomas tend to have similar chemo-sensitivity to CS whereas the highly undifferentiated tumours may show transient chemosensitivity but there is usually a very rapid regrowth of tumour within a short period of time.

Given that CS are most probably epithelial derived tumours, it is not surprising that the drugs that are active in this condition are similar to those active in endometrial carcinomas. The most active agents are the anthracyclines, the platinums, dacarbazine and the taxanes, but in addition ifosfamide is a useful drug although it carries a greater risk of toxicity and inconvenience of scheduling. A very comprehensive recent review of systemic chemotherapy in uterine sarcomas from Canada is highlighted, [54]. From a historical point of view the earlier studies used doxorubicin (Adriamycin) as a single agent or combined with dacarbazine, cyclophosphamide or both and achieving around 10% response rate [55–58]. During the late 1980s and early 1990s cisplatin was introduced and single agent activity ranged between 18 and 40% [59–63] and at the same time ifosfamide was reported by Sutton with 32% response rates [61, 62]. Some of the earlier reports are difficult to interpret as they do include both CS (MMMTs) and leiomyosarcomas (see Tables 15.4a nd 15.5).

Carcinosarcomas	Leiomyosarcomas
Platinums	Doxorubicin
Anthracyclines	Ifosfamide
Taxanes	Dacarbazine
Ifosfamide	Gemcitabine Docetaxel Trabectedin

Again during the 1980s and 1990s we moved on from single agent to combined agents and doxorubicin was combined with dacarbazine (DTIC) or cyclophosphamide [55, 56]. Single agent activity varied between 10 and 25% whereas, combined agents between 19 and 30%. Jumping a decade to the 1998 Sutton on behalf of the GOG [64] showed that ifosfamide and cisplatin had a 54% response rate compared to 36% for ifosfamide alone and this has probably been considered the standard schedule until relatively recently. The EORTC 55923 protocol used cisplatin, ifosfamide and doxorubicin and achieved a 54% response rate in CS and endometrial stromal sarcomas [65] as did a Japanese group [66] while Leyvraz used high dose ifosfamide and doxorubicin and achieved 77% response rate but the numbers were small and it must be speculated that the patients were carefully selected, furthermore routine use of growth factors was advised [67, 68]. Lorigan on behalf of the EORTC Soft Tissue and sarcoma group compared ifosfamide with doxorubicin and showed no significant difference and they are now comparing doxorubicin with ifosfamide and doxorubicin in their current trial [69].

Other more recent studies have investigated paclitaxel [70], carboplatin and paclitaxel [48, 70–72] which, not surprisingly, does show reasonable activity, and most recently Homesley, from the GOG, reported on a phase-3 trial of ifosfamide vs. ifosfamide and paclitaxel showing a small advantage to the combinationala pproach [53].

Table15.4 Single agent activity in different types of uterine sarcomas

Single agent activity				
Singlea gent	Responser ate(%)	Histologicalt ype	Author	Reference
Doxorubicin	16	Any	Omura	[45]
Doxorubicin	19	Any	Muss	[56]
DoxorubicinH D	0	CS	Gershenson	[57]
Cisplatin	19	CS	Thigpen	[60]
Cisplatin	43	CS	Gershenson	[61]
Cisplatin	3	LMS	Thigpen	[62]
Ifosfamide	32	CS	Sutton	[46, 63, 81]
Ifosfamide	17	LMS	Sutton	[83]
Ifosfamide	33	ESS	Sutton	[81]
Paclitaxel	9	LMS	Sutton	[84]
Paclitaxel	8	LMS	Gallup	[85]
Topotecan	11	LMS	Miller	[86]
Trabectedin	NS	LMS	Schoffski	[76]

Table 15.5 Response rates for different combination regimens in uterine sarcoma

Combination	Responser ate(%)	Histologicalt ype	Author	Reference
Vincristine/actinomycin/ cyclophosphamide	26	Any	Hannigan	[58]
Doxorubicin/dacarbazine	24	Any	Omura	[55]
Doxorubicin/cyclophosphamide	19	Any	Muss	[56]
Cyclophosphamide/doxorubicin/ cisplatin	76	CS	Willemse	[59]
Cisplatin/doxorubicin/dacarbazine	33	CS	Baker	[73]
Pegylated liposomal doxorubicin/ paclitaxel	19	CS	Campos	[74]
Doxorubicin/ifosfamide+ G -CSF	77	CS	Leyvraz	[67, 68]
Topotecan/paclitaxel	29	CS	Fuller	[75]
Cisplatin/ifosfamide	54	CS	Sutton	[48,64]
Cisplatin/doxorubicin/ifosfamide	54	CS	vanR ijswijk	[65]
Ifosfamide/paclitaxel	45	CS	Homesley	[53]
Carboplatin/paclitaxel	60	CS	Hoskins	[52]
Doxorubicin/ifosfamide	30	LMS	Sutton	[70,88]
Doxorubicin/ifosfamide	55	LMS	Leyvraz	[67, 68]
Mitomycin/doxorubicin/cisplatin	23	LMS	Edmonson	[87]
Docetaxel/gemcitabine	53	LMS	Hensley	[72,89]

Unfortunately, ifosfamide remains an inconvenient drug to use and is associated with considerable morbidity particularly in older patients with bulky disease. It was therefore very encouraging to read a recent phase-2 report from Hoskins in Canada which they gave their experience with carboplatin and paclitaxel [48] in addition to the smaller earlier reports of this combination [70–72]. This combination clearly shows considerable activity and there were 40 patients reported, 28 of whom were newly diagnosed and 12 relapsed. Of the 20 evaluable patients 12 responded (5 CR and 7 PR) giving a 60% response rate and of the relapsed and recurrent patients previously treated, 6 out of 11 responded (2 CR and 4 PR). Median progression-free survival was 16 and 12 months respectively for these two groups. The attraction of this schedule is that it's well-known, easily used and so much more convenient than the ifosfamide regimes. It is difficult to conceive whether there will be any larger randomised controlled studies to try and bring this into routine practise, the numbers of patients are relatively small and we will probably see other phase-2 studies giving a similar level of benefit. Nevertheless, it is very likely that this will become accepted as the standard of care over the course of the next few years.

More recent papers have looked at using liposomal doxorubicin along with paclitaxel, the combination of cisplatin, adriamycin and dacarbazine, and a non-platinum regime of topotecan with paclitaxel but have failed to make a great impact [73–75]. Trabectedin has been investigated in soft tissue sarcomas with potential interest [76]. Surgical resection of isolated lung metastases has been used selectively in sarcoma patients but it is unusual in CS to see isolated and slow-growing lungorli verle sionss uitedforthis a pproach [77–79].

In terms of further development this is likely to come from the use of targeted agents and, not surprisingly, there is an increasing and booming literature on a variety of targeted agents in these tumours. At present, none of these has reached the stage where they can be recommended for clinical use outside the context of a clinical trial, but the author anticipates that within 5 years these will become part of the standard treatment.

15.9 Conclusions

Uterine sarcomas are relatively uncommon tumours. The only curative treatment remains surgical and most experts would advise including pelvic lymphadenectomy. At present there is no convincing data to support the use of adjuvant pelvic radiation treatment when there has been complete macroscopic removal. Radiotherapy in CS remains unproven in terms of survival benefit, even though it may improve local control. However, the use of chemotherapy should strongly be considered given the fact that these tumours have a high incidence of relapse and their similarity to high risk endometrial carcinomas. The judgement may be to offer delayed rather than immediate radiation therapy for salvage. Newer and better agents are required and we need to await and see if any of the newer targeteda gentsc ane stablisha role .

References

1. McCluggage WG. Malignant biphasic uterine tumours: carcinosarcomas or metaplastic carcinomas? J Clin Pathol. 2002;55(5):460–9.
2. Hendrickson M, Longacre T, Kempson R. Pathology of uterine sarcomas. In: Coukos G, Rubin SC, editors. Cancers of uterus. New York: Marcel Dekker; 2005. p. 149–95.
3. Arrastia CD, Fruchter RG, Clark M, Maiman M, Remy JC, Macaset M, et al. Uterine carcinosarcomas: incidence and trends in management and survival. Gynecol Oncol. 1997;65: 158–63.
4. Brooks SE, Zhan M, Cote T, Baquet CR. Surveillance, Epidemiology and End Results analysis of 2677 cases of uterine sarcoma 1989–1999. Gynn Oncol. 2004;93:204–8.
5. Henson DE, Schwartz AM, Tilara A, Grimley PM, Anderson WF. Population-based analysis of pathologic data: a new approach to the investigation of uterine endometrial and ovarian endometrioid carcinomas. Arch Pathol Lab Med. 2007;131(9):1337–42.
6. Yamada D, Burger R, Brewster W, et al. Pathologic variables and adjuvant therapy as predictors of recurrence and survival for patients with surgically evaluated carcinosarcoma of the uterus. Cancer. 2000;88:2782–6.
7. Ozguroglu M, Bilici A, Ilvan S, Turna H, Atalay B, Manel N, et al. Determining predominating histologic component in malignant mixed mullerian tumors: is it worth it? Int J Gyn Oncol. 2007;18(4):809–12.
8. Kounelis S, Jones M, Papadaki H, Bakker A, Swalsky P, Finkelstein S. Carcinosarcomas (malignant mixed mullerian tumors) of the female genital tract: Comparative molecular analysis of epithelial and mesenchymal components. Hum Pathol.1998; 29:82–7.
9. Zelmanowicz A, Hildesheim A, Sherman ME, et al. Evidence for a common aetiology for endometrial carcinomas and malignant mixed Mullerian tumours. Gynecol Oncol. 1998; 69:253–7.
10. Amant F, Vergote I. Bifunctional pathway of uterine carcinosarcomas. Hum Pathol. 2003;34(3):299.
11. Amant F, Dreyer L, Makin J, Vergote I, Lindeque BG. Uterine sarcomas in South African black women: a clinicopathologic study with ethnic considerations. Eur J Gynaecol Oncol.2001; 22(3):194–200.
12. Sreenan JJ, Hart W. Carcinosarcomas of the female genital tract. A pathologic study of 29 metastatic tumors; further evidence for the dominant role of the epithelial component and the conversion theory of histogenesis. Am J Surg Pathol. 1995;5:310–3.
13. Bergman L, Beelen ML, Gallee MP, Hollema H, Benraadt J, van Leeuwen FE. Risk and prognosis of endometrial cancer after tamoxifen for breast cancer. Comprehensive Cancer Centres' ALERT Group. Assessment of liver and endometrial cancer risk following tamoxifen. Lancet. 2000;356: 881–7.
14. Curtis R, Freedman DM, Sherman ME, Fraumeni JF. Risk of malignant mixed mullerian tumors after tamoxifen therapy for breast cancer. J Nat Cancer Institute. 2004;96(1):70–2.
15. Bokhman JV. Two pathogenetic types of endometrial carcinoma. Gynecol Oncol. 1983;15(1):10–7.
16. FIGO Committee on Gynecologic Oncology. FIGO staging for uterine sarcomas. Int J Gynaecol Obstet. 2009;104:179.
17. Major FJ, Blessing JA, Silverberg SG, Morrow CP, Creasman WT, Currie JL, et al. Prognostic factors in early-stage uterine sarcoma. A Gynecologic Oncology Group study. Cancer. 1993;71:1702–9.
18. Amant F. The rationale for comprehensive surgical staging in endometrial carcinosarcoma. Gynecol Oncol. 2005;99(2): 521–2.
19. Amant F, Cadron I, Fuso L, et al. Endometrial carcinosarcomas have a different prognosis and pattern of spread compared to high risk epithelial endometrial cancer. Gyn Oncol. 2005;98:274–80.
20. Evans HL. Endometrial stromal sarcoma and poorly differentiated endometrial sarcoma. Cancer. 1982;50:2170–82.
21. Norris HJ, Taylor HB. Mesenchymal tumors of the uterus. I. A clinical and pathological study of 53 endometrial stromal tumors. Cancer. 1966;19(6):755–66.
22. Oliva E, Clement PB, Young RH. Endometrial stromal tumors: an update on a group of tumors with a protean phenotype. Adv Anat Pathol. 2000;7(5):257–81.
23. Chauveinc L, Deniaud E, Plancher C, Sastre X, Amsani F, de la Rochefordiere A, et al. Uterine sarcomas: the Curie Institute experience. Prognosis factors and adjuvant treatments. Gynecol Oncol. 1999;72(2):232–7.
24. George M, Pejovic MH, Kramar A, Gynecologic Cooperating Group of French Oncology Centers. Uterine sarcomas: prognostic factors and treatment modalities-study on 209 patients. Gynecol Oncol. 1986;24:58–67.
25. Gadducci A, Sartori E, Landoni F, Zola P, Maggino T, Cosio S, et al. The prognostic relevance of histological type in uterine sarcomas: a Cooperation Task Force (CTF) multivariate analysis of 249 cases. Eur J Gynaecol Oncol. 2002;23(4): 295–9.
26. Edwards CL. Undifferentiated Tumours. Book chapter, in Cancer of Uterus and Ovary Year Book. Chicago: Medical Publishers Inc; 1969. p. 84–94.

27. Badib AO, Vongtama V, Kurohara SS, Webster JH. Radiotherapy in the treatment of sarcomas of the corpus uteri. Cancer. 1969;24:724–9.
28. Belgrad R, Elbadawi N, Rubin P. Uterine sarcoma. Radiology. 1975;144(1):181–8.
29. Salazar O, Bonfiglio TK, Patten SF, Kellser BE, Feldstein ME, Dunne ME, et al. Uterine sarcomas: natural history, treatment and prognosis. Cancer. 1978;42:1152–60.
30. Salazar OM, Bonfiglio TA, Patten SF, Keller BE, Feldstein ML, Dunne ME, et al. Uterine sarcomas. Analysis of failures with special emphasis on the use of adjuvant radiotherapy. Cancer.19 78;42:1161–70.
31. Sorbe B. Radiotherapy and/or chemotherapy as adjuvant treatment of uterine sarcomas. Gynecol Oncol. 1985;20: 281–9.
32. Hornback NB, Omura G, Major FJ. Observations on the use of adjuvant radiation therapy in patients with stage I and II uterine sarcoma. Int J Rad Oncol Biol Phys. 1986;12(12): 2127–30.
33. Le T. Adjuvant pelvic radiotherapy for uterine carcinosarcoma in a high risk population. Eur J Surg Oncol. 2001;27(3): 282–5.
34. Chi DS, Mychalczak B, Saigo PE, Rescigno J, Brown CL. The role of whole pelvic irradiation in the treatment of early-stage uterine carcinosarcoma. Gynecol Oncol. 1997;65: 493–8.
35. Dusenbery KE, Potish RA, Agenta PA, et al. On the apparent failure of adjuvant pelvic radiotherapy to improve survival for women with uterine sarcomas confined to the uterus. Am J Clin Oncol. 2005;28:295–300.
36. Reed NS, Mangioni C, Malmstrom H, et al. First results of a randomised trial comparing radiotherapy versus- observation post operatively in patients with uterine sarcomas, an EORTC-GCG study. Europ J Cancer. 2008;44(6):808–18.
37. Wolfson AH, Brady MF, Rocereto TF, et al. A Gynecologic Oncology Group randomized trial of whole abdominal irradiation (WAI) vs. cisplatin-ifosfamide and mesna (CIM) as post surgical therapy in stage I-IV carcinosarcoma (CS) of the uterus. Gynecol Oncol. 2007;107(2):177–85.
38. Efficacy of systemic pelvic lymphadenectomy in endometrial cancer (MRC ASTEC Trialists): a randomised study. Lancet2009;373:125–36.
39. Chan JK, Wu H, Cheung MK, Shin JY, Osann K, Kapp DS. The outcomes of 27,063 women with unstaged endometrioid uterine cancer. Gynecol Oncol. 2007;106(2):282–8.
40. Kong A, Johnson N, Cornes P, Simera I, Collingwood M, Williams C, et al. Adjuvant radiotherapy for stage I endometrialc ancer. http://thecochranelibrary.com
41. Kong A, Simera I, Collingwood M, Williams C, Kitchener HK; Cochrane Gynaecological Cancer Group. Adjuvant radiotherapy for stage I endometrial cancer: systematic review and meta-analysis. Ann Oncol. 2007;18:1595–604.
42. AmantF .Pe rsonalc ommunication
43. Fiorica JV, Brunetto G, Hanjani P, Lentz SS, Mannel R, Andersen W. Phase II trial of alternating courses of megestrol acetate and tamoxifen in advanced endometrial carcinoma a Gynecologic Oncology Group study. Gynecol Oncol. 2004;92(1):10–4.
44. Crawford D, George WD, Smith DC, Stewart M, Paul J, Leake R. Cyclic sequential endocrine therapy for advanced breast cancer using a combination of tamoxifen and megestrol acetate. Oncology. 1994;51 Suppl 1:13–8.
45. Omura GA, Blessing JA, Major FJ, Lifshitz S, Mangan C, Beecham J, et al. A randomized clinical trial of adjuvant adriamycin in uterine sarcomas: a Gynecologic Oncology Group study. J Clin Oncol. 1985;3:1240–5.
46. Sutton GP, Blessing JA, Rosenshein N, Photopoulos G, DiSaia PJ. Phase II trial of ifosfamide and mesna in mixed mesodermal tumors of the uterus (A Gynecologic Oncology Group study). Am J Obstet Gynecol. 1989;161:309–15.
47. Tierney JF, Mosseri V, Stewart LA, Souhami R, Parmar MK. Adjuvant chemotherapy for soft-tissue sarcoma: review and meta-analysis of the published results of randomised clinical trials. Br J Cancer. 1995;72(2):469–75.
48. Sutton G, Kauderer J, Carson LF, Lentz S, Whitney CW, Gallion H. Adjuvant ifosfamide and cisplatin in patients with completely resected stage I or II carcinosarcomas (mixed mesodermal tumors) of the uterus. A Gynecologic Oncology Group study. Gynecol Oncol. 2005;96:630–4.
49. Pautier P, Rey A, Haie-Meder C, et al. Adjuvant chemotherapy with cisplatin, ifosfamide, and doxorubicin followed by radiotherapy in localised uterine sarcomas: Results of a case-controlled study with radiotherapy alone. Int J Gynecol Cancer.2004; 14:1112–7.
50. Manolitsas TP, Wain GV, Williams K, et al. Multimodality therapy for patients with clinical stage I and II malignant mixed Mullerian tumors of the uterus. Cancer. 2001;91: 1437–43.
51. Hogberg T, Rosenberg P, Kristensen G, de Oliveira CF, de Pont Christensen R, Sorbe B, et al. A randomised phase III study on adjuvant treatment with radiation (RT) +/–chemotherapy (CT) in early stage high risk endometrial cancer (NSGO 9505/ EORTC 55991). Proc ASCO 2007 Abstract 5503.
52. Hoskins PJ, Le N, Ellard S, Lee U, Martin LA, Swenerton KD, et al. Carboplatin plus paclitaxel for advanced or recurrent uterine malignant mixed Mullerian tumors. The British Columbia Cancer Agency experience. Gynecol Oncol. 2008;108(1):58–62.
53. Homesley H, Filiaci G, Markman M, Bitterman P, Eaton L, Kilgore LC, et al. Phase III trial of ifosfamide with or without paclitaxel in advanced uterine carcinosarcoma: a Gynecologic Oncology Group Study. J Clin Oncol. 2007;25(5):526–31.
54. Kanjeeka S, Chambers A, Kee Fung MF, Verma S. On behalf of the Cancer Care Ontario Practice Guidelines Initiative Gynecology. Cancer Disease Site Group Program in Evidence-based Care, Cancer Care Ontario, Canada. Systemic therapy for advanced uterine sarcoma: A systematic review of the literature. Gynecol Oncol. 2005;97:624–37.
55. Omura GA, Major FJ, Blessing JA, Sedlacek TV, Thigpen JT, Creasman WT, et al. A randomized study of adriamycin with and without dimethyl triazenoimidazole carboxamide in advanced uterine sarcomas. Cancer. 1983;52:626–32.
56. Muss HB, Bundy B, DiSaia PJ, Homesley HD, Fowler WC, Creasman W, et al. Treatment of recurrent or advanced uterine sarcoma. A randomized trial of doxorubicin versus doxorubicin and cyclophosphamide. (A phase II trial of the Gynecologic Oncology Group). Cancer. 1985;55:1648–53.
57. Gershenson DM, Kavanagh JJ, Copeland LJ, Edwards CL, Freedman RS, Wharton JT. High-dose doxorubicin infusion therapy for disseminated mixed mesodermal sarcoma of the uterus. Cancer. 1987;59:1264–7.
58. Hannigan EV, Elder KW, Rutledge FN. Treatment of advanced uterine sarcoma with vincristine, actinomycin D and cyclophosphamide. Gynecol Oncol. 1983;15:224–9.

59. Willemse PHB, Bouma J, Hollema H. Cisplatin in gynecologic carcinosarcoma. J Clin Oncol. 1992;10:1365. letter.
60. Thigpen JT, Blessing JA, Orr JW, DiSaia PJ. Phase II trial of cisplatin in the treatment of patients with advanced or recurrent mixed mesodermal sarcoma of the uterus: a Gynecologic Oncology Group study. Cancer Treat Rep. 1986;70:271–4.
61. Gershenson DM, Kavanagh JJ, Copeland LJ, Edwards CL, Stringer CA, Wharton JT. Cisplatin therapy for disseminated mixed mesodermal sarcoma of the uterus. J Clin Oncol. 1987;5:618–21.
62. Thigpen JT, Blessing JA, Beecham J, Homesley H, Yordan E. Phase II trial of cisplatin as first-line chemotherapy in patients with advanced or recurrent uterine sarcomas: a Gynecologic Oncology Group study. J Clin Oncol. 1991;9:1962–6.
63. Sutton GP, Blessing JA, Rosenshein N, Photopulos G, DiSaia PJ. Phase II trial of ifosfamide and mesna in mixed mesodermal tumors of the uterus (a Gynecologic Oncology Group study). Am J Obstet Gynecol. 1989;161:309–12.
64. Sutton G, Brunetto VL, Kilgore L, Soper JT, McGehee R, Olt G, et al. A phase III trial of ifosfamide with or without cisplatin in carcinosarcoma of the uterus: a Gynecologic Oncology Group study. Gynecol Oncol. 2000;79:147–53.
65. van Rijswijk REN, Vermorken JB, Reed N, Favalli G, Mendiola C, Zanaboni F, et al. Cisplatin, doxorubicin and ifosfamide in carcinosarcoma of the female genital tract. A phase II study of the European Organization for Research and Treatment of Cancer Gynecological Cancer Group (EORTC 55923). Eur J Cancer. 2003;39:481–7.
66. Yamawaki T, Shimzu Y, Hasumi K. Treatment of stage IV "high-grade" endometrial stromal sarcoma with ifosfamide, adriamycin and cisplatin. Gynecol Oncol. 1997;64(2):265.
67. Leyvraz S, Bacchi M, Lissoni A, Sessa C, Cerny T, Honegger HP. High response rate with the combination of high-dose ifosfamide and doxorubicin for the treatment of advanced gynecologic sarcomas. Proc Am Soc Clin Oncol. 1998;17: 354a.a bstract.
68. Leyvraz S, Zweifel M, Jundt G, Lissoni A, Cerny T, Sessa C, et al. Long-term results of a multicenter SAKK trial on high-dose ifosfamide and doxorubicin in advanced or metastatic gynecologic sarcomas. Ann Oncol. 2006;17:646–51.
69. Lorigan P, Verweij J, Papai Z, et al. Phase III trial of two investigational schedules of ifosfamide compared with standard-dose doxorubicin in advanced or metastatic soft tissue sarcoma: a European Organisation for Research and Treatment of Cancer Soft Tissue and Bone Sarcoma Group Study. J Clin Oncol. 2007;25(21):3144–50.
70. Curtin JP, Blessing JA, Soper JT, DeGeest K. Paclitaxel in the treatment of carcinosarcoma of the uterus: a Gynecologic Oncology Group study. Gynecol Oncol. 2001;83:268–70.
71. Duska LR, Garrett A, Eltabbakh GH, Oliva E, Penson R, Fuller AF. Paclitaxel and platinum chemotherapy for malignant Mullerian tumors of the ovary. Gynecol Oncol. 2002;85: 459–63.
72. Szlosarek PW, Lofts FJ, Pettengell R, Carter P, Young M, Harmer C. Effective treatment of a patient with a high-grade endometrial stromal sarcoma with an accelerated regimen of carboplatin and paclitaxel. Anticancer Drugs. 2000;11(4):275–8.
73. Baker T, Piver MS, Caglar H, Piedmonte M. Prospective trial of cisplatin, adriamycin and dacarbazine in metastatic mixed mesodermal sarcomas of the uterus and ovary. Am J Clin Oncol. 1991;14:246–50.
74. Campos S, Penson RT, Matulonis UA, Berkowitz RS, Duska LR, Fuller AF, et al. A phase 2 and pharmacokinetic/dynamic study of Doxil and weekly paclitaxel chemotherapy for recurrent Mullerian tumors. Proc Am Soc Clin Oncol. 2000;19:410a.a bstract.
75. Fuller AF, Penson RT, Supko JG, Matulonis UA, Berkowitz RS, Goodman AK, et al. A phase I/II and pharmacokinetic study of 96-hour infusional topotecan and paclitaxel chemotherapy for recurrent Mullerian sarcomas. Proc Am Soc Clin Oncol. 2000;19:392a. abstract.
76. Schoffski P, Wolter P, Clement P, Sciot R, De Wever I, Wozniak A, et al. Trabectedin (ET-743): evaluation of its use in advanced soft-tissue sarcoma. Future Oncol. 2007;3(4):381–92.
77. Levenback C, Rubin SC, McCormack PM, et al. Resection of pulmonary metastases from uterine sarcomas. Gynecol Oncol.1992; 45:202–5.
78. Leitao MM, Brennan MF, Hensley M, et al. Surgical resection of pulmonary and extrapulmonary recurrences of uterine leiomyosarcoma. Gynecol Oncol. 2002;87:287–94.
79. Mountain CF, McMurtrey MJ, Hermes KE. Surgery for pulmonary metastasis: a 20-year experience. Ann Thorac Surg. 1984;38:323–30.
80. Creutzberg CL, van Putten WL, Koper PC, Lybeert ML, Jobsen JJ, Warlam-Rodenhuis CC, et al. Surgery and postoperative radiotherapy versus surgery alone for patients with stage-1 endometrial carcinoma: multicentre randomised trial. PORTEC Study Group. Post Operative Radiation Therapy in Endometrial Carcinoma. Lancet. 2000; 355(9213):1404–11.
81. Sutton G, Blessing JA, Park R, DiSaia PJ, Rosenshein N. Ifosfamide treatment of recurrent or metastatic endometrial stromal sarcomas previously unexposed to chemotherapy: a study of the GOG. Obstet Gynecol. 1996;87(5 pt 1): 747–50.
82. Leath CA, Huh WK, Hyde J, et al. A multi-institutional review of outcomes of endometrial stromal sarcoma. Gynecol Oncol. 2007;105(3):630–4.
83. Sutton GP. Blessing JA. Barrett RJ. McGehee R. Phase II trial of ifosfeniide and mesna in leiomyosarcoma of the uterus: a Gynecologic Oncology Group study. Am J Obstet Gynecol 1992: 166:556-9.
84. Sutton G. Blessing. Ball H. Phase II trial of paclitaxel in leionryosarcoma of the uterus: a Gynecologic Oncology Group study. Gynecol Oncol 1999, 74:346-9.
85. Gallup DG. Blessing JA. Andersen W. Morgan MA. Evaluation of paclitaxel in previously treated leiomyosarcorna of the uterus: a gynecologic oncology group study Gynecol Oncol 2003: 89:48-51.
86. Miller DS. Blessing JA. Kilgore LC. Mannel K. Van Le L. Phase II trial of topotecan in patients with advanced, persistent or recurrent uterine leiomyosarcomas: a Gynecologic Oncology Group study. Am J Clin Oncol 2000: 23:355-7.
87. . Edmonson JH. Blessing JA. Cosin JA. Miller DS, Cohn DE. Rotmensch J. Phase II study of mitomycni. Doxoubicin, and cisplatin in the treatment of advanced uterine leiomyosarcoma: a Gynecologic Oncology Group study Gyrecol Oncol 2002: 507-10.
88. Sutton GP. Blessing JA. Malfetano JH. Ifosfanride and doxorubicin in the treatment of advanced leiomyosarcomas of the uterus: a Gynecologic Oncology Group study Gynecol Oncol 1996: 62.226-9.
89. Hensley ML. Maki R. Venkatraman E. Geller G. Lovegren M. Aghajanian C et al. Gemcitabine and docetax lel in patients with unresectable leiomyosarcoma: results of a phase II trial J Clinn Oncol 2002: 12:2824-31.

Leiomyosarcomaso fU terus

16

Nicholas Reed

16.1 Introduction

Uterine sarcomas present a challenging group of tumours to manage, but the focus in this chapter will be on uterine leiomyosarcomas (LMS) [1]. Nevertheless, historically these tumours have been lumped together with carcinosarcomas and are usually treated by Gynaecological Cancer Specialist teams rather than Soft Tissue Sarcoma Specialists. Historically, they were usually considered to be three main types of uterine sarcoma: malignant mixed Mullerian tumour (MMMT) (now known as carcinosarcoma (CS)), endometrial stromal sarcomas (ESS), LMS and a small proportion of unclassifiable high-grade tumours with sarcomatous elements. LMS have been described as malignant neoplasms differentiated as smooth muscle [2]. While they may arise in other sites such as the stomach and retroperitoneum, they account for around 30–40% of the uterine sarcomas and broad ligaments [1]. Rare primary ovarian LMS are described but will be briefly covered elsewhere, and even rarer are cervical and vaginal LMS.

Traditionalc lassification
MMMT(C S)
LMS
ESS
Undifferentiated/unclassifiable

This definition of LMS itself raises issues over how the smooth muscle phenotype is defined, but more of this shortly. In routine practice the traditional terms are still frequently employed, and therefore, the author has retained the usage of CS, ESS, LMS and undifferentiated sarcomas for the purpose of this review, but a plea is made for some form of international consensus on usage among pathologists and gynaecological oncologists. Unfortunately, although LMS may often be "pure", examples of mixed tumours have been reported, confusingly raising the possibility that the aetiology and clonality may be even more indistinct. This chapter will now focus on LMS (Table 16.1).

16.2 IncidenceandEp idemiology

Uterine sarcomas are relatively uncommon cancers accounting for between 3–8% of all uterine malignancies [1–14]; traditionally it was recognised that almost 50% were LMS. LMS make up a significant proportion of soft tissue sarcoma, being more common than non-gynaecological LMS. While in CS there may be background causation from prior exposure to radiation therapy or the use of Tamoxifen for CS, until recently there has been no known aetiology for LMS. Recent data has suggested a molecular aetiology through disturbance of the AKT/P13 kinase and mTOR pathways [15]. However, there are differences in the ages at which these patients present. LMS often occur in women of peri-menopausal age, while CSS and ESS tend to be associated with women beyond the menopause, the peak incidence being in the 60s [8–10].

N.R eed
Beatson Oncology Centre, Gartnavel General Hospital,
1053G reatW esternR oad, Glasgow G120Y N, Scotland, UK
e-mail:nic k.reed@ggc.scot.nhs.uk

N. Reed et al. (eds.), *Rare and Uncommon Gynecological Cancers*,
DOI: 10.1007/978-3-642-13492-0_16, © Springer-Verlag Berlin Heidelberg 2011

Table16. 1 Pathologyc lassifications

Oldc lassification	New classification
Carcinosarcomas (MMMT)	Carcinosarcoma or metaplastic carcinomas
Endometrial stromal sarcomas	Low grade
Leiomyosarcomas	Highgr ade
Undifferentiated or unclassifiable	Highgr ade

LMS account for 1–2% of uterine malignancies. Historically, the incidence of LMS and CS showed approximate parity with each accounting for almost half of uterine sarcomas, but recent data would suggest CS are now more frequent or being recognised more frequently, although the incidence of LMS has probably changed little [1]. It is not clear why, but this author has hypothesised better pathological diagnostic techniques and recognition, perhaps due to increased awareness and more involvement and input into tumour boards by specialist gynaecological pathologists. Immunocytochemical techniques have also greatly improved and help to sort the wheat from the chaff!

One frequently debated question is whether LMS arise from benign leiomyomas or fibroids? The answer is yes, it can happen, but it seems only very infrequently. About 1 in 800 smooth muscle tumours of uterus is an LMS, but less than 1% of women with fibroids will develop smooth muscle tumours; some studies suggest as rarely as one in 1,000 [6–8]. There is also a difference in age at diagnosis for simple leiomyoma compared to LMS; it is usually about a decade difference being early 40s for leiomyomas and early 50s for LMS. Recent data has demonstrated the potential role of the AKT-P13 kinase, mTOR and IGFR pathways and not only is this exciting for improving our understanding and aetiology, but also offers new therapeutic potential targets [15, 16].

16.3 Presentation

While CS often present with post-menopausal bleeding, LMS are most often diagnosed in peri-menopausal women. Many are found incidentally when hysterectomy is carried out for menorrhagia. There are no specific presenting symptoms for LMS. Vaginal bleeding, pain or a pelvic mass may be found. When patients have dysfunctional vaginal bleeding, they may attend a one-stop clinic for trans-vaginal scanning (TVS) and a uterine biopsy, but these may be unhelpful especially if the tumour remains intra-mural. If the diagnosis is suspected pre-operatively, full-body CT scanning must be carried out to assess any potential spread to the lungs and liver. TVS may raise suspicions of an LMS, but is not usually diagnostic.

There are important differences in the ways in which these tumours grow and metastasise with CS tending to have a higher incidence of lymphatic spread and lymph node metastases, whereas LMS are more likely to have early haematogenous spread and the first metastases may well be in the lungs or the liver [9, 11, 12, 17, 18]. While much weight is placed on the important paper by Major et al., other smaller series have suggested higher rates of pelvic and para-aortic lymph node metastases [11–14, 17, 18]. This, therefore, has important implications for the investigations, staging and surgical management of these patients. This article focuses predominantly on the clinical management of the diagnosed patient, and when the diagnosis of a sarcoma is suspected from the initial investigations, it is assumed that full radiological staging with CT and/or MRI of the chest, abdomen and pelvis will be carried out [19]. At present, there would appear to be no justification for routine ^{18}FDG-PET CT; however, where it is readily available, it may be offered. Potentially, it will be valuable in faster growing, aggressive tumours, but it may show false negative in the better differentiated, slower growing variants. There are no tumour markers of proven value as yet.

Unfortunately, many cases are only diagnosed from the pathological sections of the hysterectomy specimen, which will not usually have been planned as a cancer operation. Referral should be made to the local specialist team to advise on further management. A more difficult situation is when the tumour is diagnosed unexpectedly from a myomectomy or hysterectomy specimen in a pre-menopausal woman, with ovarian conservation. There is some debate about whether it is safe to retain the ovaries, but on balance it seems that it is not unreasonable. Ovarian castration may have potential therapeutic effect in the pre-menopausal woman, especially if the tumour is shown to be ER/PR positive. A further point of debate is whether oophorectomy should be offered at time of relapse. The less aggressive tumours with lower mitotic rates are more likely to be ER and/or PR positive [20, 21].

16.4 Pathology

The differential diagnosis of uterine LMS will include a number of conditions. They will range from simple leiomyomas, smooth muscle tumours of unknown malignant potential through to highly aggressive variants. A number of parameters are helpful in assessing risk of recurrence and these include the number of mitoses per 10 HPF (high power fields), ki 67 index, necrosis, cellular atypia and lymphovascular space invasion (LVSI). Expert gynaecological pathology opinion is strongly recommended. Most of these tumours arise in the myometrium, hence they are intramural, and about 50–75% are solitary masses. They may be more haemorrhagic and necrotic as well as be larger than simple leiomyomas which may be recognised at time of surgery and give early warning of a different diagnosis. The table below lists some of the useful differentiating features [2, 3, 5, 7, 11]. The less well-differentiated tumours prove the greatest pathological challenges.

Additionally, tumours are seen with indeterminate appearances; there are features suggestive of a smooth muscle tumour, but without the classical features of an invasive tumours. These tumours have an uncertain behaviour, hence the terminology of a STUMP – smooth muscle tumour of unknown malignant potential. These patients do need more careful follow-up as a small proportion will ultimately relapse [22].

The increased rate of diagnosis around the menopause does raise the possibility of hormonal association, but this is difficult to substantiate. However, some recent data show a new and critical role for the AKT-mTOR pathway [15] in smooth muscle transformation and leiomyosarcoma genesis and support treatment of selected sarcomas by the targeting of this pathway with new compounds or combinations of these with conventional chemotherapy agents (Hernando). Another potential target under investigation is the insulin-like growth receptor (IGFR) with studies under development in several tumour sites including LMS [16].

Leiomyoma	
Degenerating leiomyoma	Conditions that may be confused with leiomyomas
Benign metastasising leiomyoma	
Leiomyomatosispe ritonealis	
Intra-venousl eiomyomatosis	
STUMP	Unpredictable clinical behaviour
LMS	
EpithelioidL MS	
MyxoidL MS	

Alternativedi fferentiation, e.g. myxoid vs. epithelioid
Increasedc ellularity
Marked cytological atypia
Lymph node metastases
Mitotic count – (mitoses per 10 HPF)
Lymphovascular space invasion
Necrosis

16.5 SurgicalManag ement

Many of these tumours will not be recognised preoperatively and thus will be operated on by community gynaecologists because of menstrual symptoms. These tumours are commonly only detected on pathology reporting of a uterus removed for menorrhagia or simple fibroids. Furthermore, in this setting, a simple hysterectomy is likely to have been done, sparing the ovaries and without full staging as would have been done for a cancer. If suspected pre-operatively, the surgical management should involve referral to a specialist Gynaecological Oncology Surgeon for further management. This will allow careful staging procedures to be carried out including discussion of the place of lymphadenectomy; and the surgery should involve a minimum of total abdominal hysterectomy, bilateral salpingo-oophorectomy (this should at least be discussed in pre-menopausal women), careful and thorough inspection of the abdominal and pelvic contents, and sampling of fluid for cytological assessment of the washings [21, 22]. In post-menopausal women, full surgical staging is advised; however, in the younger woman keen to preserve ovaries, there is no evidence to support that conserving the ovaries is detrimental. However, when the diagnosis was not recognised pre-operatively and is only identified at pathological examination, individual discussions will ensue to debate the pros and cons of further surgical intervention, but most experts in the literature do not argue that this is needed given the uncertainties over benefit of lymph node dissection and oophorectomy. It can be argued that because the incidence of lymph node metastases is low, about 4–7% from the Gynaecology Oncology Group (GOG) experience, PLND is predicted to be of limited benefit and most experts do not advocate its use [14, 17, 18]. Nevertheless, if pelvic nodes are seen on imaging, they can be removed and referral should be made to a specialist surgeon; equally if nodes are identified at surgery, attempts should be made to remove them. Other series have suggested high rates of involvement, but these have often had small numbers. The Mayo clinic series of 208 patients indicated 93% had simple hysterectomy only and 36 of the 208 had PLND [14]. Only four of these (11%) had confirmed positive nodes. Other series from Gadducci et al., Chauvenic, Bell et al. and Dinh et al. tend to confirm that incidence of lymph nodes is low, although relatively few underwent lymphadenectomy [3–5, 11–13, 17, 18].

Specialist immunocytochemistry may be a valuable aid in the differential diagnosis of these tumours and the use of relatively simple techniques such as oestrogen and progestagen receptor (ER and PR) staining should also be carried out as this may provide therapeutic as well as prognostic guidance [20, 21]. The differential diagnosis will also include the possibility of a gastro-intestinal stromal tumour (GIST) and assessment for c-kit should be carried out. Other potentially confusing diagnoses include degenerating leiomyomas, leiomyomatosis, benign metastasising leiomyoma and disseminated peritoneal leiomyomatosis. Poorly differentiated sarcomas will additionally cause diagnostic challenges, again emphasising the skills of an expert gynaecological pathologist.

Conditions confused with LMS
Degenerating leiomyomas
Intra-venous leiomyomatosis
Benign metastasising leiomyoma
Disseminated peritoneal leiomyomatosis
ESS with myoinvasion
CS and undifferentiated sarcomas

16.6 Post-OperativeC are

16.6.1 Adjuvant Treatments

In principle, however, there are four main types of treatment that may be considered – radiation therapy, chemotherapy, hormonal therapy and, more recently, the use of biological or molecular-targeted anti-cancer agents. However, it is important to remember that these treatments may be combined or used sequentially. The article will also distinguish between the use of adjuvant treatment and the treatment for recurrent or metastatic disease.

The role of adjuvant treatments in LMS is probably less controversial, mainly because of the lack of evidence, although this has not stopped some from advocating its use!

16.6.2 Radiation Therapy

It should be stated clearly that no randomised trial has shown a survival benefit in uterine LMS. It will be demonstrated that a number of non-randomised studies and reports from large centres suggest improved local control and even a survival benefit, but there is no level one evidence. Local relapse may occur, but is usually associated with the more adverse risk factors, including incomplete local excision and poor prognostic pathological factors; furthermore, local relapse will often occur along with distant metastasis and represents a very poor prognostic sub-group with very shortened life expectancy. These tumours tend to show a pattern of distant metastatic spread with a lower incidence of lymph node metastases in the pelvis; therefore, adjuvant radiation is less likely to offer any benefit [23–32]. Historically, many of the smaller series have suggested an improvement in local control and possibly a survival benefit when adjuvant pelvic external beam radiation (EBRT) is given. However, until recently none of the larger studies has supported this and there is no randomised trial supporting the use of EBRT to the pelvis. The GOG 20 study investigating adjuvant chemotherapy with doxorubicin reported by Hornback et al. allowed use of EBRT, but it did not seem to show any benefit [29]. The large Mayo clinic series also failed to show any benefit. In this study most of the first recurrences in the irradiated patients were outside of the pelvis. A recent large retrospective series from California has suggested a survival benefit with added radiation, but no randomised trial has shown a survival benefit [33].

The only randomised trial to include LMS has been the EORTC 55874 trial [34]. This study compared adjuvant radiation therapy vs. observation in uterine sarcomas. It included 103 LMS; there was a small but non-significant reduction in local failure (22 vs. 26) and no survival advantage. Substantially more patients developed distant failure in the adjuvant radiotherapy arm (27 vs. 16). It has, therefore, been the author's policy to advise that adjuvant radiation should be withheld in women with leiomyosarcoma of the uterus where there has been complete macroscopic removal of tumour. This policy is very distressing as it is recognised that these are often young and middle-aged women with a high risk of relapse and yet we knowingly withhold adjuvant treatment, but there remains no firm evidence to give treatment which has not been shown to be of benefit. New and effective adjuvant treatments are desperately required (Tables 16.2 and 16.3).

Data extracted from EORTC 55874 series for LMS	LMS $n=99$	
	EBRT	Observe
No local recurrence	22	26
Local recurrence only	1	7
Distantme tastases	18	7
Localfollo wedbyd istant	0	2
Distantfollo wedby local	2	3
Simultaneousloc ala nddi stant	7	4
Any local recurrence	10	12
Any distant metastases	27	16

Table16. 2 EORTC558741 ocalc ontrol

Carcinosarcoma local relapse		Leiomyosarcoma local relapse	
EBRT	Obs	EBRT	Obs
39%	53%	56%	47%

Table16. 3 EORTC5 5874s urvival

Survivalye ars	CS	LMS
PFS	6.2	4.9
OS	8.5	6.7

For cases with residual disease following surgery, adjuvant radiation with or without chemotherapy should be considered and discussed at tumour boards on an individual basis. The choice of agents will be discussed in the next section. These tumours have an unpredictable behaviour ranging from highly aggressive to very indolent; some of the most aggressive tumours metastasise and lead to death within 9–18 months and yet paradoxically a further sub-group has a remarkably indolent behaviour where recurrence might take 10–15 years to manifest. These latter tumours have a greater tendency to be ER/PR positive and routine testing for ER/PR status should be considered on the initial hysterectomy specimen so that this can be offered at the appropriate time [20, 21]. Again, it is advised that these patients are considered for long-term follow-up and the case can be made for continuing annual review beyond 10 years in view of this risk. In summary, one cannot advocate any adjuvant therapies in this setting outside a clinical trial or protocol.

There is a sub-group of these tumours sometimes known as STUMP where the mitotic rate is very low; these patients have a low risk of metastatic spread and adjuvant treatment should be withheld [22]. The need for follow-up in these women remains controversial, but the author favours follow-up as a small proportion will relapse. An annual chest radiograph may be advisable, but whether it is reasonable to offer annual CT scanning is unknown and often debated at tumour boards.

16.6.3 Adjuvant Chemotherapy

In this article so far, the role of adjuvant chemotherapy has been covered only briefly [35–37]. Historically, studies have often included both CS and LMS, which has confused the picture [38–49]. Others have extrapolated from the use of chemotherapy in soft tissue sarcomas of other parts [35]. Adjuvant studies have also drawn on the experience in advanced cases, using drugs which have shown efficacy in this setting. A good recent example of this is the development of gemcitabine and docetaxel in the adjuvant setting having been shown to be active in advanced disease [50, 51]. The GOG has carried out a number of adjuvant studies in the 1980s with doxorubicin or ifosfamide [39, 41, 42], and although there was a tendency to reduction in risk of recurrence, the survival benefit was absent. In 1997, Tierney et al., on behalf of the MRC, reviewed adjuvant chemotherapy in all soft tissue sarcomas [36]. There were 264 uterine sarcomas amounting to 17% of the total within the meta-analysis, but again there was no convincing evidence to support the routine use of adjuvant chemotherapy in sarcomas. A further paper from Bramwell showed similar lack of benefit [37]. A recent Italian study which used epirubicin and ifosfamide has generated much interest in that it showed strong benefit for chemotherapy, but these were spindle cell sarcomas of the extremities [35]. We are falling into the trap of comparing apples and oranges! At this point in time, it is probably fair to say that adjuvant chemotherapy remains of unproven benefit in LMS. This is an ideal setting for further clinical studies, with conventional and newer agents. A recent report on adjuvant gemcitabine and docetaxel will be discusseds hortly [50, 51].

Other approaches that have been reported include the combination of adjuvant chemotherapy and radiation. The following have been investigated in both CS and LMS. A phase II study from Pautier, from France, of a mixture of uterine sarcomas looked at three cycles of cisplatin/doxorubicin/ifosfamide followed by external beam radiotherapy and appeared to show a significant benefit compared to historical controlled radiation alone, 76 vs. 43% progression-free survival and 100 vs. 76% 5-year overall survival [52]. A report from an Australian Group by Manolitsas looked at the sandwiched treatment of chemotherapy, radiation and chemotherapy on a background of aggressive surgery and showed 90% of patients are disease free with a combined approach compared to 47% in a group who had no combined modality [53]. However, these are small non-randomised phase II studies and it is difficult to be certain of the real benefit. What is required are well-conducted randomised clinical trials. However, history has shown that these studies, however well-designed, take longer to complete than originally planned! Shortly, we shall address newer options in advanced LMS and clearly these agents need to be incorporated into future clinical studies of adjuvant therapy in LMS.

The most recent paper from Hensley et al. may give a little encouragement [51]. Following on from their earlier papers on docetaxel and gemcitabine in relapsed disease, they treated 25 patients with stage 1–4 completely resected uterine LMS with this schedule. Of the 18 with stage 1 or 2 disease, 59% were progression-free at 2 years. This is quite intensive treatment for a relatively small gain, but represents some progress. The data need validation and should be investigated in a randomised clinical trial. The earlier reference to molecular pathways gives hints that there is potential to develop targeted agents aimed at these pathways. Several potential compounds should be considered fromf uturei nvestigation [15, 16].

In summary, this author is firmly of the view that at the time of writing (in 2009), there is no compelling evidence to support the use of adjuvant chemotherapy or radiation outside the setting of a clinical trial in a patient with no residual disease. International collaboration is needed to achieve these studies. The data from Sloan Kettering on docetaxel and gemcitabine must stillbe c onsideredinte restingb utpre mature [51].

16.7 RecurrentandA dvancedDi sease

This section will deal with patients who have recurrent or metastatic disease, but will also include those patients who present with locally advanced unresectable cancer. The latter make up a small proportion, but remain very challenging in terms of management. It is again vital to stress the significant differences between the different tumour sub-types when it comes to using systemic treatment. Some agents that are active in CS, for example, show minimal activity in LMS and vice versa. As a generalisation, the stromal sarcomas tend to have similar chemo-sensitivity to CS, whereas the highly undifferentiated tumours may show transient chemo-sensitivity, but there is usually a very rapid regrowth of tumour within a short period of time.

16.8 Recurrento rL ocallyA dvanced Leiomyosarcomas

These are very challenging tumours to treat. Firstly, they do have a much more unpredictable behaviour ranging from the highly lethal tumours which can cause death within 1–2 years to a sub-group where there is a much delayed late pattern of relapse. Surgical discussion should be considered in cases with apparently isolated relapse; this has been reviewed by Giuntoli et al. and demonstrates that selective re-operation can be highly effective [54]. This approach is best discussed at tumour boards, but in selective cases can be very rewarding. Detailed imaging and review will help to optimise this approach.

16.8.1 Hormonal Therapies

These latter tumours are sometimes strongly ER and/or PR positive and this should be checked on the initial specimen and any biopsy from recurrent tissue where possible. The use of hormonal therapy in appropriate patients will clearly be determined by the ER/PR positivity and clinical status [20, 21]. Prognostic risk factors include the number of mitoses per 10 HPF, necrosis, LVSI and tumour grade. Fewer than 10 mitoses per HPF is usually a low risk, whereas when there are more than 20 mitoses per 10 HPF, it is more predictable that there will be an early pattern of relapse and a more aggressive behaviour. At present, there is no proven benefit for adjuvant treatment in the early setting, and therefore, hormones and chemotherapy are usually conserved until relapse and the features described above are taken into account. One final point is to ensure that the tumour is not a GIST and appropriate immunocytochemical analysis for c-kit and other markers should be carried out as these tumours are treated in a very different way.

16.8.2 Chemotherapy

Most of the published trial data has come from the GOG. The GOG has investigated a number of agents through a series of phase II and III studies dating back to the early 1980s. Single agent drugs with demonstrated activity include doxorubicin, ifosfamide and dacarbazine, and older data would indicate between 17–25% response rates [38–46]. Cisplatin has less than 10% response rate [43, 44]. Omura et al. studied doxorubicin with or without dacarbazine in women with advanced or metastatic uterine sarcomas and reported response rates of 30 and 25%, respectively, among women with LMS. The activity of doxorubicin was confirmed in a subsequent phase III study by the GOG [39]. Muss et al. reported doxorubicin alone or in combination with cyclophosphamide administered to patients with advanced uterine sarcomas [41]. Twenty three patients with LMS were evaluable for response and three partial responses (response rate 13%) were observed. Lorigan et al. reported from the EORTC study of all types of STS in which doxorubicin was compared to ifosfamide in two different schedules and showed no significant difference in outcome between the two schedules [55]. Doxorubicin (Adriamycin) has consistently been shown to be the most active agent in older drug trials (Table 16.4).

Other drugs have been investigated; cisplatin was found to be an inactive drug in LMS [43, 44]; topotecan is another inactive agent in LMS [49]. In a phase II study of ifosfamide, 17.2% patients responded, while in a subsequent study, ifosfamide and doxorubicin were combined to yield a 30.3% response rate. Paclitaxel produced a response rate of 12% in another GOG trial [48, 54]. Gemcitabine has been one of the few agents with activity in these tumours with an observed response rate of 20.5% [56]. Hensley et al. combined gemcitabine with docetaxel and reported a response rate of 53% in 34 patients, some of whom hadf aileddoxorubic inthe rapy [50].

Table16. 4 Single-agent activity in different types of uterine sarcomas

Single-agenta ctivity			
Singlea gent	Responser ate(%)	Histologicalt ype	References
Doxorubicin	16	Any	Omurae ta l. [39]
Doxorubicin	19	Any	Musse ta l. [41]
Cisplatin	3	LMS	Thigpene ta l. [43, 44]
Ifosfamide	17	LMS	Suttone ta l. [42, 45]
Paclitaxel	9	LMS	Suttone ta l. [48]
Paclitaxel	8	LMS	Gallupe ta l. [54]
Topotecan	11	LMS	Millere ta l. [49]

Table16. 5 Response rates for different combination regimens in uterine sarcoma

Combination	Responser ate(%)	Histologicalt ype	References
Vincristine/actinomycin/ cyclophosphamide	26	All Ut sarc	Hannigan [40]
Doxorubicin/dacarbazine	24	All Ut sarc	Omura [39]
Doxorubicin/cyclophosphamide	19	All Ut sarc	Musse ta l. [41]
Doxorubicin/ifosfamide	30	LMS	Suttone ta l. [46]
Doxorubicin/ifosfamide	55	LMS	Leyvraze ta l. [47, 57]
Mitomycin/doxorubicin/cisplatin	23	LMS	Edmonsone ta l. [58]
Docetaxel/gemcitabine	53	LMS	Hensleye ta l. [50, 51]

16.8.3 Combination Therapy

Combining ifosfamide and doxorubicin increases the response rate to 30%, but overall survival was relatively short in these patients, usually between 9 and 12 months [47, 57]. Following from their previous study [55], the current EORTC trial 62012 is comparing single agent doxorubicin with doxorubicin plus ifosfamide and continues to recruit. This will be important as being able to withhold ifosfamide has many advantages, given its high toxicity and need for in-patient stay.

Sutton, on behalf of the GOG, reported on doxorubicin and ifosfamide with a 30% response rate in 33 patients, whereas Leyvraz et al., using the higher dose, achieved a 55% response in 17 patients, but use of growth factors was routinely given [47, 57], although a later follow-up report suggested only 48% response rate. Other combinations have added in methotrexate and etoposide, but again generally without great benefit. Single agent paclitaxel and topotecan have been very disappointing inute rineLM S [48, 49, 54].

Because of preliminary observations favouring the use of mitomycin, doxorubicin and cisplatin (MAP) chemotherapy in LMS, the GOG investigated this combination [58], but they demonstrated only moderate activity with 9% achieving a CR and 14% receiving a PR, giving an overall response rate of 23%.

All of this was relatively disappointing; however, a report from Sloan Kettering Hospital attracted interest using docetaxel and gemcitabine, including previously treated patients with a 53% response rate in 34 patients, 29 of whom had LMS [50, 51]. Neither drug individually had shown particularly high activity, but somewhat surprisingly when combined produced superior response rates indicating some form of synergy. This schedule is quite toxic and may require the use of growth factors, but nevertheless does hold promise for new combinations. Reference has already been made to the use of this combination as an adjuvant in completely resected disease stages 1 through to 4. For the future, there is considerable excitement in trabectedin (Yondelis); this has recently been reported and shows very promising results and gained EMEA approval in 2009 [59, 60]. Again, new targeted agents would be worthy of further investigation and a number of clinical trials are underway which will evaluate their benefit (Table 16.5).

16.8.4 Targeted Agents

New agents are desperately called for and the recent paper suggesting the involvement of the mTOR/AKT pathway offers clues to the potential use of this class of agents and clinical trials are underway to evaluate this as well as IGFR receptor antagonists [15, 16]. By the time this chapter is published, it is likely that it will be obsolete given the recent speed of progress.

In summary, at present, for metastatic disease single agent doxorubicin remains the treatment of choice in patients with advanced soft tissue sarcoma. Adding in ifosfamide for relapse may be considered as second line, but an alternative would be to switch to the Sloan Kettering schedule of docetaxel and gemcitabine. Newer drugs like trabectedin hold promise, but remain unproven and are not readily available yet.

16.9 LungMet astases

In some circumstances where there is a slowly growing tumour with isolated or clustered lesions in one lobe of lung or liver, pulmonary or hepatic metastasectomy may be considered. Multi-disciplinary discussion is required with expert teams in these situations [61–63]. Repeated procedures over a number of years may be attempted. Newer video assisted or laparoscopic techniques have made this simpler and safer. Radiofrequency ablation (RFA) may also be deployed in this setting [64].

16.10 Clinical Trials

Given the relative rarity of many of these tumours, it is important that we do drive standards up and one of the most important ways is to carry out clinical trials. It is strongly recommended that these tumours, where possible, should be recorded on regional or national databases so that we can learn more about them, not only both in terms of their clinical behaviour and their response to treatment, but also translational research. The author strongly believes that these tumours should not be managed by clinicians working in isolation and these are well-suited to be managed by the supra-regional networks. Their rarity makes them well-suited for this approach. It will also allow more intelligence and information about these tumours and this can only be viewed as a positive development. International collaborative groups like Gynaecological Cancer Inter Group (GCIG) and European Network of Gynaecological Oncology Trialists (ENGOT) may be able to facilitate trial development, but industry support is needed, especially in Europe, to deal with the issues of both financial and legal sponsorship and the EU clinical trials directive.

16.11 Conclusions

Uterine sarcomas are relatively uncommon tumours and LMS account for about 1–3% of uterine cancers. The only curative treatment remains surgical by hysterectomy with or without bilateral salpingo-oophorectomy, although pelvic lymph node dissection remains unproven. At present, there is no convincing data to support the use of adjuvant pelvic radiation treatment when there has been complete macroscopic removal. LMS are different tumours with different pattern of spread and different chemo-sensitivity. It is, therefore, essential that they are treated with a different approach. There is no evidence at all to support the use of adjuvant drug treatment in these patients and sadly one has to watch and wait until they relapse before treatment may be administered. There are promising new schedules becoming available for LMS and there remains the exciting potential of targeted anti-cancer agents.

References

1. Brooks SE, Zhan M, Baquet C. Surveillance, epidemiology, and end results analysis of 2677 cases of uterine sarcoma 1989–1999. Gynecol Oncol. 2004;93:204–8.
2. Hendrickson M, Longacre T, Kempson R. Pathology of uterine sarcomas. In: Coukos G, Rubin SC, editors. Cancers of uterus. New York: Marcel Dekker; 2005. p. 149–95.
3. Dinh TA, Woodruff JD. Leiomyosarcoma of the uterus. Am J Obstet Gynecol. 1982;144:817–23.
4. Dinh TA, Oliva EA, Fuller AF, Lee H, Goodman A. The treatment of uterine leiomyosarcoma. Results from a 10 year experience (1990–1999) at Massachusetts General Hospital. Gynecol Oncol. 2004;92:648–52.
5. Bell SW, Kempson RL, Hendrickson MR. Problematic uterine smooth muscle neoplasms: a clinicopathological study of 213 cases. Am J Surg Pathol. 1994;18:535–58.
6. Leibsohn S, d'Ablaing G, Misell DR, Schlaerth JB. Leiomyosarcoma in a series of hysterectomies performed for presumed uterine leiomyomas. Am J Obstet Gynecol. 1990;162:968–74.
7. Evans HL, Chawla SP, Simpson C, Finn KP. Smooth muscle neoplasms of the uterus other than ordinary leiomyoma. A study of 46 cases with emphasis on diagnostic criteria and prognostic factors. Cancer. 1988;62:2239–47.
8. Schwartz LB, Diamond MP, Schwartz MP. Leiomyosarcomas: clinical presentation. Am J Obstet Gynecol. 1993;168:180–3.
9. Major FJ, Blessing JA, Silverberg SG, Morrow CP, Creasman WT, Currie JL, et al. Prognostic factors in early-stage uterine sarcoma. A Gynecologic Oncology Group study. Cancer. 1993;71:1702–9.
10. Henson DE, Schwartz AM, Tilara A, Grimley PM, Anderson WF. Population-based analysis of pathologic data: a new approach to the investigation of uterine endometrial and ovarian endometrioid carcinomas. Arch Pathol Lab Med. 2007;131(9):1337–42.
11. Yamada D, Burger R, Brewster W, et al. Pathologic variables and adjuvant therapy as predictors of recurrence and survival for patients with surgically evaluated carcinosarcoma of the uterus. Cancer. 2000;88:2782–6.

12. George M, Pejovic MH, Kramar A, Gynecologic Cooperating Group of French Oncology Centers. Uterine sarcomas: prognostic factors and treatment modalities-study on 209 patients. Gynecol Oncol. 1986;24:58–67.
13. Gadducci A, Sartori E, Landoni F, Zola P, Maggino T, Cosio S, et al. The prognostic relevance of histological type in uterine sarcomas: a Cooperation Task Force (CTF) multivariate analysis of 249 cases. Eur J Gynaecol Oncol. 2002;23(4): 295–9.
14. Giuntoli RL, Metzinger D, DiMarco C, et al. Retrospective review of 208 patients with leiomyosarcoma of the uterus: prognostic indicators, surgical management and adjuvant therapy. Gynecol Oncol. 2003;89:460–9.
15. Hernando H, Charytonowicz E, Dudas ME, Menendez S, et al. The AKT-mTOR pathway plays a critical role in the development of leiomyosarcomas. Nat Med. 2007;13: 748–53.
16. Garber K. IGF-1: old growth factor shines as new drug target. J Natl Cancer Inst. 2005;97(11):790–2.
17. Goff BA, Rice LW, Fleischhacker D, et al. Uterine leiomyosarcoma and endometrial stromal sarcoma: lymph node metastases and sites of recurrence. Gynecol Oncol. 1993;50:105–9.
18. Amant F. The rationale for comprehensive surgical staging in endometrial carcinosarcoma. Gynecol Oncol. 2005;99(2): 521–2.
19. Cornfeld D, Israel G, Martel M, Weinreb J, Schwartz P, McCarthy S. MRI appearance of mesenchymal tumors of the uterus. Eur J Radiol. 2009 Apr 4.
20. Sutton GP, Stehman FB, Michael H, Young PC, Ehrlich CE. Estrogen and progesterone receptors in uterine sarcomas. Obstet Gynecol. 1986;68:709–14.
21. Ioffe YJ, Li AJ, Walsh CS, Karlan BY, Leuchter R, Forscher C, et al. Hormone receptor expression in uterine sarcomas: prognostic and therapeutic roles. Gynecol Oncol. 2009; 115(3):466–71.
22. Guntupalli SK, Ramirez PT, Anderson ML, Milam MR, Bodurka DC, Malpica A. Uterine smooth muscle tumour of uncertain malignant potential: a retrospective analysis. Gynecol Oncol. 2009;113(3):324–6.
23. Edwards CL. Undifferentiated tumours. In: Cancer of uterus and ovary. Chicago: Year Book, Medical; 1969. p. 84–94.
24. Badib AO, Vongtama V, Kurohara SS, Webster JH. Radiotherapy in the treatment of sarcomas of the corpus uteri. Cancer. 1969;24:724–9.
25. Belgrad R, Elbadawi N, Rubin P. Uterine sarcoma. Radiology. 1975;144(1):181–8.
26. Salazar O, Bonfiglio TK, Patten SF, Kellser BE, Feldstein ME, Dunne ME, et al. Uterine sarcomas: natural history, treatment and prognosis. Cancer. 1978;42:1152–60.
27. Salazar OM, Bonfiglio TA, Patten SF, Keller BE, Feldstein ML, Dunne ME, et al. Uterine sarcomas. Analysis of failures with special emphasis on the use of adjuvant radiotherapy. Cancer.19 78;42:1161–70.
28. Sorbe B. Radiotherapy and/or chemotherapy as adjuvant treatment of uterine sarcomas. Gynecol Oncol. 1985;20:281–9.
29. Hornback NB, Omura G, Major FJ. Observations on the use of adjuvant radiation therapy in patients with stage I and II uterine sarcoma. Int J Radiat Oncol Biol Phys. 1986;12(12): 2127–30.
30. Le T. Adjuvant pelvic radiotherapy for uterine carcinosarcoma in a high risk population. Eur J Surg Oncol. 2001;27(3):282–5.
31. Chi DS, Mychalczak B, Saigo PE, Rescigno J, Brown CL. The role of whole pelvic irradiation in the treatment of early-stage uterine carcinosarcoma. Gynecol Oncol. 1997;65:493–8.
32. Dusenbery KE, Potish RA, Agenta PA, et al. On the apparent failure of adjuvant pelvic radiotherapy to improve survival for women with uterine sarcomas confined to the uterus. Am J Clin Oncol. 2005;28:295–300.
33. Mahdavi A, Monk BJ, Ragazzo J, Hunter MI, Lentz SE, Vasilev SA, et al. Pelvic radiation improves local control after hysterectomy for uterine leiomyosarcoma: a 20-year experience. Int J Gynecol Cancer. 2009;19(6):1080–4.
34. Reed NS, Mangioni C, Malmstrom H, et al. First results of a randomised trial comparing radiotherapy versus – observation post operatively in patients with uterine sarcomas, an EORTC-GCG study. ESGO Congress. Int J Gyn Cancer. 2003;13 Suppl 1:4 (Abstr. PL12).
35. Frustaci S, Gherlinzoni F, De Paoli A, Bonetti M, Azzarelli A, Comandone A, et al. Adjuvant chemotherapy for adult soft tissue sarcomas of the extremities and girdles: results of the Italian randomized cooperative trial. J Clin Oncol. 2001;19:1238–47.
36. Tierney JF, Mosseri V, Stewart LA, Souhami R, Parmar MK. Adjuvant chemotherapy for soft-tissue sarcoma: review and meta-analysis of the published results of randomised clinical trials. Br J Cancer. 1995;72(2):469–75.
37. Bramwell VHC. Adjuvant chemotherapy for adult soft tissue sarcoma. Is there a standard of care? J Clin Oncol. 2001; 19:1235–7.
38. Kanjeeka S, Chambers A, Kee Fung MF, Verma S, on behalf of the Cancer Care Ontario Practice Guidelines Initiative Gynecology. Cancer Disease Site Group Program in Evidence-based Care, Cancer Care Ontario, Canada. Systemic therapy for advanced uterine sarcoma: a systematic review of the literature. Gynecol Oncol. 2005;97:624–37.
39. Omura GA, Major FJ, Blessing JA, Sedlacek TV, Thigpen JT, Creasman WT, et al. A randomized study of adriamycin with and without dimethyl triazenoimidazole carboxamide in advanced uterine sarcomas. Cancer. 1983;52:626–32.
40. Hannigan EV, Elder KW, Rutledge FN. Treatment of advanced uterine sarcoma with vincristine, actinomycin D and cyclophosphamide. Gynecol Oncol. 1983;15:224–9.
41. Muss H, Omura GA, Blessing JA, Major FJ, Lifshitz S, Mangan C, et al. A randomized clinical trial of adjuvant adriamycin in uterine sarcomas: a Gynecologic Oncology Group study. J Clin Oncol. 1985;3:1240–5.
42. Sutton GP, Blessing JA, Rosenshein N, Photopoulos G, DiSaia PJ. Phase II trial of ifosfamide and mesna in mixed mesodermal tumors of the uterus (a Gynecologic Oncology Group study). Am J Obstet Gynecol. 1989;161:309–15.
43. Thigpen T, Blessing JA, Wilbanks GD. Cisplatin as second-line therapy in the treatment of patients with advanced or recurrent leiomyosarcoma of the uterus. A phase II trial of the gynecologic oncology group. Am J Clin Oncol. 1986;9: 18–20.
44. Thigpen JT, Blessing JA, Beecham J, Homesley H, Yordan E. Phase II trial of cisplatin as first-line chemotherapy in patients with advanced or recurrent uterine sarcomas: a Gynecologic Oncology Group study. J Clin Oncol. 1991;9:1962–6.
45. Sutton GP, Blessing JA, Barrett RJ, McGehee R. Phase II trial of ifosfamide and mesna in leiomyosarcoma of the uterus: a Gynecologic Oncology Group study. Am J Obstet Gynecol.1992; 166:556–9.

46. Sutton GP, Blessing JA, Malfetano JH. Ifosfamide and doxorubicin in the treatment of advanced leiomyosarcomas of the uterus: a Gynecologic Oncology Group study. Gynecol Oncol.1996;62:226 –9.
47. Leyvraz S, Bacchi M, Lissoni A, Sessa C, Cerny T, Honegger HP. High response rate with the combination of high-dose ifosfamide and doxorubicin for the treatment of advanced gynecologic sarcomas. Proc Am Soc Clin Oncol. 1998;17:354a (Abstr).
48. Sutton G, Blessing JA, Ball H. Phase II trial of paclitaxel in leiomyosarcoma of the uterus: a Gynecologic Oncology Group study. Gynecol Oncol. 1999;74:346–9.
49. Miller DS, Blessing JA, Kilgore LC, Mannel R, Van Le L. Phase II trial of topotecan in patients with advanced, persistent or recurrent uterine leiomyosarcomas: a Gynecologic Oncology Group study. Am J Clin Oncol. 2000;23:355–7.
50. Hensley ML, Maki R, Venkatraman E, Geller G, Lovegren M, Aghajanian C, et al. Gemcitabine and docetaxel in patients with unresectable leiomyosarcoma: results of a phase II trial. J Clin Oncol. 2002;12:2824–31.
51. Hensley ML, Ishill N, Soslow R, et al. Adjuvant gemcitabine plus docetaxel for completely resected stages I-IV high grade uterine leiomyosarcoma. Results of a prospective study. Gynecol Oncol. 2009;112(3):563–7.
52. Pautier P, Rey A, Haie-Meder C, et al. Adjuvant chemotherapy with cisplatin, ifosfamide, and doxorubicin followed by radiotherapy in localised uterine sarcomas: results of a case-controlled study with radiotherapy alone. Int J Gynecol Cancer.20 04;14:1112–7.
53. Manolitsas TP, Wain GV, Williams K, et al. Multimodality therapy for patients with clinical stage I and II malignant mixed Mullerian tumors of the uterus. Cancer. 2001;91: 1437–43.
54. Gallup DG, Blessing JA, Andersen W, Morgan MA. Evaluation of paclitaxel in previously treated leiomyosarcoma of the uterus: a gynecologic oncology group study. Gynecol Oncol. 2003;89:48–51.
55. Lorigan P, Verweij J, Papai Z, et al. Phase III trial of two investigational schedules of ifosfamide compared with standard-dose doxorubicin in advanced or metastatic soft tissue sarcoma: a European Organisation for Research and Treatment of Cancer Soft Tissue and Bone Sarcoma Group Study. J Clin Oncol. 2007;25(21):3144–50.
56. Look KY, Sandler A, Blessing JA, Lucci III JA, Rose PG. Phase II trial of gemcitabine as second-line chemotherapy of uterine leiomyosarcoma: a gynecologic oncology group (GOG) study. Gynecol Oncol. 2004;92:644–7.
57. Leyvraz S, Zweifel M, Jundt G, Lissoni A, Cerny T, Sessa C, et al. Long-term results of a multicenter SAKK trial on high-dose ifosfamide and doxorubicin in advanced or metastatic gynecologic sarcomas. Ann Oncol. 2006;17:646–51.
58. Edmonson JH, Blessing JA, Cosin JA, Miller DS, Cohn DE, Rotmensch J. Phase II study of mitomycin, doxorubicin, and cisplatin in the treatment of advanced uterine leiomyosarcoma: a Gynecologic Oncology Group study. Gynecol Oncol.2002; :507–10.
59. Schoffski P, Wolter P, Clement P, Sciot R, De Wever I, Wozniak A, et al. Trabectedin (ET-743): evaluation of its use in advanced soft-tissue sarcoma. Future Oncol. 2007;3(4): 381–92.
60. Amant F, Coosemans A, Renard V, Everaert E, Vergote I. Clinical outcome of ET-743 (Trabectedin; Yondelis) in high-grade uterine sarcomas: report on five patients and a review of the literature. Int J Gynecol Cancer. 2009;19(2): 245–8.
61. Levenback C, Rubin SC, McCormack PM, et al. Resection of pulmonary metastases from uterine sarcomas. Gynecol Oncol.1992; 45:202–5.
62. Leitao MM, Brennan MF, Hensley M, et al. Surgical resection of pulmonary and extrapulmonary recurrences of uterine leiomyosarcoma. Gynecol Oncol. 2002;87:287–94.
63. Mountain CF, McMurtrey MJ, Hermes KE. Surgery for pulmonary metastasis: a 20-year experience. Ann Thorac Surg. 1984;38:323–30.
64. Gillams AR, Lees WR. Radiofrequency ablation of lung metastases: factors influencing success. Eur Radiol. 2008; 18(4):672–7.
65. Giuntoli II RL, Garrett-Mayer E, Bristow RE, Gostout BS. Secondary cytoreduction in the management of recurrent uterine leiomyosarcoma. Gynecol Oncol. 2007;106(1):82–8.

MucinousT umourso ft heU terineC orpus

17

Nicholas Reed

Mucinous tumours can arise in the uterus but are uncommon and account for less than 5% in most series. It is said that they may account for between 1 and 9% of uterine cancer, the percentage being higher where there are mixed tumours with mucinous and other cell types but mucinous predominates. Pure mucinous tumours are far less common and probably do represent around 1%. The differential diagnoses will include an endocervical tumour or metastatic deposits from a gastrointestinal tumour or ovarian mucinous tumour. There are similarities to mucinous endocervical tumours. Rare primary mucinous tumours do exist and may have a signet ring appearance. This again may add to the confusion with metastatic disease. Once again the importance of access to experienced pathologists is critical [1–11].

17.1 Presentation

Most present in the classical way with post-menopausal bleeding. The usual ages of presentation are 45–60 years and they are usually considered along with the type 1 endometrial cancer [2, 3]. Some experts believe they are even a variant of endometrioid endometrial carcinoma. This is supported by there being a history of prior oestrogen exposure, in up to 40% in some series. The initial investigations will be as for any woman presenting with post-menopausal bleeding. It may be difficult to recognise a mucinous tumour from the initial diagnostic sample, and therefore, the final pathology will only be determined once hysterectomya nds tagingha sbe enc arriedout [5–9].

N.R eed
BeatsonO ncologyC entre, GartnavelG eneralH ospital, 1053 GreatW esternR oad, Glasgow, ScotlandG 120Y N, UK
e-mail:nic k.reed@ggc.scot.nhs.uk

17.2 SurgicalManag ement

Since they are often thought to be "low risk" tumours on initial investigations, many will be operated on by community gynaecologists and thus undergo total hysterectomy, bilateral salpingo-oophorectomy and washings. It is unlikely that nodal sampling or dissection will be done as a routine. The importance of immunocytochemistry to confirm the diagnosis and to exclude metastatic disease is highly relevant. It is usually stated that to be recognised as a mucinous variant, at least 50% of the cell population should contain intracytoplasmic mucin. Given their relatively low risk of aggressive behaviour, there seems little reason to recommend a more aggressive surgical approach.

17.3 Post-OperativeManag ement

Because of their uncommonness, there is little evidence-based literature to support the use of adjuvant treatments. Given their low-risk behaviour, it is probably reasonable to withhold re-operating to remove the pelvic nodes. We can extrapolate from other endometrial carcinomas and use the same kind of risk criteria to assist in recommending any adjuvant treatment. These patients should be discussed at the local tumour board or multidisciplinary team meeting so that the benefit of additional expert advice can be offered. The consensus view is that they behave like endometrioid endometrial carcinomas, and most are surgical stage

N. Reed et al. (eds.), *Rare and Uncommon Gynecological Cancers*,
DOI: 10.1007/978-3-642-13492-0_17,

1 and have minimally invasive features together with low-grade pathology and so fall into low-risk groups. Therefore, on these grounds it will usually be advised to omit any adjuvant treatment. This decision will need to be taken on an individual basis and should be part of the tumour board discussions.

Adjuvant radiation treatment would probably only be considered if the tumour is incompletely excised and there remains residual disease in the pelvis. There are no real data on the role of chemotherapy; so the dilemma is whether to treat as a standard endometrioid endometrial cancer or whether schedules used for mucinous gastrointestinal tumours might have advantages. The standard options would lie between cisplatin and doxorubicin or carboplatin and paclitaxel. Alternatively the concept is being investigated by several international gynaecological trial groups where carboplatin and paclitaxel are being compared to oxaliplatin and capecitabine. Given the rarity of mucinous tumours of the endometrium, it is unlikely that any prospective randomised trials will ever be developed but at least they should be registered locally, if not nationally, so that a true estimate of their frequency maybe a chieved.

References

1. Tiltman AJ. Mucinous carcinoma of the endometrium. Obstet Gynecol. 1980;55:244–7.
2. DiSaia PJ, Creasman WT. Clinical gynecologic oncology. 6th ed. St. Louis: Mosby; 2002.
3. Acharya S, Hensley ML, Montag AC, et al. Rare uterine cancers. Lancet Oncol. 2005;6(12):961–71.
4. Creasman WT, Odicino F, Maisonneuve P, et al. Carcinoma of the corpus uteri: FIGO 6th Annual Report on the Results of Treatment in Gynecological Cancer. Int J Gynaecol Obstet. 2006;95 Suppl 1:S105–43.
5. Ross JC, Eifel PJ, Cox RS, Kempson RL, Hendrickson MR. Primary mucinous adenocarcinoma of the endometrium. A clinicopathologic and histochemical study. Am J Surg Pathol. 1983;7:715–29.
6. Park KJ, Bramlage MP, Ellenson LH, Pirog EC. Immunoprofile of adenocarcinomas of endometrium, endocervix and ovary with mucinous differentiation. Appl Immunohistochem Mol Morphol. 2009;17(1):8–11.
7. Giordano G, D'Adda T, Gnetti L, et al. Endometrial mucinous microglandular adenocarcinoma: morphologic, immunohistochemical features, and emphasis in the human papillomavirus status. Int J Gynecol Pathol. 2006;25(1): 77–82.
8. Mendivil A, Schuler KM, Gehrig P. Non-endometrioid adenocarcinoma of uterine corpus: a review of selected histological subtypes. Cancer Control. 2009;16(1):46–52A.
9. McMeekin DS, Filiaci VL, Thigpen JT, Gallion HH, Fleming GF, Rodgers WH. The relationship between histology and outcome in advanced and recurrent endometrial cancer patients participating in first-line chemotherapy trials: A Gynecologic Oncology Group study. Gynecol Oncol. 2007;106:16–22.
10. Young RH. From krukenberg to today: the ever present problems posed by metastatic tumors in the ovary part I. Historical perspective, general principles, mucinous tumors including the krukenberg tumor. Adv Anat Pathol. 2006;13:205–27.
11. Young RH. From krukenberg to today: the ever present problems posed by metastatic tumors in the ovary part II. Historical perspective, general principles, mucinous tumors including the krukenberg tumor. Adv Anat Pathol. 2007;14:149–77.

18 Clear Cell Cancers of Uterus

Nicholas Reed

18.1 Incidence and Epidemiology

Clear cell cancers (CCC) of the endometrium are uncommon, accounting for between 1 and 5% of all endometrial cancers. They usually occur in the older age group and tend to have features more consistent with type II endometrial cancer [1–5]. Thus they may not have the classically associated history of obesity, diabetes or exogenous oestrogen exposure.

18.2 Clinical Presentation

They most typically present with post menopausal bleeding but do not usually share the characteristics of type 1 endometrioid endometrial cancer with obesity, diabetes and hypertension. They usually occur in an older age group.

18.3 Imaging and Diagnostic Work Up

Post-menopausal bleeding is the usual mode of presentation, and referral for gynaecological assessment is made, increasingly to a one-stop clinic where trans-vaginal scan (TVS) and Pipelle or endometrial biopsy are undertaken [6, 7]. When a CCC is diagnosed, referral should be made to a surgical gynaecological oncologist to assess fitness for surgery including lymphadenectomy. Serum tumours markers have not been proven to be of value at present. Imaging may be helpful to assess extent of myometrial invasion and presence of lymph node metastases in pelvis, but para-aortic nodes should also be imaged. As with serous endometrial cancers (SEC), there is a significantly higher risk of extra-uterine spread even when there is limited myometrial invasion; this may be omental infiltration or pelvic and/or para-aortic lymph node infiltration. For a fuller discussion the reader is referred to the chapter on imaging. The choice of imaging test may depend on local availability; however, MR scanning is generally better at showing endometrial and myometrial infiltration but CT scanning will be better at looking for upper abdominal lymphadenopathy. More recently, newer techniques such as ^{18}F-PET CT, where available, may be considered an alternative option. This may also help in the planning of the surgical procedure. Another technique under development is MR imaging with ultra-small iron oxide particles (USPIO), which has the potential to identify early nodal invasion. To date sentinel lymph node assessment has yet to establish a role in endometrial cancer. [7–10]. The reasons for this more extended imaging protocol are discussed later but reflect the fact that like serous cancers, CCC can show high levels of extra-uterine disease whilst having minimal myometrial disease.

18.4 Pathology

Clear cell carcinomas are so named as they have clear cytoplasm; this is due to the presence of glycogen in the cell. Commonly, there is a mixed pattern with serous and/or endometrioid elements. The distinctive hobnail appearance is seen when cells have discharged the glycogen and lost the cytoplasm leaving a "naked" nucleus. Nuclear atypia and frequent mitoses are common

N. Reed
Beatson Oncology Centre, Gartnavel General Hospital, 1053 Great Western Road, Glasgow G12 0YN, Scotland, UK
e-mail: nick.reed@ggc.scot.nhs.uk

N. Reed et al. (eds.), *Rare and Uncommon Gynecological Cancers*,
DOI: 10.1007/978-3-642-13492-0_18,

Table 18.1 Comparison of molecular markers in CCC uterus

	CCC	SEC
P53	Low/negative	Positive
ER/PR	Low/negative	Low/negative
Ki67	High	High
PTEN	Intermediate	Low/rare

features. Many of the published series have lumped CCC together with serous endometrial carcinomas (SEC) because of several common features of their behaviour [11–18]. Whilst there are some strong similarities between the pattern of spread and clinical behaviour of uterine serous cancers, there are important differences in their molecular biology. P53 for example is usually negative but these tumours do have a high ki67 index. There is often loss of PTEN, which is unusual in endometrioid endometrial cancers. ER and PR status is usually negative [2, 3, 19] (Table 18.1).

More than three quarters will show deep myometrial invasion and at least 25% will show lymphovascular space invasion. Forty percent will have extra-uterine spread at the time of initial diagnosis but as with uterine serous cancers, the depth of invasion does not necessarily correlate with the presence of extra-uterine disease. One series reported 17% lymph node metastases. Occasional patients may have disease confined to a polyp and stage 1 patients do carry a better prognosis [11–18, 20]. Mixed tumours are common with both endometrioid and serous components, but there is as yet no consistent approach to define what percentage of clear cell component is needed to call it a CCC or a mixed tumour. Some series have used 10, 2 or 50% as the necessary minimum, but international consensus would be desirable for consistency. This is discussed in the pathology chapter. The GOG pathology committee has proposed that at least 50% of a tumour must contain clear cell elements. This consistency in reporting may help to allow international comparisons.

18.5 SurgicalA ssessment and Management

When a localised CCC is recognised at the initial assessment, referral should be discussed with a surgical gynaecological oncologist for the definitive procedure. There is a strong belief that these CCCs should be treated in a different manner from endometrioid endometrial cancer. There is no doubting that the overall survival for these tumours is lower than for endometrioid cancers [20–23]. This different pattern of spread must be taken into account when planning the surgical procedure. They are more aggressive in their clinical behaviour and there is a greater risk that they may be associated with extra-uterine spread at the time of presentation and as already stressed, more than three quarters will show myometrial invasion and at least 25% will show lymphovascular space invasion. Over 40% will have extra-uterine spread at the time of initial diagnosis but as with uterine serous cancers, the depth of invasion does not necessarily correlate with the presence of extra-uterine disease. Lymph node metastases are more common, occurring in up to 17% [18]. Occasional patients may have disease confined to a polyp and if confirmed as stage 1 they carry a much better prognosis [20–30].

The recent review by Thomas [28, 29] combining the experience from two major centres is the largest reported clinical series with 99 patients. Sixty-nine patients (70%) were thought to have optimal cytoreduction with no macroscopic residual disease and yet, after pathological analysis, only 33 (48%) were confirmed as stage 1. Of the 36, 21 had occult cervical involvement, 12 had lymphatic dissemination and seven had positive peritoneal cytology. This nicely summarises the problems of a tumour which can "silently" involve other organs. Other series have shown similar patterns of spread [22, 23, 25–30].

The clinical behaviour of CCC and SEC justify a different approach surgically. Given the risks of occult extra-uterine disease, when the initial diagnostic workup suggests a clear cell carcinoma, comprehensive surgical staging should include hysterectomy, bilateral salpingo-oophorectomy and omentectomy and the taking of peritoneal washings as standard practice, plus pelvic lymphadenectomy (PLND). There is no level 1 evidence to support this but a number of surgical series have confirmed the risks of nodal spread even with "early" myometrial infiltration [11–18, 24]. An assessment of the para-aortic nodes should be included as part of the staging operation. Some experts advocate that para-aortic sampling with frozen section or para-aortic node dissection (PAND) should be carried out initially to help plan the remainder of the operation. When extensive para-aortic disease is present, there remains some controversy as to whether the procedure should be completed or abandoned and chemotherapy initiated and a later attempt made at surgical debulking.

There is further debate about what to do if there is significant extra-pelvic disease where maximal cytoreduction cannot be achieved. This is discussed late in this section. Thomas reported a significant difference in progression-free survival of 17 vs. 7 months for those in whom optimal surgery could not be achieved [28, 29]. Overall survival was 40 vs. 18 months. Other series have suggested that a maximal debulking effort should be attempted [22, 26–29, 31]. Neo-adjuvant chemotherapy is not yet considered a standard of care in endometrial cancers but is currently being explored in a number of centres. There is increasing interest in the use of neo-adjuvant chemotherapy in locally advanced unresectable endometrial cancer to try and reduce tumour volume and make a delayed primary procedure more effective. This concept has now been shown to be safe in ovarian cancer in a large EORTC-GCG study [32] and has been reported by the Flemish group and is the subject of a trial by the Flemish Gynaecological Oncology Group [33, 34]. Their experience has now been reported in a recent paper from Amant et al. from Leuven and has shown that neo-adjuvant chemotherapy followed by delayed primary surgery is a safe alternative approach for the more advanced SECs and it is likely that this could be extrapolated to CCC [35].

Several recent papers have advocated that this aggressive and comprehensive surgical approach may avoid the need for adjuvant treatment for stage 1 cancers [31]; this is discussed further in the adjuvant treatment section. Amant and colleagues from the Flemish Gynaecological Oncology Group are conducting a phase 2 study of adjuvant chemotherapy vs. no adjuvant treatment to try and address this topic based on their earlier reports [33, 34]. Their study incorporates comprehensive surgical staging and resection and randomisation to adjuvant chemotherapy or no treatment. In the meantime it must be recommended that the standard of care for a fit patient is to refer to a specialist gynaecological oncology surgeon for comprehensive surgical staging and pelvic clearance.

Future ideas will include improvements in imaging techniques to identify advanced cancers pre-operatively, and increasing interest in the use of neo-adjuvant chemotherapy in locally advanced endometrial cancer to try and reduce tumour volume and make a delayed primary procedure more effective and safer, as has been shown in ovarian cancer.

18.6 AdjuvantPo st-Operative Treatments

Post-operative review of the histology at a tumour board and multidisciplinary discussion will help to advise on further post-operative care. Pathology review is crucial as there are often mixed elements and the treatment maybe influenced by the final decision. There are diagnostic pitfalls which a more experienced pathologist is likely to avoid. These tumours, in common with serous cancers, are cytologically high-grade neoplasms and furthermore, there may be mixed patterns. Hendrickson discusses some of the practical difficulties in distinguishing CCC and serous cancers and compares their adverse clinical behaviour, which ultimately suggests that confusion of these two types may in fact have relatively little clinical consequence [36]. Not surprisingly, prognosis is related to the degree of invasion and those tumours confined to the endometrium or with minimal myometrial invasion do best. As is seen in discussions regarding adjuvant therapy, stage 1 cancers are associated with 75–79% five-year survival which does differ greatly from endometrioid cancers whereas for stage 2 and beyond there is a greater discrepancy with far worse outcome for CCC [37–42]. In one series from Touboul et al. [39], clear cell pathology was an independent prognostic risk factor.

There is a paradox in that whilst most of the major textbooks have some detailed discussion and debate about the pathology of CCC, most have very little to say on the clinical management! A recent review article from Mendivil et al. summarises much of the recent approaches to diagnosis and management [3]. Much will depend on the primary surgical procedure and if PLND has not been performed, discussion will take place to consider a repeat surgical procedure to remove the nodes vs. the option of radiation. Unfortunately many of these patients are older and frailer and thus may not be optimal candidates for more extensive surgery which in itself may have been part of the rationale for limiting surgery to a simple TAH and BSO in the first instance.

Kwon et al have even proposed that for both CCC and SEC with stage 1 disease where optimal surgical staging including both PLND and PAND has been carried out, no adjuvant treatment is required [31]. Level 1 evidence to support adjuvant treatment is difficult to obtain but chemotherapy, radiation and combined sequential or synchronous chemo-radiation should be discussed at the tumour board.

18.6.1 External Beam Radiation Therapy

Much intense debate rages about the whole value of adjuvant radiation in all types of endometrial cancer. However, very little has been published on the role of external beam radiation therapy (EBRT) and vaginal brachytherapy (VBT) in CCC and most opinions are extracted from major reviews or large trials, which have included small numbers of CCC [37–46]. The whole field is highly charged with opinion determined by the reviewer's own interpretation of the literature! A moderate contemporary view would recommend that adjuvant EBRT can be avoided in low-risk endometrial cancers, and probably also in intermediate-risk endometrial cancer since there is no survival benefit but only a reduction in local failure rate [46–48]. For high-risk cancers, there are no randomised trial data, but from meta-analyses, Cornes and Johnson [46] and Lee et al. [47] have shown that there may be survival benefits in up to 10% for adjuvant radiation even when PLND is carried out; these are the first reports to suggest that a survival benefit may occur when EBRT is given. Previously many authorities remained concerned that combining adjuvant radiation and PLND only increases risk of late morbidity. It has already been suggested that for early stage CCC, adjuvant treatment may be omitted after PLND.

Thus, the best the reviewer can do is to extrapolate from the small mixed pathology series and from high-risk cancers and try and estimate the level of benefit against any risk. The most educated interpretation is that adjuvant radiation is useful when the patient is unable to undergo PLND but is of unproven benefit in patients who have undergone PLND and should probably be withheld if there is no residual disease, but would be advised in the case of positive pelvic nodes or residual disease present.

Where EBRT has been used it does seem to produce a lower relapse rate. Two studies which looked at the role of EBRT in CCC confirmed lower rate of relapse. Cirsano et al. reviewed 38 patients with CCC, 22 of whom received varying types of post-operative radiation but there were no local recurrences within the radiation fields [22]. In another series by Thomas, 22 patients who underwent comprehensive surgery were reviewed of whom 11 had post-operative EBRT; there was only one recurrence at the vaginal cuff [28]. Kwon et al in their mixed series of CCC and SEC also had one vaginal cuff recurrence that was salvaged by radiation. Thus, from small numbers of patients who generally had optimal surgery, it would seem that adjuvant EBRT with or without VBT may protect against relapse but others feel that it is not required and the risks of systemic disease are higher, hence the need for systemic therapy which is discussed next.

Thomas et al., Craighead et al. and Murphy et al. all showed that when pelvic EBRT is given, there are fewer pelvic or vaginal relapses [28, 37, 41]. However, when sub-optimal surgical staging was carried out, failure to deliver adjuvant radiation was associated with higher failure rate. Thomas et al state that if lymphatic assessment is sub-optimal and repeat PLND not pursued, pelvic EBRT is needed to reduce risk of local relapse [28, 29].

Other recent papers [44, 48] have looked at whole abdominal irradiation (WAI) and radionuclide therapy with radioactive phosphorus (^{32}P). The GOG compared WAI to chemotherapy with AP chemotherapy and confirmed the superiority of the latter. Many feel that the technical complexities and morbidity of WAI make it unattractive as an option. Hoosier and Indiana Universities have reported on radionuclide therapy with phosphorus and whilst the results seem attractive, it may be argued that the crucial inclusion of comprehensive surgical staging was the key determinant [48]. There are also additional practical challenges with administering intra-cavitary colloids.

18.6.2 Brachytherapy

VBT remains controversial but paradoxically where it has been used does seem to reduce local failure rates. Given that intra-peritoneal or lymph node spread are more common, vaginal recurrence would seem less likely to occur, but several series have shown in serous cancers and CCC that this happens and when VBT is used there seems to be a benefit with reduced vaginal relapse. The author has chosen to use VBT routinely in hispra cticeforC CCa nds erousc ancers [28, 31, 43].

In summary, there is an impression that adjuvant EBRT maybe avoided if comprehensive staging has been carried out although some may recommend VBT as an adjuvant. When PLND is not performed and it is not planned to surgically intervene, EBRT at least reduces local relapse rate and may even improve survival. The addition of adjuvant chemotherapy with radiation is uncertain in CCC.

18.6.3 Chemo-Radiotherapy

However, newer data from the Scandinavian trial NSGO 9505 indicates an improvement in PFS and a trend towards an improvement in OS using sequential chemotherapy and radiation [49]. Their study included 1C G3 and occult stage 2 G3 cancers. Patients received an anthracycline and platinum-based therapy in most cases although latterly carboplatin and paclitaxel were permitted. The data support the use of combined modality adjuvant therapy in "high-risk" stage 1 patients although it is reported that there was no benefit seen in CCC and SEC cancers; numbers, however, were small. The definitive paper awaits publication; it is difficult to know if this is a statistical fluke or a genuine finding, it is certainly counter-intuitive. The PORTEC 3 trial in G3 high risk endometrial cancers is comparing EBRT alone vs. EBRT with concomitant cisplatin chemotherapy followed by four cycles of carboplatin and paclitaxel, and has opened in 2008. The recently presented GOG 184 study (Homesley) investigated adjuvant therapies in stage 3 and 4 endometrial cancers, and included 18% with CCC or SEC [50]. It evaluated volume-directed radiation and adjuvant chemotherapy with cisplatin and doxorubicin (CD) with or without paclitaxel (CDP). Final results are still awaited but the abstract at SGO in 2008 reported that in stage 3 endometrial carcinoma, the addition of paclitaxel to cisplatin and doxorubicin did not reduce locoregional and systemic relapse rates following maximum surgical cytoreduction and radiation. However a sub-group of patients with gross residual disease benefited from CDP. The RTOG have also shown that concomitant chemoradiation with weekly cisplatin followed by adjuvant carboplatin and paclitaxel can be safely delivered [51].

18.7 AdjuvantC hemotherapy

By and large, the use of chemotherapy as an adjuvant has emerged from experience in advanced disease. The author is not aware of any specific studies of chemotherapy in CCC; thus, any experience must be extrapolated from other subtypes. Hogberg has written a nice recent review on this topic [52]. The experience also derives predominantly from the trials in relapsed disease, which are extrapolated into the adjuvant setting. Three trials have compared chemotherapy vs. radiation but all are in the setting of mixed tumours, with only small numbers of CCC. These have used Adriamycin (doxorubicin) and cisplatin and compared with pelvic EBRT [53, 54] or in GOG 120 [44] vs. WAI. The Italian and Japanese studies failed to show any survival benefit; with hindsight and modern practice we can suggest that by today's standards the doses and intensity of the regime were less intensive. Today, the community standard is increasingly carboplatin and paclitaxel despite the lack of level one evidence, but there is of course a huge experience in ovarian cancer where this regime is widely used. A small minority continue to prescribe AP. A proposed European lead study will compare chemotherapy vs. no additional treatment in medium high-risk stage 1 or 2 who have undergone surgery including lymphadenectomy with negative nodes. This may answer the question of whether chemotherapy without radiation improves survival. It is a great shame that the PORTEC 3 trial did not have a third arm with chemotherapy alone; this would have addressed more questions although the trial does not mandate PLND!

18.7.1 Relapsed/Advanced Local Disease

Very early studies of chemotherapy in endometrial cancers used doxorubicin (A) as a single agent [55], whilst later series looked at cisplatin (P) before comparing doxorubicin (A) with cisplatin and doxorubicin (AP) [56–59]. Two studies showed AP to be better than A alone. Historically doxorubicin and cisplatin (AP) have been considered the standard treatments but have quite high morbidity and side effects. The current GOG study follows on from the comparison of AP vs. Taxol AP [60] and is comparing TAP with carboplatin and paclitaxel (TC). Increasingly the combination of carboplatin and paclitaxel is becoming standard treatment and extrapolation may be made from the use of these agents in ovarian cancers. There is huge experience with these drugs especially in ovarian cancers and they are generally well tolerated even in older patients. It should be remembered that the endometrial cancer population often has significant co-morbidity in comparison to the ovarian cancer population and thus avoidance of cisplatin and doxorubicin is advantageous. So, is there evidence to support the use of carboplatin and paclitaxel? There is now considerable literature mainly from single centres and phase 2 studies but it does support the use of this combination in endometrial cancer [61–64]. There is very little specific literature on CCC of endometrium, however. For a fuller discussion on clear cell ovarian cancers, the reader is advised to refer to the relevant chapters where important contributions are found on the differences between CCC in the Far East compared to Europe and the Americas [65, 66]. This will also include a discussion of the merits of conventional chemotherapy vs. novel approaches.

18.8 Follow-UpPr otocols

Follow-up of these patients generally is very similar to common forms of endometrial carcinomas and there are no useful or reliable tumour markers. There is no established place for routine scanning and imaging would normally be done only if there is a clinical indication. Most clinicians would suggest a check up at 4–6 weeks to confirm the follow-up plan and any need for adjuvant treatment. If no adjuvant therapy is advised, a more cautious follow-up would be proposed to detect any localised recurrence and offer salvage therapy. In the Kwon paper [31], one patient relapsed locally and was salvaged with treatment. Most series in endometrial cancers show a salvage rate in excess of 80% for localised vaginal vault relapse, but whether this can be extrapolated to CCC is unknown. Regular examinations at three months are advised for the first year and then four-monthly for year two. Thereafter six-monthly appointments are offered up to five years when it is usual to discharge patients

18.9 RelapsedDi sease

The management of relapsed disease will be determined by the type of previous adjuvant treatments, the time interval, the age and performance status of the patient and the sites and extent of disease. Initial staging scans will include CT or MR scanning but PET CT scanning may offer the best re-staging especially when radical salvage therapy is being considered. If there has been no prior radiation and disease is confined to the pelvis, then adjuvant radiation with VBT with or without chemotherapy should be offered. However, given the more aggressive behaviour pattern it is more likely that the patient will have systemic disease and therefore chemotherapy should be offered. Given that these tumours are usually ER/PR negative there is unlikely to be any significant role for hormonal treatments. Cisplatin and doxorubicin [55–59] or carboplatin and paclitaxel are likely to be standard chemotherapeutic options [60–64]. The current GOG study (no. 209) is comparing Taxol AP (TAP) vs. carboplatin and paclitaxel and the EORTC completed a study of TAP vs. AP but no results are available at the time of writing (protocol 55984). Improved response rates are seen with the addition of paclitaxel as in GOG 177 study but to deliver TAP may require use of growth factors and many feel this is unacceptable [60]. This is rarely needed with carboplatin and paclitaxel, and of course there is great experience with this combination in ovarian cancer. None of these makes specific reference to CCC of the uterus but they make up a higher proportion of the studies since they have a higher rate of relapse and thus are candidates for systemic therapy

Other drugs that may be considered would include ifosfamide and docetaxel but for progression after standard treatments entry into clinical trials with phase I agents are often the best options. The potential for investigation of newer targeted agents should be considered. The epothilones and topo-isomerase inhibitors are worthy of clinical trials. In Japan, a combination of cisplatin and irinotecan is considered to be more active in epithelial ovarian CCC and is currently being compared with carboplatin and paclitaxel [65, 66]. The new targeted agents are prime candidates for investigation and study although given the rarity of CCC, it may be difficult to do separate studies. Correlation with translational science may help identify new targets and in turn new targeted agents. Currently the most interest is being generated in mTOR pathway inhibitors but yet again, whether they have potential activity in CCC is uncertain. A recently published review on attitudes to management of CCC from SGO members has just been published and the reader is recommended to refer to this [67].

References

1. Abeler VM, Kjorstad KE, Berle E. Carcinoma of the endometrium in Norway: a histopathological and prognostic survey of a total population. Int J Gynecol Cancer. 1992; 2:9–22.
2. Acharya S, Hensley ML, Montag AC, et al. Rare uterine cancers. Lancet Oncol. 2005;6(12):961–71.

3. Mendivil A, Schuler KM, Gehrig PA. Non-endometrioid adenocarcinoma of the uterine corpus: a review of selected histological subtypes. Cancer Control. 2009;16(1):46–52.
4. Cirisano FR, Robboy SJ, Dodge RK, et al. Epidemiologic and surgicopathologic findings of papillary serous and clear cell endometrial cancers when compared to endometrial carcinoma. Gynecol Oncol. 1999;74:385–94.
5. Matthews RP, Hutchinson-Colas J, Maiman M, et al. Papillary serous and clear cell type lead to poor prognosis of endometrial carcinoma in black women. Gynecol Oncol. 997;65(2):206–12.
6. Scottish Intercollegiate Guidelines Network (SIGN). Investigation of post-menopausal bleeding (SIGN publication no. 61). SIGN, Edinburgh. http://www.sign.ac.uk. Accessed Sept 2002.
7. Smith-Bindman R, Kerlikowske K, Feldstein VA, et al. Endovaginal ultrasound to exclude endometrial cancer and other endometrial abnormalities. JAMA. 1998;280(17): 1510–7.
8. Kinkel K, Kaji Y, Yu KK, et al. Radiologic staging in patients with endometrial cancer: a meta-analysis. Radiology. 1999; 212:711–8.
9. Horowitz NS, Dehdashti F, Herzog TJ, et al. Prospective evaluation of FDG-PET for detecting pelvic and para-aortic lymph node metastasis in uterine corpus cancer. Gynecol Oncol.2004;95:546 –51.
10. Rockall AG, Sohaib SA, Harisinghani MG, et al. Diagnostic performance of nanoparticle-enhanced magnetic resonance imaging in the diagnosis of lymph node metastases in patients with endometrial and cervical cancer. J Clin Oncol. 2005;23:2813–21.
11. Abeler VM, Kjorstad KE. Clear cell carcinoma of the endometrium: a histological and clinical study of 97 cases. Gynecol Oncol. 1991;40:207–17.
12. Abeler VM, Vergote IB, Kjørstad KE, et al. Clear cell carcinoma of the endometrium: prognosis and metastatic pattern. Cancer.19 96;78(8):1740–7.
13. Christopherson WM, Alberhasky RC, Connelly PJ. Carcinoma of the endometrium: I. A clinicopathologic study of clear cell carcinoma and secretory carcinoma. Cancer. 1982;49:1511–23.
14. Creasman WT, Kohler MF, Odicino F, Maisonneuve P, Boyle P. Prognosis of papillary serous, clear cell, and grade 3 stage I carcinoma of the endometrium. Gynecol Oncol. 2004;95: 593–6.
15. Hendrickson MR, Ross J Eifel P, et al. Uterine papillary serous carcinoma: a highly malignant form of endometrial carcinoma. Am J Surg Pathol. 1982;6:93–108.
16. Ronnett B, Seidman JD, Zaino RJ, Ellenson LH and Kurman RJ. Pathology of Endometrial Hyperplasia and Carcinoma. Chapter in Cancers of uterus. Ed Coukos G and Rubin SC. Pub Marcel Dekker New York. 2005: 93–147.
17. Kanbour-Shakir A, Tobon H. Primary clear cell carcinoma of the endometrium. A clinicopathologic study of 20 cases. Int J Gynecol Pathol. 1991;10:67–78.
18. Kurman RJ, Scully RE. Clear cell carcinoma of the endometrium, an analysis of 21 cases. Cancer. 1976;37:872–82.
19. Lax S, Pizer ES, Ronnett BM, Kurman RJ. Clear cell carcinoma of the endometrium is characterised by a distinctive profile of p53, ki 67, estrogen and progesterone receptor expression. Hum Pathol. 1998;29(6):551–8.
20. Matthews RP, Hutchinson-Colas J, Maiman M, Fruchter RG, Gates EJ, Gibbon D, et al. Papillary serous and clear cell type lead to poor prognosis of endometrial carcinoma in black women. Gynecol Oncol. 1997;65(2):206–12.
21. Alektiar KM, McKee A, Lin O, et al. Is there a difference in outcome between stage I–II endometrial cancer of papillary serous/clear cell and endometrioid FIGO Grade 3 cancer? Int J Radiat Oncol Biol Phys. 2002;54:79–85.
22. Cirisano Jr FD, Robboy SJ, Dodge RK, et al. The outcome of stage I-II clinically and surgically staged papillary serous and clear cell endometrial cancers when compared with endometrioid carcinoma. Gynecol Oncol. 2000;77(1):55–65.
23. McMeekin DS, Filiaci VL, Thigpen JT, Gallion HH, Fleming GF, Rodgers WH. The relationship between histology and outcome in advanced and recurrent endometrial cancer patients participating in first-line chemotherapy trials: a Gynecologic Oncology Group study. Gynecol Oncol. 2007;106:16–22.
24. Silverberg SG, De Giorgi LS. Clear cell carcinoma of the endometrium. Clinical, pathologic and ultra-structural findings. Cancer. 1973;31:1127–40.
25. Sakuraji N, Hareyama H, Todo Y, et al. Prognostic significance of serous and clear cell adenocarcinoma in surgically staged endometrial carcinoma. Acta Obstet Gynecol Scand. 2000;79:311–6.
26. Memarzadeh S, Holschneider CH, Bristow RE, Jones NL, Fu YS, Karlan BY, et al. FIGO stage III and IV uterine papillary serous carcinoma: impact of residual disease on survival. Int J Gynecol Cancer. 2002;12(5):454–8.
27. Bristow RE, Duska LR, Montz FJ. The role of cytoreductive surgery in the management of stage IV uterine papillary serous carcinoma. Gynecol Oncol. 2001;81:92–9.
28. Thomas M, Mariani A, Wright JD, et al. Surgical management and adjuvant therapy for patients with uterine clear cell carcinoma: a multi-institutional review. Gynecol Oncol. 2008;108(2):293–7.
29. Thomas MB, Mariani A, Cliby WA, Keeney GA, Podratz KC, Dowdy SC. Role of systematic lymphadenectomy and adjuvant therapy in stage I uterine papillary serous carcinoma. Gynecol Oncol. 2007;107(2):186–9.
30. Amant F, Moerman P, Neven P, Timmerman D, Van Limbergen E, Vergote I. Endometrial cancer: a review. Lancet.2005; 366:491–505.
31. Kwon J, Abrams J, Sugimoto A, Carey MS. Is adjuvant therapy necessary for stage IA and IB uterine papillary serous carcinoma and clear cell carcinoma after surgical staging? Int J Gynecol Cancer. 2008;18:820–4.
32. Vergote I, Trop CG, Amant F, Kristensen G, Sardi JE, Ehlen T, Johnson N, Verheijen R, van der Burg MEL, Lacave AJ, Benedetti-Panici PL, Kenter GG, Casado A, Mendiola C, Coens C, Verleye L, Stuart G, Pecorelli S and Reed NS. EORTC-GCG/NCIC-CTG randomised trial primary debulking surgery with neoadjuvant chemotherapy or in Stage IIIc and IV ovarian, fallopian tube and primary peritoneal cancer. IJGC 2008
33. Despierre E, Moerman P, Vergote I, Amant F. Is there a role for neoadjuvant chemotherapy in the treatment of stage IV serous endometrial carcinoma? Int J Gynecol Cancer. 2006;16 Suppl 1:273–7.
34. Amant F, Despierre E, Vandenput I. Residual tumor after neoadjuvant chemotherapy and interval debulking surgery for advanced endometrial cancer. Gynecol Oncol. 2009 Apr 25. Epub ahead of print

35. Vandenput I, Van Calster B, Capoen A, Leunen K, Neven P, Moerman Ph, et al. Neoadjuvant chemotherapy followed by interval debulking surgery in patients with serous endometrial cancer with transperitoneal spread (stage IV): a new preferred treatment? Br J Cancer. 2009;101:244–9.
36. Hendrickson M, Longacre T. Pathology of uterine cancers. In: Gershenson D, McGuire W, Gore M, Quinn MA, Thomas G, editors. Gynecologic cancer – controversies in management. Philadelphia: Elsevier; 2004. p. 209–28.
37. Murphy KT, Rotmensch J, Yamada SD, et al. Outcome and patterns of failure in pathologic stages I-IV clear-cell carcinoma of the endometrium: implications for adjuvant radiation therapy. Int J Radiat Oncol Biol Phys. 2003;55(5):1272–6.
38. Martinez AA, Weiner S, Podratz K, et al. Improved outcome at 10 years for serous-papillary/clear cell or high-risk endometrial cancer patients treated by adjuvant high-dose whole abdomino-pelvic irradiation. Gynecol Oncol. 2003;90: 537–46.
39. Touboul E, Belkacemi Y, Buffat L, et al. Adenocarcinoma of the endometrium treated with combined irradiation and surgery; a study of 437 patients. Int J Radiat Oncol Biol Phys. 2001;50:81–97.
40. Alvarez Secord A, Havrilesky LJ, Bae-Jump V, et al. The role of multimodality adjuvant chemotherapy and radiation in women with advanced stage endometrial cancer. Gynecol Oncol.2007;107(2) :285–91.
41. Craighead PS, Sait K, Stuart GC, et al. Management of aggressive histologic variants of endometrial carcinoma at the Tom Baker cancer centre between 1984 and 1994. Gynecol Oncol. 2000;77:248–53.
42. Aquino-Parsons C, Lim P, Wong F, Mildenberger M. Papillary serous and clear cell carcinoma limited to endometrial curettings in FIGO stage 1a and 1b endometrial adenocarcinoma: treatment implications. Gynecol Oncol. 1998;71: 83–6.
43. DuBeshter B, Estler K, Altobelli K, McDonald S, Glantz C, Angel C. High-dose rate brachytherapy for stage I/II papillary serous or clear cell endometrial cancer. Gynecol Oncol. 2004;94(2):383–6.
44. Randall ME, Filiaci VL, Muss H, Spirtos NM, Mannel RS, Fowler J, et al. Randomized phase iii trial of whole-abdominal irradiation versus doxorubicin and cisplatin chemotherapy in advanced endometrial carcinoma: a Gynecologic Oncology Group Study. J Clin Oncol. 2006;24(1):36–44.
45. Creutzberg CL, van Putten WL, Koper PC, Lybeert ML, Jobsen JJ, Warlam-Rodenhuis CC, et al. Surgery and postoperative radiotherapy versus surgery alone for patients with stage-1 endometrial carcinoma: multicentre randomised trial. PORTEC study group. Post operative radiation therapy in endometrial carcinoma. Lancet. 2000;355(9213):1404–11.
46. Cornes P, Johnson N. Survival risks and benefits with adjuvant therapy for endometrial cancer: systematic review and meta-analysis. Eur J Cancer Suppl. 2007;5(4):312. Abstr5004.
47. Lee CM, Szabo A, Shrieve DC, MacDonald OK, Gaffney DK. Frequency and effect of adjuvant radiation therapy among women with stage I endometrial adenocarcinoma. JAMA.20 06;295:389–97.
48. Fakiris AJ, Moore DH, Reddy SR, Look KY, Yiannoutsos CT, Randall ME, et al. Intraperitoneal radioactive phosphorus (32P) and vaginal brachytherapy as adjuvant treatment for uterine papillary serous carcinoma and clear cell carcinoma: a phase II Hoosier Oncology Group (HOG 97-01) study. Gynecol Oncol. 2005;96:818–23.
49. Hogberg T, Rosenberg P, Kristensen G, de Oliveira CF, de Pont Christensen R, Sorbe B, Lundgren C, Salmi T, Andersson H, Reed NS. A randomized phase-III study on adjuvant treatment with radiation (RT) ± chemotherapy (CT) in early-stage high-risk endometrial cancer (NSGO-EC-9501/EORTC 55991). Proc Am Soc Clin Oncol. 2007; Abstr 5503.
50. Homesley HD, Filiaci V, Gibbons SK, et al. Randomized phase III trial in advanced endometrial carcinoma of surgery and volume-directed radiation followed by cisplatin and doxorubicin with or without paclitaxel: a Gynecologic Oncology Group study. Gynecol Oncol. 2008;108:S1.
51. Greven K et al. Final analysis of RTOG 9708: adjuvant postoperative irradiation combined with cisplatin/paclitaxel chemotherapy following surgery for patients with high-risk endometrial cancer. Gynecol Oncol. 2006;103(1):155–9.
52. Hogberg T. Adjuvant chemotherapy in endometrial cancer: overview of randomised trials. Clin Oncol. 2008;20:463–9.
53. Susumu N et al. Randomized phase III trial of pelvic radiotherapy versus cisplatin-based combined chemotherapy in patients with intermediate- and high-risk endometrial cancer: a Japanese Gynecologic Oncology Group study. Gynecol Oncol.2008; 108(1):226–33.
54. Maggi R, Lissoni A, Spina F, Melpignano M, Zola P, Favalli G, et al. Adjuvant chemotherapy vs radiotherapy in high-risk endometrial carcinoma: results of a randomised trial. Br J Cancer.2006; 95:266–71.
55. Thigpen JT, Buchsbaum HJ, Mangan C, Blessing JA. Phase 2 trial of Adriamycin in the treatment of advanced or recurrent endometrial carcinoma: a Gynaecologic Oncology Group Study. Cancer Treat Rep. 1979;63:21–7.
56. Thigpen JT, Blessing JA, Lagasse JD, et al. Phase 2 trial of cisplatin as second line chemotherapy in patients with advanced or recurrent endometrial carcinoma: a Gynecologic Oncology Group Study. Am J Clin Oncol. 1984;7:253–5.
57. Blessing TJT, JA HHD, et al. Phase 2 trial of cisplatin as first line chemotherapy in patients with advanced or recurrent endometrial carcinoma: a Gynecologic Study Group study. Gynecol Oncol. 1989;33:68–70.
58. Thigpen JT, Blessing JA, Homesley HD, et al. Phase 2 trial of doxorubicin ± cisplatin in advanced or recurrent endometrial carcinoma; a Gynaecologic Oncology Group Study. Proc ASCO. 1993;12:261.
59. Aapro M, Bolis G, Chevalier B, et al. Doxorubicin versus doxorubicin and cisplatin in endometrial carcinoma: a randomised trial of the EORTC gynaecological cancer cooperative group (GCCG). Ann Oncol. 1994;5(8):98–0490.
60. Fleming G, Brunetto V, Cella D, et al. Phase III trial of doxorubicin plus cisplatin with or without paclitaxel plus filgrastim in advanced endometrial carcinoma: a Gynecologic Oncology Group study. J Clin Oncol. 2004;22:2159–66.
61. Hoskins P, Swenerton KD, Pike JA, Wong F, Lim P, Acquino-Parsons C, et al. Paclitaxel and carboplatin, alone or with irradiation, in advanced or recurrent endometrial cancer: a phase II study. J Clin Oncol. 2001;19:4048–53.
62. Lupe K, Kwon J, D'Souza D, et al. Adjuvant paclitaxel and carboplatin chemotherapy with involved field radiation in advanced endometrial cancer: a sequential approach. Int J Radiat Oncol Biol Phys. 2007;67:110–6.

63. Mazgani M, Le N, Hoskins PJ. Re-use of carboplatin and paclitaxel in patients with relapsed endometrial cancer-the British Columbia Cancer Agency experience. Gynecol Oncol.2008;111:47 4–7.
64. Papadimitriou CA, Bafaloukos D, Bozas G, Kalofonos H, Kosmidis P, Aravantinos G, Fountzilas G, Dimopoulos MA; Hellenic Co-operative Oncology Group. Paclitaxel, epirubicin, and carboplatin in advanced or recurrent endometrial carcinoma: a Hellenic Co-operative Oncology Group (HeCOG) study. Gynecol Oncol. 2008;110(1): 87–92.
65. Takano M, Kikuchi Y, Yaegashi N, et al. Adjuvant chemotherapy with irinotecan hydrochloride and cisplatin for clear cell carcinoma of the ovary. Oncol Rep. 2006;16(6):1301–6.
66. Takano M, Sugiyama T, Yaegashi N, Suzuki M, Tsuda H, Sagae S, et al. Progression-free survival and overall survival of patients with clear cell carcinoma of the ovary treated with paclitaxel-carboplatin or irinotecan-cisplatin: retrospective analysis. Int J Clin Oncol. 2007;12(4):256–60.
67. Olawaiye AB, Boruta DM. Management of women with clear cell endometrial cancer. A Society of Gynecologic Oncology (SGO) review. Gynecol Oncol. 2009;113(2):277–83.

Part IV

Cervix and Vulval Cancers

Small Cell and Neuroendocrine Cancerso ft heC ervix

19

Nicholas Reed

19.1 Introduction

Neuroendocrine (NE) cell carcinomas of the cervix are uncommon and constitute 1–2% of cervix cancers. They were first identified in the 1970s [1] but major progress occurred after a consensus conference on the topic in 1997 [2]. This proposed a more formal classification. More recent experience has proposed a new WHO classification of NE cancers although this is not usually applied for cervical cancers [3, 4]. They constitute small cell cancers, large cell variants as well as typical and atypical carcinoids. This chapter will focus mainly on small cell cancers and their variants rather than carcinoids. Well differentiated NE cancers in the cervix are extremely rare and should be managed by teams experienced in managing neuroendocrine tumours (NETs). Metastatic disease should be excluded before labelling as a primary carcinoid or NET of cervix. They are likely to behave like any other well differentiated NET and there is plenty of guidance available on this topic from UKINET and ENETS [5, 6]. However, small cell cancers and their variants are most typically managed by gynaecological cancer multidisciplinary teams, as they usually present with gynaecological symptoms.

One of the principal challenges in managing small cell tumours is distinguishing them from metastatic small cell disease arising at another site, in particular with a bronchial origin; and from other small round cell tumours which may have a subtly similar appearance. This topic is well discussed for lung small cell cancers in a recent review by Renshaw [7]. There are some differences in the immunocytochemical profile, but the method of presentation and age may be relevant. The reader is advised to refer to the chapter 3 by McCluggage and Millan where some of these important issues are covered in detail. Some other references are provided for the reader on pathology and prognostic factors [8–13]. Carcinoids and undifferentiated sex cord tumours may also cause confusion. The literature suggests that small cell cancers are commoner peri-menopausally although recent personal experience seems to suggest they are becoming more prevalent in younger women, i.e., under the age of 30, even though older data suggest that the average age of diagnosis is close to 50 years. This diagnosis should always be considered in a younger woman presenting with advanced disease. The SEER data paper from McCusker gives some insights into the epidemiological differences between squamous and nonsquamous cervix cancers [14].

It is important to distinguish pure small cell tumours from those tumours that may contain NE differentiation; NE differentiation may be a feature of poorly differentiated squamous cell cancers. The presence of one small focus is insufficient to label as a small cell carcinoma. Finally when a pure small cell cancer is seen, it is necessary to exclude a metastatic process from another primary, most typically in the lung.

Furthermore these tumours may sometimes be associated with the ectopic production of neuropeptides which may give distinctive clinical syndromes including hypercalcaemia, hypoglycaemia, Cushing's syndrome, hyponatraemia (SIADH) and myaesthenic syndromes but not as commonly as in small cell ovarian cancers. There are parallels with ovarian small cell cancers where the two main sub-types have different patterns of behaviour (SCCOHT vs. SCCOPT). The reader is referred to chapter 13 dicussed but SCCOHT occurs in younger women while SCCOPT is more common in older women.

N.R eed
Beatson Oncology Centre, Gartnavel General Hospital,
1053G reatW esternR oad, Glasgow G120Y N, Scotland, UK
e-mail:nic k.reed@ggc.scot.nhs.uk

N. Reed et al. (eds.), *Rare and Uncommon Gynecological Cancers*,
DOI: 10.1007/978-3-642-13492-0_19, © Springer-Verlag Berlin Heidelberg 2011

These tumours are often very highly aggressive and carry a poor prognosis and unless they are diagnosed at a very early stage, they usually are associated with early death. Most series report less than 30% five-year survival and many are dead within 2 years despite treatment [14–17]. Distressingly, they are often young women with young families, and social support for the bereaved is an essential component of care.

19.2 Presentation

The presentation is usually with abnormal vaginal bleeding and mimics squamous cell cancers, usually with no distinguishing features [13]. Cervical screening may occasionally identify small cell cancers. The mean age at diagnosis is 50 years in contrast to 52 years for squamous cell cancers although this author believes that more recent experience might suggest a shift to younger age at diagnosis. The literature suggests about 41% have stage 1 disease as opposed to 51% for squamous cell cancers, however, small cell tumours have a higher incidence of lymph node metastases. There does seem to be a greater risk of earlier blood-borne and lymphatic spread. It is highly likely that clinical staging will underestimate the stage compared to newer radiological imaging techniques. A strong case can be made for ^{18}FDG PET-CT in these rare tumours. Tumour markers are of limited use, although neuron-specific enolase (NSE) may be of use in serial measurement of individual cases.

19.3 Pathology

These were first described much earlier than ovarian small cell cancers, the first recognised report being in 1976 [1, 2]. Historically there is confusion over the terminology used in what we now call small cell cancer of cervix. This was addressed by a consensus conference that helped to resolve some of the issues [8–12]. Small cell carcinoma of the cervix is uncommon; it is said to account for up to 2% of cervix cancers. The incidence is said to have risen over the past 20 years but whether this is a true rise or simply better recognition and use of new immunocytochemical techniques is unclear. They seem to occur more frequently in younger women with cervix cancers; in a woman under thirty with a poorly differentiated squamous carcinoma, a small cell/neuroendocrine tumour should be considered. Some poorly differentiated squamous cancers may have NE features with patchy immunocytochemical profile. The presence of chromogranin, synaptophysin and CD56 is usually considered necessary to make a diagnosis of small cell carcinoma [18]. Several recent papers including a review from Carlson in Boston have shown the potential value of TTF-1 in differentiating small cell cancers of ovary, cervix and lung [19–21]. This probably represents the aggressive end of the spectrum of squamous cancers rather than an NE cancer. HPV 18 seems to be most commonly associated (in about 50% of cases) and HPV 16 less so, in contrast to squamous epithelial cancers of cervix [22–25]. Primary carcinoids and paragangliomas of the cervix are described in the literature but are exceedingly rare. A carcinoid tumour found in the cervix is most likely to be metastatic and a search for other disease is advised.

A workshop meeting in 1997, reported by Albores-Saavedra [2] proposed that cervix (neuro)-endocrine cancers be classified into the four following categories. This is based on the pathological classification used in pulmonary NETs but is not consistent with the newer WHO classification of NETS which mainly focuses on gastro-entero-pancreatic NETs [3, 4]. The paradox is that the term carcinoid is familiar to many and thus in practice it may be easier to retain this term for clinical usage, and it will be referred to in this article.

Specialist pathological review is required with access to comprehensive immunocytochemical profile which should include staining for immunohistochemical NE markers, p53, p16, p14 and cyclin D1 [17, 18]. Immunohistochemical staining for CD 56, synaptophysin, NSE and chromogranin A may be helpful. It is proposed that p16 is up-regulated or accumulated in the small cell cancers of the uterine cervix, probably caused by infection with human papillomavirus. p14 inactivation is of high prevalence and detection rate of p53 is similar to that in other histologic types of cervicalc arcinomas.

- Typical(c lassical)c arcinoid
- Atypicalc arcinoid
- Largec ellne uroendocrine
- Smallc ell(oa tc ell)ne uroendocrine

19.4 Staging

Blood should be taken for full haematological and biochemical profile. This must include serum calcium. Full staging including imaging with CT, MRI or PET CT to include the chest is essential in order to exclude a primary intra-pulmonary tumour. Connor in the accompanying chapter gives an excellent overview of imaging in cervix cancers. Given that these are very metabolically active cancers, ^{18}FDG PET CT scanning seems particularly attractive for staging purposes. Nevertheless even this cannot guarantee to rule out an occult primary small cell tumour of the lung. Serum tumour markers are of limited benefit. For well differentiated NETs a "gut hormone profile" should be sent for analysis. This will normally include chromogranins A and B, gastrin, neurotensin, somatostatin, VIP, glucagons and pancreatic polypeptide. NSE and B-HCG may be useful for monitoring if initially raised but are infrequently raised at diagnosis. Somatostatin receptor imaging with Octreoscan is again only of value in well differentiated tumours [5, 6]. PET CT would seem to offer greater potential.

19.5 TreatmentOp tions

The management of these cases generates a great deal of debate and discussion and there are some experts who feel that surgery has little role to play. As one might predict, there are few published data to substantiate any viewpoint. The main message is that multimodality therapy is necessary and teams should work closely to manage individual patients [26–48]. Much of the debate has evolved from the management of small cell lung cancer (SCLC). In this condition extensive disease at presentation is common, hence chemotherapy with radiation is the key treatment involved. In limited disease SCLC there is generally little role for surgery although a few studies have claimed survival advantages. For limited disease, chemotherapy and radical radiation are standard, usually followed by prophylactic cranial irradiation (PCI) in patients achieving remission [35]. These approaches have helped to formulate the management of small cell cancer of cervix. In cervix small cell cancers, the mean survival is much poorer than for squamous tumours, 36% vs. 71% five-year survival [7, 12, 14, 26–38]. Patients with advanced disease at presentation will rarely survive longer than a year to 18 months. This will not match the optimal results in SCLC. The concepts for managing rare cancers are well discussed and reviewed [44, 45].

19.6 LocalisedDi sease

19.6.1 The Role of Surgery

Since most cases will not be recognised as small cell cervix cancer initially, patients will be referred to gynaecology through the usual channels of referral, and if disease is localised to the cervix, stage 1A and 1B, early 2A and 2B, primary surgical management will be advised. Hence the first discriminant is to determine if the disease is localised or extensive. There is no exact cut off size and this will vary from centre to centre, but often when the cervix tumour is greater than 4 cms, referral for primary chemo-radiation will be made. Some surgeons do not see the size of the tumour as an obstacle to primary surgery, but this may be perceived as short-sighted since we are trying to avoid delivering triple modality therapy with its attendant increased risk of late toxicity. However, this category may be the exception as there is a view that these patients need multi-modality therapy. Consideration should be given to neo-adjuvant chemotherapy to try and downsize the tumour and lead to a discussion of delayed primary surgery or subsequent chemo-radiation. In squamous cell cancers, the case for neo-adjuvant chemotherapy remains unproven and there is even less evidence in small cell cancers.

However, the best results in the recent literature have come from a combination of surgery, radiation and chemotherapy [26–34, 36–43]. Some of the early reports [14–17] suggested that radiation alone was better than surgery, but this has been surpassed by modern combined modality approach. The importance of new imaging techniques to optimally stage the patient and plan the treatment is vital. Initial staging which shows extra pelvic disease would suggest that a primary radical surgical procedure is inappropriate; a combination of CT or MR and PET CT will be recommended depending upon local availability. Small tumours should be considered for a radical hysterectomy and pelvic lymph node dissection, followed by chemotherapy and radiation either concomitantly or sequentially

[27, 32, 33, 36, 38]. The issue of para-aortic node sampling or lymphadenectomy (PALND) remains unresolved. Many would advocate sampling but there is no evidence base to substantiate routine PALND. However several series, in which primary chemotherapy and radiation have been used, have seen isolated first relapses in the para-aortic area, often just above the upper border of the radiation field, raising the issue of whether there is any justification for either para-aortic nodal dissection or extending the radiation fields.

19.6.2 Adjuvant Therapy

Adjuvant treatments should probably include both chemotherapy and radiation. There are no randomised trials to support this but in the series which have been reported, when post-operative chemotherapy was omitted, there were high relapse rates and most patients were dead within 3 years [26–34, 36–43]. Conversely, when chemotherapy was given, distant relapse rates were lower and better survival was seen but there was a risk of greater local failure. For unexplained reasons, in their review of ovarian small cell cancers, Harrison et al. reported better survival when both radiation and chemotherapy were delivered [49]. It is not unreasonable to extend this adjuvant approach to small cell cervix cancers.

In the adjuvant setting a minimum of four cycles of chemotherapy is given. The choice of agents normally reflects what is used in SCLC. Chan reported that vincristine, doxorubicin and cyclophosphamide or cisplatin and etoposide are effective adjuvant therapies after hysterectomy [41]. Currentlye itherc isplatino rc arboplatin and etoposide are deployed; other agents have been used, but these seem to achieve the best results.

19.6.3 Primary Chemo-Radiation

One of the first series to report combined chemo-radiation was from Hoskins et al. who reported 28% three-year survival. They used concomitant cisplatin and etoposide with involved field pelvic radiation plus or minus para-aortic nodal irradiation in the first phase. They subsequently modified the schedule to use carboplatin and paclitaxel and regularly included para-aortic irradiation and PCI, with nearly 60% three-year survival. This more than doubled their three-year survival rates. The main prognostic determinant was radiological stage, with 80% of stage 1 and 2 vs. 38% of stage 3 and 4 disease free at three years [50].

Standard doses of radiation are prescribed and vary with local protocols but generally, pelvic radiation using the pelvic brick or box technique is used to deliver 45–52 Gray in 25–28 fractions. There is no evidence to support intensity modulated radiation therapy (IMRT) but it is increasingly being adopted without any evidence base in squamous cell cervix cancer. Brachytherapy is added and the technique is determined by whether or not there has been prior surgery; colpostats or ovoids are applied if there has been surgery, and full insertion is done if uterus is intact. Doses and number of insertions should normally conform to local practice for squamous cell cancers.

19.6.4 Multi-Modality Therapy

A more recent review from New York found only 17 patients in 17 years; the majority (72%) underwent RHND, and 22% had primary definitive radiation, eleven RT alone and one concomitant chemoradiation. This was given in the form of cisplatin and etoposide with radiation followed by two more cycles. Again staging and extent of disease were principal prognostic factors. For all patients estimated PFS and OS were 22% and 30%, with median time to progression of 9 months and 14 months OS. However for early disease stage 1 and 2, the time to progression was 10 months compared to 4 months for more advanced stages, where there were no long-term survivors [51]. The relatively poor overall results most probably reflect the long time span over which they were collected and treated.

Siva presented a poster at ASCO 2006 reporting the experience of two Scottish centres [52]. A total of 21 patients were eligible for the analysis with a median age of 33 years (range 22–74). Nine patients were FIGO stage 1B, 3 were 2A and 4 were 2B, 3 were 3B and 2 with metastatic disease. Surgery was performed in 13 patients [11 radical hysterectomy/pelvic lymphadenectomy, 1 radical hysterectomy and 1 total abdominal hysterectomy]. Chemotherapy was given to 16 patients [Neo-adjuvant 6, Adjuvant 9, Concurrent 3]. Fourteen of these patients received combination chemotherapy containing platinum and etoposide. One received a non-platinum combination. Fourteen also received radiotherapy [10 pelvic radiotherapy and brachytherapy, 3 pelvic only, 1 brachytherapy only, 2 PCI]. Two patients died of progressive disease shortly after diagnosis without any specific anti-cancer treatment, two patients were disease free after a follow-up of 40 and 53 months, respectively, and one was lost to follow-up 7 years after diagnosis. Median relapse free survival (RFS) was 16 months. Two-year RFS was 25%. The sites of relapse were as follows: liver 4, chest 4, para-aortic 4, brain 3, neck 3, local 2, abdomen 1. Twelve patients received salvage therapy after relapse [5 – responded, 2 – not assessed and 5 – progressed]. Seven were alive after a median follow-up of 40 months (range 17–90). Median survival was 28 months and the three-year overall survival was 45%. It is believed that these results are attributable to the use of aggressive combination therapy of surgery, chemotherapy and radiotherapy.

19.7 ExtensiveDi sease

The larger tumours which may not be suitable for surgical resection should probably be managed with initial chemotherapy. This parallels the treatment of SCLC. For those presenting with extra pelvic disease, primary chemotherapy is the treatment of choice. PET CT is likely to be an important tool in staging and serial PET CT may give prognostic information. Drug combinations similar to those used in SCLC are prescribed, such as cisplatin or carboplatin and etoposide combination. Early trials used a variety of agents including the CAVE regimen, with generally poor responses, and it was not until the modern agents used in SCLC were introduced that better results were first seen. Up to 6 cycles are prescribed with careful monitoring and an interval scan after 3 cycles to assess response. The patient should then be discussed again at the tumour board to consider whether to follow with radical hysterectomy or radical radiation or both. PET CT is most probably the imaging modality of choice before contemplating radical surgery. Surgery should not be considered if there is continuing evidence of extra pelvic disease.

While these tumours may show a high level of chemo- or radio-sensitivity early relapse is frequent and associated with an aggressive and usually lethal pattern. Patients who relapse are most unlikely to be salvaged. In the series of extensive disease generally less than 20% are alive at 3 years. Patterns of relapse may be unusual with lymph node metastases in the para-aortic area as first site and may occasionally be an isolated site of relapse, which strengthens the argument for lymphadenectomy at the time of initial surgery [32, 40, 42]. Alternatively, as recommended by Hoskins and others, extended field irradiation may prevent this but at the cost of additional morbidity.

Early relapse is common and usually aggressive, but occasional cases may recur 2–3 years later and if the patient is of good PS, reconsideration of surgery must be done and chemotherapy must be given. If the time interval exceeds 12–18 months, re-challenging with platinum and etoposide is worth considering. Isolated pelvic masses may require further surgery or radiation depending on prior treatment. The CAV(E) regime incorporating cyclophosphamide, doxorubicin and vincristine may be used and is a good choice in the poorer-performance patient. Topotecan and other camptothecins may be considered for relapse but have not been extensively tested in first line setting in cervical SCC.

For patients who achieve a complete remission, especially if they presented with extensive disease, consideration should be given to PCI as used in extensiveSC LC.

19.8 LargeC ellV ariant of Small Cell Cancer

Large cell variants are more challenging and again there is a paucity of publications in the literature. There are a few pathology papers mainly from the last 10 years [53–56]. In general they are treated along the same lines, with primary surgery and adjuvant therapy for earlier small volume disease, and primary chemotherapy and radiation plus or minus surgery for more extensive disease. Again platinum and etoposide are likely to be the preferred agents.

19.9 Conclusions

These are uncommon cancers and there is clearly much further work to be done in terms of the optimal investigations, staging and management of these tumours.

Because of their rarity, a case can be made for regional centres to look after these rare cancers. These centres should develop agreed protocols and there should be a local database and internationally agreed protocols for their management so that more information can be gained about the optimal care. Opportunities for translational research and new clinical trials can only be reachedbys uchc ollaboration.

References

1. Albores-Saavedra J, Larraza O, Poucell S, Rodriguez Martinez H. Carcinoid of the uterine cervix: additional observations on a new tumor entity. Cancer. 1976;38:2328–42.
2. Albores-Saavedra J, Gersell D, Gilks CB, Henson DE, Lindberg G, Santiago H, et al. Terminology of endocrine tumors of the uterine cervix: results of a workshop sponsored by the College of American Pathologists and the National Cancer Institute. Arch Pathol Lab Med. 1997;121:34–9.
3. Rindi G, Capella C Solcia E. Introduction to a revised clinicopathological classification of neuroendocrine tumors of the gastroenteropancreatic tract. Q J Nucl Med. 2000;44(1): 13–21.
4. Klöppel G, Perren A, Heitz PU. The gastroenteropancreatic neuroendocrine cell system and its tumors: the WHO classification. Ann N Y Acad Sci. 2004;1014:13–27.
5. Ramage JK, Davies AH, Ardill J, Bax N, Caplin M, Grossman A, et al. Guidelines for the management of gastroenteropancreatic neuroendocrine (including carcinoid) tumours. Gut. 2005;54 Suppl 4:v1–16.
6. Rindi G, de Herder W, O'Toole D, Wiedenmann B. Consensus Guidelines for the management of patients with digestive neuroendocrine tumors: the second event and some final considerations. Neuroendocrinology. 2008;87:5–7.
7. Renshaw AA, Haja J, Lozano RL, Wilbur DC. Distinguishing carcinoid from small cell carcinoma of the lung: correlating cytologic features and performance in the College of American pathologists Non-Gynecologic Cytology programme. Arch Pathol Lab Med. 2005;129(5):614–8.
8. Gersell DJ, Mazoujian G, Mutch DG, Rudloff MA. Small cell undifferentiated carcinoma of the cervix. A clinicopathological, ultrastructural and immunocytochemical study of 15 cases. Am J Surg Pathol. 1988;12:684–98.
9. Silva E, Gershenson D, Sneige N, Brock WA, Saul P, Copeland LJ. Small cell carcinoma of the uterine cervix: pathology and prognostic factors. Surg Pathol. 1989;2: 105–15.
10. Miller B, Dockter M, el Torky M, Photopulos G. Small cell carcinoma of the cervix: a clinical and flow-cytometric study. Gynecol Oncol. 1991;42:27–33.
11. Abeler VM, Holm R, Nesland JM, Kjørstad KE. Small cell carcinoma of the cervix. A clinicopathologic study of 26 patients. Cancer. 1994;73:672–7.
12. Alfsen GC, Kristensen GB, Skovlund E, Pettersen EO, Abeler VM. Histologic subtype has minor importance for overall survival in patients with adenocarcinoma of the uterine cervix: a population based study of prognostic factors in 505 patients with non-squamous cell carcinomas of the cervix. Cancer. 2001;92:2471–83.
13. Conner MG, Richter H, Cesar A, Hameed A, Albores-Savada J. Small cell carcinoma of cervix: a clinicopathologic and immunohistochemical study of 23 cases. Ann Diagn Pathol.2002; 6:345–8.
14. McCusker ME, Cote TR, Clegg LX, Tavassoli FJ. Endocrine tumors of the uterine cervix: incidence, demographics, and survival with comparison to squamous cell carcinoma. Gynecol Oncol. 2003;88(3):333–9.
15. van Nagell Jr JR, Donaldson ES, Wood EG, Maruyama Y, Utley J. Small cell cancer of the uterine cervix. Cancer. 1977;40:2243–9.
16. Scully RD, Aguirre P, DeLellis RA. Argyrophilia, serotonin, and peptide hormones in the female genital tract and its tumors. Int J Gynecol Pathol. 1984;3:51–70.
17. van Nagell Jr JR, Powell DE, Gallion HH, Elliott DG, Donaldson ES, Carpenter AE, et al. Small cell carcinoma of the uterine cervix. Cancer. 1988;62:1586–93.
18. Horn LC, Lindner K, Szepankiewicz G, Edelmann J, Hentschel B, Tannapfel A, et al. p16, p14, p53, and cyclin D1 expression and HPV analysis in small cell carcinomas of the uterine cervix. Int J Gynecol Pathol. 2006;25(2): 182–6.
19. Agoff SN, Lamps LW, Philip AT, Amin MB, Schmidt RA, True LD, et al. Thyroid transcription factor-1 is expressed in extrapulmonary small cell carcinomas but not in other extrapulmonary neuroendocrine tumors. Mod Pathol. 2000;13(3): 238–42.
20. Ordóñez NG. Value of thyroid transcription factor-1 immunostaining in distinguishing small cell lung carcinomas from other small cell carcinomas. Am J Surg Pathol. 2000;24(9): 1217–23.
21. Carlson JW, Nucci MR, Brodsky J, Crum CP, Hirsch MS. Biomarker-assisted diagnosis of ovarian, cervical and pulmonary small cell carcinomas: the role of TTF-1, WT-1 and HPV analysis. Histopathology. 2007;51:305–12.
22. Mannion C, Park WS, Man YG, Zhuang Z, Albores-Saavedra J, Tavassoli FA. Endocrine tumors of the cervix: morphologic assessment, expression of human papillomavirus, and evaluation for loss of heterozygosity on 1p, 3p, 11q, and 17p. Cancer. 1998;83(7):1391–400.
23. Ambros RA, Park JS, Shah KV, Kurman RJ. Evaluation of histologic, morphometric, and immunohistochemical criteria in the differential diagnosis of small cell carcinomas of the cervix with particular reference to human papillomavirus types 16 and 18. Mod Pathol. 1991;4(5):586–93. Erratum in: Mod Pathol 1992 Jan;5(1):40.
24. Herrington CS, Graham D, Southern SA, Bramdev A, Chetty R. Loss of retinoblastoma protein expression is frequent in small cell neuroendocrine carcinoma of the cervix and is unrelated to HPV type. Hum Pathol. 1999;30(8):906–10.
25. Stoler MH, Mills SE, Gersell DJ, Walker AN. Small-cell neuroendocrine carcinoma of the cervix. A human papillomavirus type 18-associated cancer. Am J Surg Pathol. 1991;15(1):28–32.
26. Boruta II DM, Schorge JO, Duska LA, Crum CP, Castrillon DH, Sheets EE. Multimodality therapy in early-stage neuroendocrine carcinoma of the uterine carcinoma of the uterine cervix. Gynecol Oncol. 2001;81:82–7.

27. Sheets EE, Berman ML, Hrountas CK, Liao SY, DiSaia PJ. Surgically treated, early-stage neuroendocrine small-cell cervical carcinoma. Obstet Gynecol. 1988;71:10–4.
28. O'Hanlan KA, Goldberg GL, Jones JG, Runowicz CD, Ehrlich L, Rodriguez-Rodriguez L. Adjuvant therapy for neuroendocrine small cell carcinoma of the cervix: review of the literature. Gynecol Oncol. 1991;43:167–72.
29. Morris M, Gershenson DM, Eifel PJ, Silva EG, Mitchell MF, Burke TW, et al. Treatment of small cell carcinoma of the cervix with cisplatin, doxorubicin, and etoposide. Gynecol Oncol. 1992;47:62–5.
30. Lewandowski GS, Copeland LJ. A potential role for intensive chemotherapy in the treatment of small cell neuroendocrine tumors of the cervix. Gynecol Oncol. 1993;48:127–31.
31. Perrin L, Ward B. Small cell carcinoma of the cervix. Int J Gynecol Cancer. 1995;5:200–3.
32. Sevin BU, Method MW, Nadji M, Lu Y, Averette HA. Efficacy of radical hysterectomy as treatment for patients with small cell carcinoma of the cervix. Cancer. 1996;77:1489–93.
33. Sevin BU, Lu Y, Bloch DA, Nadji M, Koechli OR, Averette HE. Surgically defined prognostic parameters in patients with early cervical carcinoma. A multivariate survival tree analysis. Cancer. 1996;78:1438–46.
34. Kim YB, Barbuto D, Lagasse LD, Karlan BY. Successful treatment of neuroendocrine small cell carcinoma of the cervix metastatic to regional lymph nodes. Gynecol Oncol. 1996;62:411–4.
35. Auperin A, Arriagada R, Pignon JP, Le Pechoux C, Gregor A, Stephens RJ. Prophylactic cranial irradiation for patients with small-cell lung cancer in complete remission. Prophylactic Cranial Irradiation Overview Collaborative Group. N Engl J Med. 1999;341:476–84.
36. Chang TC, Lai CH, Tseng CJ, Hsueh S, Huang KG, Chou HH. Prognostic factors in surgically treated small cell cervical carcinoma followed by adjuvant chemotherapy. Cancer. 1998;83:712–8.
37. Weed JC, Shoup B, Tawfik O. Small cell carcinoma of the cervix: a clinical study of 15 patients and review of the literature. Prim Care Update Ob Gyn. 1998;5:159.
38. Lim FK, Chong SM, Sethi V. Small cell neuroendocrine carcinoma of the cervix with involvement of multiple pelvic nodes – a successfully treated case by multimodal approach. Gynecol Oncol. 1999;72:246.
39. Delaloge S, Pautier P, Kerbrat P, Castaigne D, Haie-Meder C, Duvillard P, et al. Neuroendocrine small cell carcinoma of the uterine cervix: what disease? what treatment? Report of ten cases and a review of the literature. Clin Oncol (R Coll Radiol).2000;12:3 57–62.
40. Straughn Jr JM, Richter HE, Conner MG, Meleth S, Barnes MN. Predictors of outcome in small cell carcinoma of the cervix – a case series. Gynecol Oncol. 2001;83:216–20.
41. Chan JK, Loizzi V, Burger RA, Rutgers J, Monk BJ. Prognostic factors in neuroendocrine small cell cervical carcinoma: a multivariate analysis. Cancer. 2003;97:568–74.
42. Ishida GM, Kato N, Hayasaka T, Saito M, Kobayashi H, Katayama Y, et al. Small cell neuroendocrine carcinomas of the uterine cervix: a histological, immunohistochemical, and molecular genetic study. Int J Gynecol Pathol. 2004;23(4): 366–72.
43. Viswanathan AN, Deavers MT, Jhingran A, Ramirez PT, Levenback C, Eifel PJ. Small cell neuroendocrine carcinoma of the cervix: outcome and patterns of recurrences. Gynecol Oncol.2004; 93:27–33.
44. Plaxe SC. Chasing zebras: the study and treatment of rare diseases. Gynecol Oncol. 2006;100:227–8.
45. Levels of Evidence and Grades of Recommendation. http://www.cebm.net/levels_of_evidence.asp#levels.
46. Crowder S, Tuller E. Small cell carcinoma of the female genital tract. Semin Oncol. 2007;34(1):57–63.
47. Chen J, MacDonald OK, Gaffney DK. Incidence, mortality and prognostic factor of small cell carcinoma of the cervix. Obstet Gynecol. 2008;111:1394–402.
48. Reed NS. Small cell cancers of the ovary and cervix. Eur J Oncol Suppl. 2007;5(5):255–8.
49. Harrison ML, Hoskins P, du Bois A, Quinn M, Rustin GJS, Ledermann JA, et al. Small cell of the ovary, hypercalcemic type – analysis of combined experience and recommendation for management. A GCIG study. Gynecol Oncol. 2006;100:233–8.
50. Hoskins PJ, Swenerton KD, Pike JA, Lim P, Aquino-Parsons C, Wong F, et al. Small-cell carcinoma of the cervix: fourteen years of experience at a single institution using a combined-modality regimen of involved-field irradiation and platinum-based combination chemotherapy. J Clin Oncol. 2003;21:3495–501.
51. Siva M, Mahmood R, Kakumanu S, Sadozye A, Reed N. Small cell neuroendocrine carcinoma of uterine cervix: the Scottish experience Journal of Clinical Oncology, 2006 ASCO Annual Meeting Proceedings Part I. 2006;24(18S) (20S uppl):15026.
52. Zivanovic O, Leitao MM, Park KJ, Zhao Z, Diaz JP, Konner J, et al. Small cell neuroendocrine carcinoma of the cervix: analysis of outcome, recurrence pattern and the impact of platinum-based combination chemotherapy. Gynecol Oncol. 2009;112:590–3.
53. Albores-Saavedra J, Martinez-Benitez B, Luevano E. Small cell carcinomas and large cell neuroendocrine carcinomas of the endometrium and cervix: polypoid tumors and those arising in polyps may have a favorable prognosis. Int J Gynecol Pathol. 2008;27(3):333–9.
54. Gilks CB, Young RH, Gersell DJ, Clement PB. Large cell carcinoma of the uterine cervix. A clinicopathologic study of 12 cases. Am J Surg Pathol. 1997;21:905–14.
55. Rhemtula H, Grayson W, van Iddekinge B, Tiltman A. Large cell neuroendocrine carcinoma of the uterine cervix. A clinicopathologic study of five cases. S Afr Med J. 2001;91: 525–8.
56. Sato Y, Shimamoto T, Amada S, Hayashi T. Large-cell neuroendocrine carcinoma of the uterine cervix. A clinicopathologic study of six cases. Int J Gynecol Pathol. 2003;22: 226–30.

Primary Malignant Melanoma oft heV ulvaandV agina

20

Catriona Hardie and Nadeem Siddiqui

20.1 Introduction

Malignant melanoma is an aggressive disease which affects both skin and mucosal surfaces. Primary malignant melanoma of the female lower genital tract, including vulva and vagina, is a rare entity. This disease accounts for only approximately 5–10% of all vulvar malignancies [1]. Primary vaginal melanoma is an even less common variant. Due to the scarcity of malignant melanoma at these sites, there is little evidence-based literature to guide clinicians in the appropriate management of patients. In contrast to this, there has been a threefold increase in cutaneous melanoma in recent years [2] with many advances in diagnosis and treatment. This has meant that, inevitably, clinical trials involving cutaneous malignant melanoma have been used to draw parallels with disease of the vulva and vagina. This is a contentious issue and one which affects the way these tumours are both staged and managed a ppropriately.

20.2 Demographicsand A etiology

Caucasian females have an increased relative risk (RR 2.6) of vulvar melanoma [1], although this does not apply to vaginal disease. Disease occurs in an older population than cutaneous melanoma (30–40 years), with a recent large multivariate analysis suggesting a median age at diagnosis of 68 years [3] in vulvar melanoma. Vaginal melanoma has been shown to occur in a slightly younger age group of approximately 58ye ars [4].

Aetiological factors relating to melanoma of the female genital tract are less well understood than their cutaneous counterparts. Genital tract melanomas are not exposed to ultraviolet radiation, therefore sun exposure does not contribute to the aetiology unlike cutaneous melanoma. In fact, in stark contrast to cutaneous melanoma, the incidence of this disease has remaineds tatic [5].

20.3 ClinicalPr esentation

The clinical presentation of vulvar and vaginal melanoma is non-specific, and can include the presence of a mass, pigmented skin change or itch. Women who present with suspicious pigmented lesions should undergo examination and full thickness biopsy. Locally advanced disease may be suggested by pain, bleeding or vaginal discharge.

20.4 HistopathologicalSub types

There are three histological subtypes of vulvar melanoma which have been described in substantial detail by a large Swedish Group [6]. These consist of mucosal lentiginous melanomas, superficial spreading melanoma and nodular melanomas. Mucosal lentiginous are the most common subtype, although nodular types are more aggressive with earlier metastasis evident [6].

Nodular melanoma is the most common subtype describedinv aginalme lanoma [7].

C.H ardie(✉) and N. Siddiqui
Department of Gynaecological Oncology, Glasgow Royal Infirmary, 84C astleSt reet, Glasgow G40SF , UK
e-mail:c atriona.hardie@hotmail.co.uk

N. Reed et al. (eds.), *Rare and Uncommon Gynecological Cancers*,
DOI: 10.1007/978-3-642-13492-0_20, © Springer-Verlag Berlin Heidelberg 2011

20.5 Staginga ndPr ognosis

Vulvar cancers are surgically staged. Debate has existed over the appropriateness of different staging systems in vulvar and vaginal melanoma. The International Federation of Gynaecology and Obstetrics (FIGO) staging system has previously been used, but this classification system applies only to squamous carcinoma of the lower genital tract. FIGO staging for vulvar and vaginal cancer is shown in Table 20.1 and 20.2. Staging systems for cutaneous melanoma which are now commonly applied to genital tract melanoma include those

Table20. 1 FIGOs tagings ystemof v aginalc ancer

Vulvarc ancer		
Carcinoma of the vulva (FIGO 2008)		
Stage 0		Deleted
StageI		Tumourc onfined to the vulva
	IA	Lesions ≤2 cm in size, confined to the vulva or perineum and with stromal invasion ≤1.0m m[a], no nodal metastasis
	IB	Lesions > 2 cm in size or with stromal invasion > 1.0 mm[a], confined to the vulva or perineum, with negative nodes
Stage II		Tumour of any size with extension to adjacent perineal structures (1/3 lower urethra, 1/3 lower vagina, anus) with negative nodes
Stage III		Tumour of any size with or without extension to adjacent perineal structures (1/3 lower urethra, 1/3 lower vagina, anus) with positive nodes
	IIIA	(i) With 1 lymphnodal metastases(≥ 5 mm), or (ii) 1-2 lymphnodal metastases(< 5 mm)
	IIIB	(i) With 2 or more lymphnodal metastases (≥ 5 mm), or (ii) 3 or more lymphnodal metastases(< 5 mm)
	IIIC	With positive nodes with extracapsular spread.
Stage IV		Tumour invades other regional (2/3 upper urethra, 2/3 upper vagina), or distant structures
	IVA	Tumour invades any of the following: (i) upper urethral and/or vaginal mucosa, bladder mucosa, rectal mucosa, or fixed to pelvic bone, or (ii) fixed or ulcerated femoral-inguinal lymph nodes
	IVB	Any distant metastasis including pelvic lymph nodes

[a]The depth of invasion is defined as the measurement of the tumour from the epithelial-stromal junction of the adjacent most superficial dermal papilla to the deepest point of invasion

Table 20.2 FIGOs taging:v aginalc ancer

Stage 0	Carcinoma in situ; intraepithelial neoplasia grade III
Stage I	Carcinoma limited to the vaginal wall
Stage II	Carcinoma involves subvaginal tissue but without extension to pelvic side wall
Stage III	Carcinoma extends to pelvic side wall
Stage IVa	Tumour invades bladder +/or rectal mucosa +/ or direct extension beyond true pelvis
StageI Vb	Distantm etastasis

Table 20.3 Comparison of staging systems for cutaneous melanoma

Staging level	Clark	Breslow thickness (mm)	Chung
I	Confined to epidermis	<0.75	Confined to epidermis
II	Invades basal layer epidermis	0.76–1.5	<1m mi nvasion dermis or lamina propria
III	Invades papillary dermis	1.5–2.5	1.0–2.0m m invasion into subepithelial tissue
IV	Invades reticular dermis	2.26–3.0	>2 mm invasion to fibrous tissue
V	Invades subcutaneous fat	>3.0	Invades subcutaneousf at

based on depth of local invasion (Clark [8], Chung [9]) and lesion thickness (Breslow [10]), which are compared in Table 20.3. Chung et al. [9] modified the Clark [9] system to specifically incorporate anatomy of the vulva. In general terms, more locally invasive and thicker tumours have a worse prognosis. Recently, the cutaneous melanoma tumour node metastasis (TNM) staging system has been revised, but this has not been incorporated into staging of lower genital tract melanoma [11]. Interestingly, a prospective Gynaecologic Oncology group (GOG) trial of vulvar melanoma has shown, though, that TNM staging has a better correlation with survival outcome than FIGO staging [12]. Staging has not yet been addressed prospectively in those patients with vaginal melanoma.

In comparison to other malignancies, there have been few centres which have accrued sufficient numbers of patients to identify true prognostic factors related to melanoma of the vulva and vagina. Prognosis for lower genital tract melanoma is generally poor, regardless of the treatment delivered [13]. Multivariate analysis has shown that increased age, later stage disease and nodal metastasis are adverse prognostic factors in vulvar melanoma [3]. Other negative prognostic factors related to vulvar disease include ulcerated disease, centrally located tumours, increased mitotic activity and DNA ploidy [13, 14]. The only prognostic factor which is significant for patients with vaginal melanoma is tumour size [15].

20.6 Role of Primary Surgery

Primary surgery remains pivotal in controlling, or even curing, vulvar melanoma. However, there are no prospective randomised controlled trials (RCTs) to guide the extent of primary surgery which is required here. Historically, patients underwent radical surgery and bilateral inguinofemoral lymph node dissection [16]. Recently though, reports have shown that radical surgery has no survival benefit over more conservative local resection with clear margins [17, 18], potentially preserving normal tissue and overall function. Based on cutaneous melanoma retrospective studies, vulvar melanoma margins should be 1 cm if the tumour is less than 1 mm thick, and 2 cm if it is 1–4 mm thick. The margin of depth should be 1 cm in all cases, though [19].

The impact of surgery on vaginal melanoma is not well understood. There are limited conflicting retrospective clinical data. Some authors suggest an improved survival with exenterative surgery [20], and they would advocate this more aggressive surgical procedure as vaginal melanoma can metastasise earlier than its cutaneous counterpart [21]. This is in contrast to other reports that suggest no significant survival benefit in radical vs. conservative surgery [7, 15].

Utilisation of improved imaging techniques is useful in the preoperative assessment of patients with vaginal melanoma. Positron emission tomography (PET)-CT is more accurate than CT or MRI alone in detecting metastatic disease in cutaneous melanoma [22]. PET-CT is also an accurate way to determine extent of disease in patients with vaginal melanoma. This can potentially upstage disease, and alter surgical management and treatment depending on PET-CT findings [23].

20.7 Assessment of Lymph Node Status

Groin lymph node status is the most significant prognostic factor in vulvar malignancy [24]. Specifically, in vulvar melanoma, five-year survival rates for those patients with positive nodes vs. those with negative nodes are significantly poorer [3]. Currently, there are no non-invasive investigations which can accurately assess nodal status prior to surgery. Studies evaluating the accuracy of PET-CT, MRI and ultrasound with histology after sentinel node surgery are needed. Recommended treatment in squamous cell malignancy includes inguinofemoral lymph node dissection which carries significant associated morbidity [25, 26], and only up to 35% of patients will actually have positive nodes in early stage disease [27]. In contrast, cutaneous melanoma is treated with local excision and selective regional node dissection.

The role of sentinel lymph node biopsy was originally described in 1977 [28]. Melanoma invariably metastasises via the lymphatics. The first affected lymph node is the sentinel node, and this can be located by a hand-held γ probe and confirmed as the sentinel node using blue dye staining. It is then removed for histological examination. There is no consensus on whether this procedure is appropriate for use in patients affected by melanoma of the vulva or vagina. There is some recent evidence which has shown it to provide useful prognostic information in the management of patients with early stage vulvar malignancy [29, 30] and melanoma [31, 32]. Some evidence suggests that sentinel node detection is highly accurate in identifying those vulvar cancer patients with positive nodes in whom it may be appropriate to perform inguinofemoral lymph node dissection [33, 34]. However, this may not necessarily pertain to melanoma itself. Evidence suggests that small micrometastases in the sentinel node have no prognostic relevance in melanoma, which can result in upstaging disease and performing unnecessary lymphadenectomy in patients [35, 36]. The multicentre selective lymphadenectomy trial (MSLT-1) showed no significant survival difference in those patients who underwent regional lymphadenectomy if the sentinel node was positive [37]. Additionally, there is no current role for adjuvant therapy in those sentinel node positive patients with vulvar or vaginal melanoma without clinical trials. However, although the removal of a positive sentinel node may not significantly improve long-term survival, this does reduce the chance of recurrent disease in the affected lymph node basin. Additionally, if patients are counselled that the sentinel node biopsy is normal, they can be reassured that metastatic disease in the regional lymph nodes is unlikely.

20.8 Roleo fA djuvantT herapy

The role of adjuvant radiotherapy in the treatment of lower genital tract melanoma is unproven. There may be some advantage in its utilisation in patients with vulvar disease, including melanoma, if there are confirmed positive surgical margins or in those with positive lymph nodes [38, 39]. Larger studies are required, though. Radiotherapy treatment may achieve a locoregional response in a select group of patients with vaginal melanoma [40], but there is no evidence for its routine use. There is no current role for chemotherapy in lower genital tract melanoma outside the setting of a clinical trial.

There are currently randomised Phase III trials of more novel therapeutic agents underway. The use of adjuvant interferon alpha-2b in treating cutaneous melanoma has been examined in a meta-analysis and may benefit select subsets of patients [41]. Although the recent EORTC 18991 trial showed an improvement in a subgroup of patients with microscopic disease, the differences were small and this was not evident in those with gross nodal involvement [42]. Relapse-free intervals and survival therefore remain poor. The GOG in the USA have a phase II study of dasatinib in melanomas of the vulva and vagina harbouring mutations of c-kit.

20.9 Conclusion

Malignant melanoma of the vulva and vagina encompasses a rare group of malignancies occurring in an older population than does cutaneous melanoma. These tumours have an overall poor prognosis, and there remains a lack of consensus in the current published literature on how they should be treated. Surgery does remain the gold standard of treatment, and local excision with a margin of between 1 and 2 cm rather than more radical excision does not reduce survival in patients. Sentinel lymph node biopsy may provide prognostic information but there is still not sufficient evidence for its routine clinical use. The use of adjuvant therapy in melanoma of the vulva and vagina remains unproven, but with larger clinical trials investigating the use of novel chemotherapeutic agents in cutaneous melanoma, it would be anticipated that these findings may be extrapolated to those patients with lower genital tract melanoma in due course.

References

1. Weinstock MA. Malignant melanoma of the vulva and vagina in the United States: Patterns of incidence and population-based estimates of survival. Am J Obstet Gynecol. 1994;171:1225–30.
2. Garbe C, Leiter U. Melanoma epidemiology and trends. Clin Dermatol.2009; 27(1):3–9.
3. Sugiyama VE, Chan JK, Shin JY, et al. Vulvar melanoma: a multivariate analysis of 644 patients. Obstet Gynecol. 2007;110(2 Pt 1):296–301.
4. Hauspy J, Nevin A, Harley I, et al. Paraneoplastic syndrome in vaginal melanoma: a case report and review of the literature. Int J Gynecol Cancer. 2007;17:1159–63.
5. Ragnarsson-Olding BK, Johansson H, Rutqvist L-E, et al. Malignant melanoma of the vulva and vagina. Cancer.1993; 71:1893–7.
6. Ragnarsson-Olding BK, Nilsson BR, Kanter-Lewensohn LR, et al. Malignant melanoma of the vulva in a nationwide, 25 year study of 219 Swedish females: Clinical observations and histopathological features. Cancer. 1999;86:1273–84.
7. Reid GC, Schmidt RW, Roberts JA, et al. Primary melanoma of the vagina: a clinicopathologic analysis. Obstet Gynecol. 1989;74:190–9.
8. Clark WH, From L, Bernadino EA, et al. The histogenesis and biologic behavior of primary human malignant melanoma of the skin. Cancer Res. 1969;29:705–26.
9. Chung AF, Woodruff JM, Lewis JL. Malignant melanoma of the vulva: a report of 44 cases. Obstet Gynecol. 1975;45: 638–46.
10. Breslow A. Thickness, cross-sectional areas and depth of invasion in the prognosis of cutaneous melanomas. Ann Surg.1970; 172:902–8.
11. Balch CM, Buzaid AC, Soong SJ, et al. Final version of the American Joint Committee on Cancer staging system for cutaneous melanoma. J Clin Oncol. 2001;19:3635–48.
12. Phillips GL, Bundy BN, Okagaki T, et al. Malignant melanoma of the vulva treated by radical hemivulvectomy: a prospective study of the Gynecologic Oncology Group. Cancer. 1994;73:2626–32.
13. Scheistroen M, Trope C, Koern J, et al. Malignant melanoma of the vulva: evaluation of prognostic factors with emphasis on DNA ploidy in 75 patients. Cancer. 1995;75(1): 72–80.
14. Wechter ME, Gruber SB, Haefner HK, et al. Vulvar melanoma: a report of 20 cases and review of the literature. J Am Acad Dermatol. 2004;50:554–62.

15. Tjalma WA, Monaghan JM, de Barros Lopes A, et al. Primary vaginal melanoma and long-term survivors. Eur J Gynaecol Oncol. 2001;22:20–2.
16. Morrow CP, Rutledge F. Melanoma of the vulva. Obstet Gynecol.1972;39:7 45–52.
17. Verschraegen CF, Benjabpidal M, Supakarapongkul W, et al. Vulvar melanoma at the M.D. Anderson Cancer Center: 25 years later. Int J Gynecol Cancer. 2001;11:359–64.
18. Trimble EL, Lewis Jr JL, Williams LL, et al. Management of vulvar melanoma. Gynecol Oncol. 1992;45:254–8.
19. Irwin WP, Legallo RL, Stoler MH, et al. Vulvar melanoma: a retrospective analysis and literature review. Gynecol Oncol.2001;83:457 –65.
20. Van Nostrand KM, Lucci JA, Schell M, et al. Primary vaginal melanoma: improved survival with radical pelvic surgery. Gynecol Oncol. 1994;55:234–7.
21. Skowronek J, Roszak A. A case of metastatic malignant melanoma of the vagina with a background of primary vaginal melanoma: clinical case. Ginekol Pol. 1997;68:390–3.
22. Mohr P, Eggermont AM, Hauschild A, et al. Staging of cutaneous melanoma. Ann Oncol. 2009;20(6):vi14–21.
23. Oudoux A, Rousseau T, Bridji B, et al. Interest of F-18 fluorodeoxyglucose positron emission tomography in the evaluation of vaginal malignant melanoma. Gynecol Oncol. 2004; 95(3):765–8.
24. Stehman FB, Look KY. Carcinoma of the vulva. Obstet Gynecol.2006;107(3):719–33.
25. Rouzier R, Haddad B, Dubernard G, et al. Inguinofemoral dissection for carcinoma of the vulva: effect of modifications of extent and technique on morbidity and survival. J Am Coll Surg. 2003;196(3):442–50.
26. Gould N, Kamelle S, Tillmanns T, et al. Predictors of complications after inguinal lymphadenectomy. Gynecol Oncol. 2001;82(2):329–32.
27. Burger MP, Hollema H, Emanuels AG, et al. The importance of the groin node status for the survival of T1 and T2 vulval carcinoma patients. Gynecol Oncol. 1995;57:327–34.
28. Cabanas RM. An approach for the treatment of penile carcinoma. Cancer. 1977;39:456–66.
29. Van der Zee AGJ, Oonk MH, De Hullu JA, et al. Sentinel node dissection is safe in the treatment of early-stage vulvar cancer. J Clin Onc. 2008;26(6):884–9.
30. Johann S, Klaeser B, Krause T, et al. Comparison of outcome and recurrence-free survival after sentinel lymph node biopsy and lymphadenectomy in vulvar cancer. Gynecol Oncol.2008;110:32 4–8.
31. Kettlewell S, Moyes C, Bray C, et al. Value of sentinel node status as a prognostic factor in melanoma: prospective observational study. BMJ. 2006;332:1423–5.
32. Carlson GW, Murray DR, Lyles RH, et al. The amount of metastatic melanoma in a sentinel lymph node: does it have prognostic significance? Ann Surg Oncol. 2003;10:575–81.
33. Puig-Tintoré LM, Ordi J, Vidal-Sicart S, et al. Further data on the usefulness of sentinel lymph node identification and ultrastaging in vulvar squamous cell carcinoma. Gynecol Oncol.2003; 88:29–34.
34. Terada KY, Shimizu DM, Jiang CS, et al. Outcomes for patients with T1 squamous cell cancer of the vulva undergoing sentinel node biopsy. Gynecol Oncol. 2006;102: 200–3.
35. Spanknebel K, Coit DG, Bieligk SC, et al. Characterization of micrometastatic disease in melanoma sentinel lymph nodes by enhancing pathology: recommendations for standardizing pathological analysis. Am J Surg Pathol. 2005;29: 305–17.
36. Van Akkooi AC, de Wilt JH, Verhoef C, et al. Clinical relevance of melanoma micrometastases (<0.1mm) in sentinel nodes: are these nodes to be considered negative? Ann Oncol.2006; 17:1578–85.
37. Morton DL, Thompson JF, Cochran AJ, et al. Sentinel node biopsy or nodal observation in melanoma. N Engl J Med. 2006;355:1307–17.
38. Parthasarathy A, Cheung MK, Osarin K, et al. The benefit of adjuvant radiation therapy in single-node-positive squamous cell vulvar carcinoma. Gynecol Oncol. 2008;103:1095–9.
39. Agrawal S, Kane JM, Guadagnolo BA, et al. The benefits of adjuvant radiation therapy after therapeutic lymphadenectomy for clinically advanced, high-risk, lymph node-metastatic melanoma. Cancer. 2009;115(24):5836–44.
40. Irwin Jr WP, Bliss SA, Rice LW, et al. Malignant melanoma of the vagina and locoregional control: radical surgery revisited. Gynecol Oncol. 1998;71:476–80.
41. Wheatley K, Ives N, Hancock B, et al. Does adjuvant interferon-alpha for high risk melanoma provide a worthwhile benefit? A meta-analysis of the randomised trials. Cancer Treat Rev. 2003;29:241–62.
42. Eggermont AM, Suciu S, Santinami M, et al. Adjuvant therapy with pegylated interferon alfa-2b versus observation alone in resected stage III melanoma: final results of EORTC 18991, a randomised phase III trial. Lancet. 2008;372(9633): 117–26.

Gynecologic Cancers in Pregnancy: Guidelines of an International ConsensusM eeting

21

Frédéric Amant, Kristel Van Calsteren, M.J. Halaska, J. Beijnen, L. Lagae, M. Hanssens, L. Heyns, L. Lannoo, P. Ottevanger, W. Van den Bogaert, L. Ungar, I. Vergote, and A. du Bois

21.1 Introduction

The estimation of the worldwide cancer burden indicates that gynecologic cancers (i.e., cancer of the vulva, vagina, cervix uteri, uterine corpus, ovary, and fallopian tube) account for 19% of the 5.1 million estimated new cancer cases and 2.9 million cancer deaths in 2002 [143]. They account for 22% of all new cancer cases among women in developing countries compared to 15% of all new cases among women in developed countries. Overall incidence distinguishes developed from developing countries; also, the incidence of the gynecologic cancers is remarkably different. Endometrial cancer and ovarian cancer are the most frequent gynecologic malignancies in developed countries, and increasing age of the populations in those countries will even increase the relative frequency of both entities related to cervical cancer. Both the availability of population-screening programs and HPV immunization, especially in developed countries, will add to this disparity. In contrast, cancer of the cervix is the second most common cancer among women worldwide due to the fact that it is the most common gynecologic cancer in the developing world [143]. In unscreened populations, the peak risk of invasive cervical cancers occurs earlier than for most adult cancers, peaking or reaching a plateau from about 35–55 years of age [67]. The increase starts in the second decade and early in the

F.A mant (✉)
Gynaecologic Oncology, Leuven Cancer Institute (LKI), UZ Gasthuisberg,K atholiekeU niversiteitLe uven, Belgiuma nd

Division of Gynaecological Oncology, Department of Obstetrics and Gynaecology, UZ Gasthuisberg, Katholieke UniversiteitLe uven, Herestraat49 , 3000 Leuven, Belgium
e-mail:fre deric.amant@uz.kuleuven.ac.be

K. Van Calsteren, L. Heyns, and I. Vergote
Gynaecologic Oncology, Leuven Cancer Institute (LKI), UZ Gasthuisberg,K atholiekeU niversiteitLe uven, Belgium

M.J.H alaska
Division of Oncogynaecology, Department of Gynaecology and Obstetrics Charles University in Prague, 2nd Medical Faculty, CzechR epublic

J.B eijnen
Department of Pharmacy and Pharmacology, The Netherlands CancerIns titute/SlotervaartH ospital, Amsterdam, TheN etherlands

L.L agae
Department of Pediatrics, UZ Gasthuisberg, Katholieke UniversiteitLe uven, Belgium

M. Hanssens and L. Lannoo
Department of Obstetrics, UZ Gasthuisberg, Katholieke UniversiteitLe uven, Belgium

P.O ttevanger
Department of Medical Oncology, Radboud University NijmegenM edicalC entre, Nijmegen, TheN etherlands

W. Van den Bogaert
Department of Radiation Oncology, Leuven Cancer Institute (LKI), UZ Gasthuisberg, Katholieke Universiteit Leuven, Leuven,B elgium

L.U ngar
GynaecologicO ncology, NationalC ancerI nstitute, Budapest, Hungary

A.duB ois
Department of Gynaecology and Gynaecologic Oncology, HSK,D r.H orstSc hmidtK linik, Wiesbaden, Germany

Frédéric Amant is clinical researcher for Research Foundation-Flanders (F.W.O.); Kristel Van Calsteren is aspirant for Research Foundation-Flanders (F.W.O.). Lieven Lagae is holder of the UCB Chair in Cognitive Dysfunctions in Childhood.

N. Reed et al. (eds.), *Rare and Uncommon Gynecological Cancers*,
DOI: 10.1007/978-3-642-13492-0_21, © Springer-Verlag Berlin Heidelberg 2011

third decade [67]. This partial overlap with the reproductive era renders pregnant women susceptible to cervical cancer. In contrast, endometrial, vulvar, and ovarian cancers are diagnosed less frequently in the reproductive era.

Cancer affecting the reproductive system during pregnancy is a complex situation that endangers at least two lives, those of the pregnant woman and the fetus. The tremendous therapeutic challenge implicated by this coincidence on one hand and the sparse experience of individual clinicians on the other hand demands clinical guidance. However, literature data on cancers of the pelvic female reproductive system during pregnancy mainly consist of anecdotal case reports or small series only. We expected that gathering and summarizing all available data could help to provide a useful tool in this situation. Therefore, we organized an International Consensus meeting on 3rd July 2008 in Leuven, Belgium.

Experts were selected in order to cover the fields of gynecologic oncology, medical oncology, clinical pharmacology, obstetrics, pediatrics, and radiation oncology. A basic manuscript and a CD-ROM including 263 articles was sent to all participants before the meeting. These articles were identified during a PUBMED search looking for keywords including pregnancy, offspring, cancer, chemotherapy, radiotherapy, cervical, vulvar, endometrial, and ovarian. Articles before 1990 were only included if considered important. Some articles were hand searched based on reference lists. Cancers diagnosed in the postpartum are excluded. Malignant trophoblastic disease was regarded as a distinct and well-described entity and was not included.

All participants were assigned to comment on and review the topic of their experience. This new manuscript served as a basis for discussion during the meeting. The discussion during the meeting resulted in a new version that circulated six times. All participants agreed with the final recommendations. Questions we sought to answer in particular include the identification of stages that exclude pregnancy preservation as a safe option, requirements for safe surgery for pelvic cancer during pregnancy, alternative surgical treatment options that aim to preserve the pregnancy, choice of chemotherapy, timing of delivery, and the neonatal outcome.

We focus firstly on imaging and cancer treatment modalities during pregnancy, subsequently on monitoring of the pregnancy and neonatal outcome and finally on organ pathology.

21.2 ImagingandOnc ological Treatment Modalities During Pregnancy

The risk of fetal damage (for example, by surgery related hypoxia, radiation, or chemotherapy) and hence the possibility to stage and treat cancer during pregnancy will largely depend on the exposure period in pregnancy. With regard to this, the pregnancy can be divided into three stages: fertilization/implantation, organogenesis, and the fetal phase.

During the first 10 days post-conception (fertilization/implantation) cells are omnipotent and can develop in the three different embryological layers. Viability will depend on the number of cells that is killed during treatment and this will result in an "all-or-nothing" phenomenon. When sufficient cells remain the embryo will unaffectedly develop normally. However, when too many cells are damaged, miscarriage will occur.

The most vulnerable phase expands from 10 days until 8 weeks after conception (organogenesis). The potential for fetal damage is the highest during this period but varies depending on the agents used. The use of radiation or cytotoxic drugs during the organogenesis will increase the risk for fetal malformations, but a background risk of 3% is inevitable [26]. Therefore, radiation or chemotherapy until 10 weeks' gestational age (= duration of amenorrhea) is contraindicated. However, some systems including the eyes, genitals, hematopoietic system, and the central nervous system continue to develop afterwards. We propagate a 2–4-week "safety period" in order to allow treatment from 12–14 weeks' pregnancy (i.e., 10–12 weeks after conception). Proper dating is crucial to plan safe treatment. During the second and third trimesters, radiotherapy and chemotherapy can be administered relatively safely [26, 83]. Chemotherapy is administered until a gestational age of 35 weeks or preferably, an interval of at least 3 weeks before delivery is aimed for. When the interval is too short, there is a risk for delivery-related maternal/fetal infection or bleeding, whereas an inadequate elimination of cytotoxic drugs by the immature fetal organs may contribute to an increased fetal risk.

21.2.1 Imaging and Diagnosis During Pregnancy

Staging should be as comprehensive as in nonpregnant women. Ultrasonography and magnetic resonance imaging are relatively safe and widely used during pregnancy [118, 136]. The safety for the latter however is not proven [136]. In contrast to previous belief, gadolinium-enhanced magnetic resonance imaging is also possible during pregnancy [171]. X-ray studies expose the fetus to radiation and the highest dosages are generatedb yc omputedt omography(Table 21.1).

Although the fetal doses do not reach the threshold dose for deterministic effects, stochastic effects need to be considered since fetuses have a high proportion of dividing cells [83]. In children this results in a higher lifetime risk for cancer after exposure to radiation [22]. The risk for childhood cancer is highest after abdominopelvic imaging (but not other sites) with exposure during the third trimester [43, 94]. Positron emission tomography combined with computed tomography exposed the fetus to 19 mGy and might be considered if it is the only tool to make a proper diagnosis [176]. Staging examinations during pregnancy are possible but fetal protection with abdominal shielding is advised.

The incidence of adnexal masses during pregnancy varies from 2.3 to 4.1% [20, 61]. The diagnosis and characterization of the adnexal mass is mainly based on sonography findings and less on serum tumor markers such as alpha-fetoprotein, CA 125, human chorion gonadotropin, and inhibin as these fluctuate during pregnancy and are less specific [61]. An expert sonographer needs to characterize the lesion. Nulliparity and treatment for infertility increase the risk for a pathologic mass [86, 117]. Ultrasound-guided aspiration of the cyst should be avoided, as the sensitivity of diagnosis from aspiration is only 70% [103] and the recurrence rate of cyst is around one third [66]. Cyst aspiration is not reliable for diagnosis, but may worsen the prognosis in case of early ovarian cancer [113, 167]. Furthermore, approximately 90% of lesions diagnosed during the first trimester of pregnancy will disappear spontaneously. Pathologic lesions are most frequently benign and include teratoma, cystadenoma, endometrioma, ovarian cysts, or leiomyomas. It is estimated that approximately 6% of all operated adnexal masses are malignant,[61] including epithelial (49–75%), sex cord stromal (9–16%) and germ cell tumors (6–40%) [61, 124].

The sentinel lymph node procedure with ^{99m}Tc can safely be performed during pregnancy. Studies in breast cancer show that after injection of 18.5 MBq ^{99m}Tc the fetal dosage approximately ranges from 0.0 to 0.05 mGy, which is far below the deterministic threshold dosage [56, 87]. This is mainly due to the low dosages that are administered and due to the fact that ^{99m}Tc is captured in the lymph nodes during a period during which radioactivity decreases considerably. The exposure after sentinel node procedure is in the same level as few day dosages of natural background irradiation [56, 87, 130]. In vulvar cancer, a dosage of 60 or 80 MBq is often used to detect the sentinel lymph node. Approximately 80% of a theoretical dosage of 100 MBq remains in the pelvis (injection location and some lymph nodes). The distance from the fetus is at least 10 cm. In this situation, fetal exposure can be estimated to be 100 μSv (or 0.1 mGy). According to the International Commission on Radiological Protection (ICRP) [56], fetal risk starts from 100 mSv (or megagray). The fetal exposure is thus 1,000 times lower and the fetal risk is negligible when a sentinel node procedure is used for vulvar cancer (Ate Van der Zee, personal communication) [166].

Table 21.1 Approximate fetal absorbed doses during imaging studies [8]. The threshold dose for fetal damage is estimated to vary between 10 and 20 cGy

Procedure	Fetaldos e(cGy)	Procedure	Fetal dose (cGy)
Chest X-ray (PA and lateral)	0.00006	Lumbosacral spine	0.2–0.6
Abdominal X-ray	0.15–0.26	Mammography	0.01–0.04
PelvicX -ray	0.2–0.35	CTt horax	0.01–1.3
Intravenousp yelography	0.4–0.9	CTa bdomen	0.8–3
Bariume nema	0.3–4	CTpe lvis	2.5–8.9
Dorsals pine	<0.001	Tc bone scan	0.15–0.20
Lumbars pine	0.4–0.6		

Anaphylactic reaction to patent blue has been described [4, 36]. However, treatment of this side effect during pregnancy is hazardous and fetal well-being is put into danger. The use of patent blue for the detection of the sentinel node is therefore not recommended.

21.2.2 Surgery During Pregnancy

Overall 0.75–2% of pregnant women will undergo surgery during pregnancy. Most common indications include cholecystitis, appendicitis, and ovarian cysts. Anesthesia is safe during pregnancy if physiologic adaptations are considered [121]. The most important recommendations are summarized in Table 21.2. Adequate maternal monitoring is crucial preventing hypoxia, hypotension, and hypoglycemia. Pregnant patients should be positioned in left lateral tilt to prevent caval compression. Preoperative fetal monitoring is always difficult to interpret and is only useful if clinically relevant. Fetal monitoring during surgery for gynecologic cancers is mostly not feasible. A cardiotocography, Doptone, or ultrasound just before and after the surgery may be useful to exclude direct fetal damage associated with surgery. With regard to fetal resuscitation, the local policy needs to be followed.

Table 21.2 Recommendations for maternal and fetal surveillance when pregnant women are operated

Anesthesia	Position: pregnant patients in left lateral tilt Prevent hypoxia, hypotension and hypoglycemia Adequate postoperative analgesia
Fetal monitoring	Screening ultrasonography before surgery Assessment of fetal well-being immediately pre and post-surgery
Uterine monitoring	Pre- and post-surgery
Lung maturation	Dexamethasone or betamethasone 24 h before interventions between 24–34 weeks
Tocolytic drugs	Case-related: to be discussed with obstetrician Consider when uterine manipulation is expected Should be started in case of preterm labor
Thrombosis prophylaxis	Low molecular weight heparin recommended
Laparoscopy	Opent echnique Limit pressure (max 15 mmHg) and time (<90 min) of pneumoperitoneum

Cohen-Kerem et al. reviewed over 12,000 cases of surgery during pregnancy [32]. The data suggest that surgery does not increase the risk for miscarriage and congenital anomalies. Only in cases of peritonitis fetal loss rate was increased. However, most of the reported surgeries did not include the reproductive tract or were indicated for cancer treatment. The latter may involve procedures like lymphadenectomies which are not included in most reports. Therefore, conclusions should be interpreted cautiously.

Surgery might slightly increase preterm delivery but numbers are difficult to interpret since no comparison was made with a normal pregnant population.

There is no literature supporting the prophylactic use of tocolysis in cases of surgery during pregnancy. When signs of preterm labor are present perioperatively, tocolytic agents like nifedipine, atosiban, or indomethacin (<32 weeks) should be considered [59, 104, 138, 175].

Jackson et al. concluded that laparoscopic surgery during pregnancy is safe and effective when performed in experienced hands [80]. The CO_2 pneumoperitoneum and CO-production during electrocoagulation does not seem to be hazardous to the fetus as long as the maximal pressure (normal 10–13 mmHg, max 15 mmHg) and operation time (25–90 min) are respected [2, 80, 104, 138, 175]. Open laparoscopy (opening of the peritoneum under direct visualization instead of using the Verres needle) is mandatory in order to avoid uterinepe rforation.

21.2.3 Systemic Anticancer Treatment During Pregnancy

Most anticancer drugs exhibit a narrow therapeutic window with small margins between toxic and therapeutic exposure. Inter-individual pharmacokinetic and pharmacodynamic variabilities are usually substantial and may be augmented by pregnancy [157]. During pregnancy multiple changes in physiology occur, affecting the major pharmacokinetic processes of a drug: absorption, distribution, metabolism, and excretion (ADME) [92]. This may have therapeutic and toxic consequences for both the pregnant woman and the fetus. Due to ADME changes, the pregnant patient may be exposed to subtherapeutic or toxic drug levels and an unwanted amount of drug may be delivered to the fetus. Obviously, these situations should be prevented, particularly in oncology where patients are treated with strong-acting, mutagenic, and teratogenic chemotherapeutics. The pharmacodynamic (antitumor activity/toxicity) consequences of all these physiological changes that theoretically lead to changes in drug exposure of pregnant patients are difficult to predict without pharmacokinetic data. Preclinical data evaluating exposure to a given dose in pregnant animals are also scarce but even if available, it is questionable how this information can reliably be translated to the clinic. Only one report compared maternal doxorubicin levels during and after pregnancy [160]. The results in a single case point to a lower drug exposure and decreased tissue toxicity when doxorubicin is administered during pregnancy. Despite the putative, emerging pharmacokinetic changes of chemotherapeutics during pregnancy, there are, however, so far no indications that pregnant cancer patients when treated with standard height–weight-based dosed chemotherapy are at higher risk for reduced efficacy or more toxicity than nonpregnant patients treated with the same drugs and dosages.

The effect on the fetus is another aspect of chemotherapy during pregnancy. The term "placental barrier" is a misnomer and false notion since the placenta is not a true barrier for the transfer of most substances from mother to fetus [152]. Instead the placenta is the entry through which the fetus is exposed to chemicals. Placental transfer of drugs from the maternal to the fetal side occurs predominantly via passive diffusion and to a lesser extent via active transport and facilitated diffusion. The amount and rate of transfer is primarily determined by the concentration gradient of the drug between the maternal and fetal circulation and placental blood flow. Besides the physicochemical properties of drugs such as lipid solubility and polarity, molecular weight and protein binding are also critical for placental transfer. Uncharged, low-molecular weight (<500 Da), lipid-soluble and unbound compounds can easily cross the human placenta. This implies that it can be expected that apart from the classic chemotherapeutic agents, new small targeted molecules also freely cross the placenta and reach the fetal circulation. Cardiac output is elevated through the second trimester and into later stages of the third trimester. The placenta will receive a gradually increasing proportion of total blood volume. Drug delivery to the placenta may therefore increase over the course of pregnancy. Recently it has been recognized that substrate-transporting proteins are present in the fetus-derived epithelial cells that make up the exchange border between the fetal and maternal blood compartment. These ATP energy-requiring transporters work against a concentration gradient and transport, for instance, nutrients into the fetal circulation. They can, however, also pump drugs including anticancer agents. The transporters are located in the syncytiotrophoblast plasma membrane, at the interface of the maternal and fetal circulations. Dependent on their location, apical or basolateral, they actively pump substrates from maternal to fetal (e.g., the organic cation transporter, OCTN), or fetal to maternal circulation (e.g., P-glycoprotein; P-gp). P-gp has received a great deal of attention in this respect. In the placenta it is located in apical trophoblast cells of the brush-border membrane. The *Mdr1a/Mdr1b* (P-gp) knockout mouse model has proved to be a useful tool for elucidating the contributions of placental P-gp in drug pharmacology, e.g., for paclitaxel [149]. It is suggested that P-gp in the placenta protects the fetal circulation for paclitaxel entrance. The same holds for the breast cancer resistance protein (BCRP), another member of the ATP-binding cassette family of drug transporters. BCRP restricts the passage of topotecan and mitoxantrone to the fetus [82]. Other identified placental transporters are the multidrug resistance proteins (MRPs), OCTNs, monocarboxylate transporters (MCTs) etc. [152]. The human placenta contains phase I (Cyt P450) and II (transferases) drug-metabolizing enzymes. Clinical relevance is, however, poorly understood [152]. Concomitant administration of drugs that block these transporters or modulate the metabolizing enzymes harbors the risk of leading to unintended exposure of the fetus to chemotherapy, and thus, alertness is advised when drug combinations are used.

Specific cytotoxic drug effects are difficult to describe since combinations are frequently used and since co-medications including steroids, analgesics, anti-emetics, and growth factors are administered as well. How chemotherapeutics should be dosed in pregnant women is uncertain and needs further research. Up till now the same schemes are used as in nonpregnant women. Table 21.3 compares combinations used in nonpregnant and pregnant women. Cytotoxic drugs used in gynecologic cancer include platin, paclitaxel, bleomycin, etoposide, and vinblastine.

Table 21.3 Recommended combinations of chemotherapy in nonpregnanta ndpre gnantw omen

	Nonpregnant	Pregnant
Ovarian cancer		
Epithelial	Paclitaxel-carboplatin	Paclitaxel-carboplatin
Germc ell	Bleomycin-etoposide-cisplatin	Paclitaxel-carboplatin or cisplatin-vinblastine-bleomycin
Cervicalc ancer	Platin-based	Paclitaxel-cisplatin Paclitaxel-carboplatin

Based on 37 reported cases, we calculate that cisplatin exposure resulted in moderate bilateral hearing loss in 1 of 37 (2.7%) and ventriculomegaly e causa ignota in 1 of 37 (2.7%) [15, 25, 48, 49, 55, 69, 74, 85, 89, 90, 96, 99, 126, 128, 135, 140, 150]. This latter patient received one cycle of bleomycin, cisplatin, and etoposide at a gestational age of 26 weeks. Apart from significant manipulation of the uterus to remove the uterus and the development of a pelvic hematoma requiring blood transfusion that might have been associated with fetal hypoxia, a direct neurotoxic effect must be considered [48]. In another case, maternal sepsis following bleomycin, cisplatin, and etoposide administration occurred, resulting in preterm labor [135]. The premature neonate (1,190 g) developed respiratory distress syndrome, myelosuppression, hearing impairment, and alopecia. Although cisplatin might have contributed to the sensorineural hearing loss, prematurity and the postnatal treatment with gentamycin were confounding factors. Taking these considerations into account, administration of cisplatin and cisplatin-containing regimens during pregnancy resulted in absence of congenital anomalies and normal neurological development in 35 of 37 (95%).

Carboplatin has been administered during pregnancy in eight cases (of which four had carboplatin in association with paclitaxel) and a normal neonatal outcome was noted in each [70, 75, 107, 114, 133, 153]. Based on a better toxicity profile, we recommend carboplatin instead of cisplatin if evaluated in the respective tumor entity. Until more data are available on the pharmacokinetics during pregnancy, we recommend dosing as usual for ovarian tumors in nonpregnant women (AUC 5–7.5). AUC is based on the glomerular filtration rate, with an upper safety limit of carboplatin of 800 mg [46]. Dose escalations can be planned according to blood counts subsequently.

Twenty case reports were found documenting the outcome after the use of taxanes during pregnancy: 13 on paclitaxel [13, 52, 54, 63, 75, 95, 101, 107, 114, 150] and seven on docetaxel [40, 53, 90, 122, 134, 146]. In 17 of 20 cases, taxanes were administered after other cytotoxic drugs (patients with breast cancer) or in combination with other cytotoxic drugs (patients with ovarian or lung cancer). Except for one case of hydrocephalia in a patient given docetaxel with doxorubicin-cyclophosphamide but with normal outcome of the child after 28 months [134], no fetal or neonatal problems after use of taxanes during pregnancy have been observed.

At least nine cases of a combination of bleomycin, cisplatin, and etoposide (BEP) during pregnancy for treatment of germ cell tumors have been described [15, 48, 69, 74, 85, 89, 99, 135]. Although reports describe a normal neonatal outcome, one child with a significant ventriculomegaly with cerebral atrophy was born after one cycle of BEP and one case of hearing impairment (see discussion above) [48, 135]. Based on this poor neonatal outcome and given the paclitaxel activity in germ cell tumors [105, 106], paclitaxel and carboplatin can be administered [75]. Vinca alkaloids are already in use for a long time and many reports cite their use as being relatively safe in pregnancy [26, 39, 57]. Also vinblastine may replace etoposide since cisplatin-vinblastine-bleomycin (PVB) has been used in four cases without maternal or fetal complications [27, 29, 100, 116]. Based on a possible fetal risk and the high risk of leukemia after etoposide administration, PVB or TC is advised in pregnant women with germ cell tumors (instead of BEP).

New targeted therapy is not recommended for pregnant patients with pelvic cancers due to the limited experience and the fact that large randomized phase III trials are still awaited to prove their efficacy.

21.2.4 Radiotherapy During Pregnancy

Therapeutic pelvic irradiation induces severe or lethal consequences and is not consistent with preservation of the pregnancy.

Table 21.4 Most important supportive drugs and their fetal safety profile [93–95]

Supportive drugs	Fetal safety data
Anti-emetics	
Metoclopramide/alizapride	Metoclopramide can be used in all stages of pregnancy. Its methoxy-2-benzamide-derivate, alizapride, is probably also safe
5-HT antagonists (granisetron, tropisetron, ondansetron)	Should not be withheld because of the pregnancy. Animal data suggest low risk. Case reports on ondansetron show its effectiveness in the control of vomiting in pregnancy and no adverse effects were observed in the children
NK1 antagonist (aprepitant)	Should not be withheld because of the pregnancy. No human data available, animal data suggest low risk
Corticoids	Can be used after the first trimester of pregnancy. Prednisolone or hydrocortisone are preferred
Growth factors	
Granulocyte colony-stimulating factors (pegfilgrastim, filgastrim, lenograstim)	Should not be withheld because of the pregnancy. Is crossing the placenta
Erythropoietins	Should not be withheld because of the pregnancy. Is probably not crossing the placenta
Pain-medication	
Paracetamol	Drug of preference (till 4 g/d)
Nonsteroidal anti-inflammatory drugs	Can be used between 12 and 32 weeks of gestation

21.2.5 Supportive Therapy and Symptom Control in the Pregnant Patient

Supportive treatment for chemotherapy can be given mainly according to the general recommendations [65]. Regarding the use of corticoids, methylprednisolone or hydrocortisone are extensively metabolized in the placenta and little crosses into the fetal compartment. They are therefore preferred over dexa- or betamethasone [21]. Repeated antenatal exposure to dexa- or betamethasone resulted in animal models in decreased body and brain weight and delay in the maturation time-table [3]. In addition, nonhuman primates given repeated doses of dexamethasone showed impaired postnatal growth, as well as impaired glucose tolerance, hyperinsulinemia, increased systolic and diastolic blood pressures, and an exaggerated cortisol response to mild stress [41]. Also in the National Institutes of Health Consensus, the concern on impaired fetal growth, suppression of pituitary-adrenal function, and long-term neurodevelopmental and behavioral problems following repeated courses of steroids was stated [119]. More children with attention problems, and higher rates of cerebral palsy have been described [38, 170].

Granulocyte colony-stimulating factor (G-CSF) and erythropoietin have been used safely in pregnant patients and their use should follow current guidelines for growth factor support during chemotherapy [127]. A list of the most important supportive drugs and their safety profile is presented in Table 21.4.

21.3 Monitoring Pregnancy and Neonatal Outcome

21.3.1 Monitoring of the Pregnancy, Complicated with a Gynecologic Cancer

In general, the mother and fetus should be monitored with the standard prenatal care. As treatment options will be dependent on the gestational age, it is very important to have a correct dating of the pregnancy. We advise performing a careful fetal examination by ultrasonographic screening before treatment is started, to ensure there are no preexisting fetal anomalies. Further ultrasound scans should be performed every 2–3 weeks to evaluate the fetal growth, development, and wellbeing. In the case of abnormal findings, more stringent monitoring of the fetus or even preterm delivery might be necessary. Pregnancy-related complications should be treated according to the standard obstetrical care.

Delivery should take place in a hospital with a neonatal care unit. When possible, the delivery should be delayed until 35–37 weeks and beyond and preferably should not be before 32 weeks. If the parents wish to save the pregnancy, one should attempt to reach at least the 28th week of pregnancy. Sequelae associated with preterm birth, of which neurodevelopmental impairments and cerebral palsy are the most important, increase with decreasing gestational age [8, 45, 112, 172]. The risk for long-term neurologic sequelae should be avoided if possible and discussed with the parents. When delivery is planned before 34 weeks, fetal lung maturation must be considered [37].

The placenta should be examined for metastases, but fetal involvement has never been described for these cancers [5, 24]. If treatment is to continue postpartum, breast-feeding during chemotherapy is contraindicated, as most of the agents used can be excreted in breast milk.

21.3.2 Neonatal and Long-Term Outcome After In Utero Exposure to Chemotherapy

Available studies on the outcome of the offspring lack both a detailed methodology and a systematic examination. Furthermore, only a selection of children has been investigated and no data are available on children who were lost to follow-up. Data on the long-term outcome of these children are very limited. This study is very complex since many confounding factors have to be taken into account.

Concerning the follow-up of the children after intrauterine exposure to chemotherapy during pregnancy, some methodological issues need to be considered. There exists a large body of experience in long-term follow up of children born "at risk." Prematurity, low birth weight,[81] smoking,[123] alcohol,[91] weight (gain) of the mother before and during pregnancy[142], and stress [164] have all been identified as contributing factors in the cognitive and emotional development of children. In general, these factors explain the variability seen in normal people in the higher cognitive and regulatory functions, such as impulsivity, attention, decision making, and self-regulation. Most of these functions are believed to be generated in the frontal lobes. In extreme cases, such as in the fetal alcohol syndrome, these prenatal factors can also cause disease. This field in developmental medicine is now called DOHaD: "developmental origins of health and disease" [147] and one of the most important challenges is to find the timing and the mechanisms by which these factors influence normal brain maturation ("fetal programming"). No doubt that one has to look for gene × environment interactions (e.g., in smoking: Langley et al. [93]).

It is clear that other known environmental factors (including birth weight, prematurity, alcohol, and stress) should be taken into account in the models that need to be developed. Previous research also guides us on which brain functions should be examined in more detail and the focus should be on so-called frontal functions.

There is no clear one-to-one relationship between results on neuropsychological testing and the everyday performance in school and normal life. This distinction between the neuropsychological and the behavioral levels (following the model by Frith [51]) is important to interpret the data that will be obtained. For instance, long-term follow-up on the effects of stress during pregnancy have shown very specific effects on self-regulation functions at the age of 18 years (such as a different response profile in a gambling task), but the large majority of the these young adults were attending university or high school and had a "normal life" [108].

The effect of in utero exposure to chemotherapy was assessed in 84 children with a median follow-up period of 18 years (range 6–29 years). Although the methodology was poorly described, the authors concluded that 84 children and 12 children from the second generation had a normal development [10]. Zemlikis et al. described one twin pregnancy exposed to cyclophosphamide [178]. One twin member was born with congenital malformations and developed thyroid cancer at the age of 11 and a neuroblastoma at the age of 14. The twin sister, however, was healthy. In the largest and recent literature review on this topic, Cardonic and Iacobucci described 376 cases of in utero exposure to chemotherapy [26]. In this series 5% intrauterine deaths and 1% neonatal deaths were registered. All but three deaths occurred with maternal hematological malignant disease. Two of these three had been exposed to idarubicin for breast cancer. The authors encountered 11 cases of congenital malformation of which 9 were exposed to chemotherapy in the first trimester. More recent publications also described no particular problems when chemotherapy was administered after the first trimester [28, 137]. Hahn et al. described 57 patients who were treated for breast cancer during pregnancy [68]. The telephone or mail was used to contact the parents/guardian or teacher. Respiratory problems were the most important neonatal complications ($n=10$). One child suffered from a subarachnoidal bleeding and three congenital anomalies were registered. Forty children were observed until the age of 2 till 157 months. Medical problems that were reported at that time included allergy, eczema, asthma, and upper respiratory infections and 2 of the 18 children who went to school needed special attention [68]. One small study systematically applied a battery of neuropsychological testing in 10 children. Morbidity after intrauterine exposure to cytotoxic drugs mainly appeared to be related to preterm neonates [161]. If possible, delivery should be planned after 35 weeks' gestational age. This strategy has been shown to be beneficial [137].

Echocardiographic follow-up data suggest a normal cardiac function in children who were exposed to cytotoxic drugs in utero [10, 110]. In a small series, Van Calsteren et al. utilized echocardiographic quantification of cardiac function using both conventional and newer techniques [161]. In all children, a normal cardiac performance without morphological abnormalities could be observed. However, a trend towards a lower wall thickness and left ventricular mass was recorded. The authors believe this could be due to chemotherapy as this influences myocyte replication and growth. Whether the different methodology that was used can explain the difference is a subject for further study.

The limited data are relatively reassuring and do not show an excessive increased risk for congenital malformations after intrauterine exposure to chemotherapy during the second and third trimesters. Long-term follow-up data are urgently needed. Especially systematic follow-up, neuropsychological testing, and cardiac function will inform us on the cognitive and cardiac function, fertility, and the occurrence of secondary malignancies or germ cell mutations.

21.4 OrganPat hology

21.4.1 Pre-Invasive Cervical Cancer

Abnormal cervical cytology complicates approximately 5% of pregnancies. Both cervical glands and stroma undergo physiologic alterations during pregnancy resulting in an increased cervical volume, stromal edema, glandular hyperplasia, and an increased vascularization that alter cytologic [16, 111] and colposcopic interpretation [16]. However, if the cytologist and colposcopist are aware of the pregnant state, their reliability is not decreased [16, 44, 162]. Moreover, a colposcopy-guided biopsy should not be postponed since the colposcopic/cytologic concordance can be worse in the postpartum [47]. Indications for colposcopy are the same as for nonpregnant patients and also the same morphological alterations in case of abnormality are present. Progression or missed diagnosis of microinvasive disease until the postpartum period was noted in 0.0, 1.1, 2.4, 8.0 and 9.7% of cases [1, 33, 129, 141, 168, 174]. Since these results will vary interindividually, treatment for CIN 2–3 lesions might be postponed until the postpartum when diagnosed by an experienced colposcopist. There is only very limited indication for conization in pregnancy in patients in whom the above-mentioned measures cannot rule out invasive disease. Then, conization refers to the excision of the transformation zone and a thickness of at least 5 mm is recommended. In the presence of pre-invasive disease, a vaginal delivery is allowed. However, this will not increase regression rates when compared to cesarean section.

21.4.2 Invasive Cervical Cancer

The incidence of cervical cancer during pregnancy is estimated to be around 1.2/10,000 [132]. Pelvic examinations during antenatal care contribute to the fact that pregnant women have a two- to threefold higher probability of being diagnosed in an operable stage of disease [177]. The treatment of cervical cancer during pregnancy is determined by the gestational age, stage of disease, and the wish of the patient to preserve the pregnancy.

The limited experience with an invasive cervical cancer diagnosed during pregnancy renders every treatment proposal experimental. Therefore, when pregnancy is not desired, standard treatment is executed. Radical hysterectomy of a pregnant uterus is possible. From the second trimester onwards, removal of the fetus by hysterotomy will improve the accessibility of the pelvis. Dissection of the anatomic structures is not more difficult during pregnancy. Sufficient experience is advised given the increased blood supply. Alternatively, chemoradiation can be used. Radiation of the pelvis during the first trimester will result in spontaneous abortion. During the second trimester, abortion may be protracted and may interfere with the radiotherapy. Surgical evacuation (hysterotomy or suction curettage) prior to the start with chemoradiotherapy will facilitate subsequent chemoradiotherapy.

When pregnancy is desired, the experimental nature of the cancer treatment during pregnancy and the potential risks should be discussed with the patient concerned. Treatment depends on the gestational age and stage of disease.

During the first trimester, a conservative approach is proposed to reach the second trimester.

During the second trimester, stage of disease will determine the treatment strategy. Stage Ia1 disease is treated by a flatc onebiops y [173].

From stage Ia2 on, interventions including lymphadenectomy, neoadjuvant chemotherapy (NACT), and trachelectomy during pregnancy can be considered.

A lymphadenectomy is performed during gestation when pregnancy- or fertility-saving surgery is possible. Pelvic lymphadenectomy is performed in order to identify high-risk disease that would exclude a pregnancy-saving policy. A retroperitoneal laparotomic approach or laparoscopy [7, 72] could potentially help to minimize uterine manipulation and hence contractility. The pathologist should be aware of the pregnant state, as decidual changes in the pelvic lymph nodes maymimic ma lignantdis ease [9, 23, 31, 35, 73].

NACT during pregnancy can be used to stabilize or reduce the size of cervical cancer [12, 25, 58, 84, 102, 128, 139, 156]. Chemotherapy for cervical cancer should be platinum based but the addition of paclitaxel will increase response rates [19]. During pregnancy, paclitaxel-carboplatin q3w is proposed and the number of cycles is guided by the presence of fetal maturity. However, a minimum of two and a maximum number of four cycles is advised. When only one cycle of chemotherapy is needed to attain fetal maturity, a waiting policy is preferred.

Trachelectomy has been described as an abdominal [158] or vaginal procedure [163]. Experience during pregnancy is however very limited and the technique requires sufficient surgical skills and may be associated with large volumes of blood loss (irrespective of the approach), and the risk of pregnancy loss is considerable [158]. The experimental nature of this approach needs to be discussed.

An algorithm for stage IA2–IB1<2 cm is presented in Fig. 21.1. In the absence of nodal metastasis, NACT followed by conservative surgery (e.g., trachelectomy) can be considered. However, standard treatment depends on the local policy and is radical hysterectomy or chemoradiation (Fig. 21.1, IA2–IB1 <2 cm).

An algorithm for stage IB1 2–4 cm tumors is presented in Fig. 21.2. Lymphadenectomy is mandatory but can be performed after NACT. The potential to preserve the pregnancy depends mainly on the nodal status and the response to NACT.

An algorithm for stage IB2–IIB is presented in Fig. 21.3. For these tumors, fertility-sparing surgery has not been sufficiently evaluated. Definitive treatment is performed after delivery. NACT during pregnancy can be applied until fetal maturity, preferably >35 weeks. Cesarean section is followed by final treatment. In case of a good response (residual tumor less than 4 cm), fertility-sparing surgery can be applied in experienced hands in an experimental setting or standard treatment can be used. Standard treatment is mandatory in nonresponders. Thus, for stage IB2–IIB, lymphadenectomy

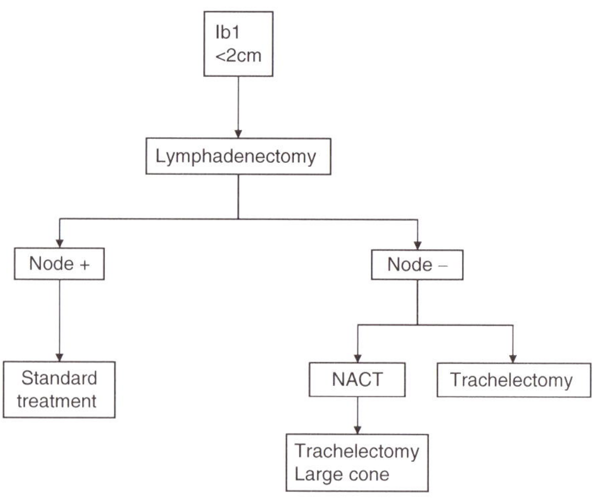

Fig. 21.1 Algorithm for treatment of cervical cancer stage Ib1, <2 cm treated during the second trimester of pregnancy in patients wishing to preserve the pregnancy and fertility

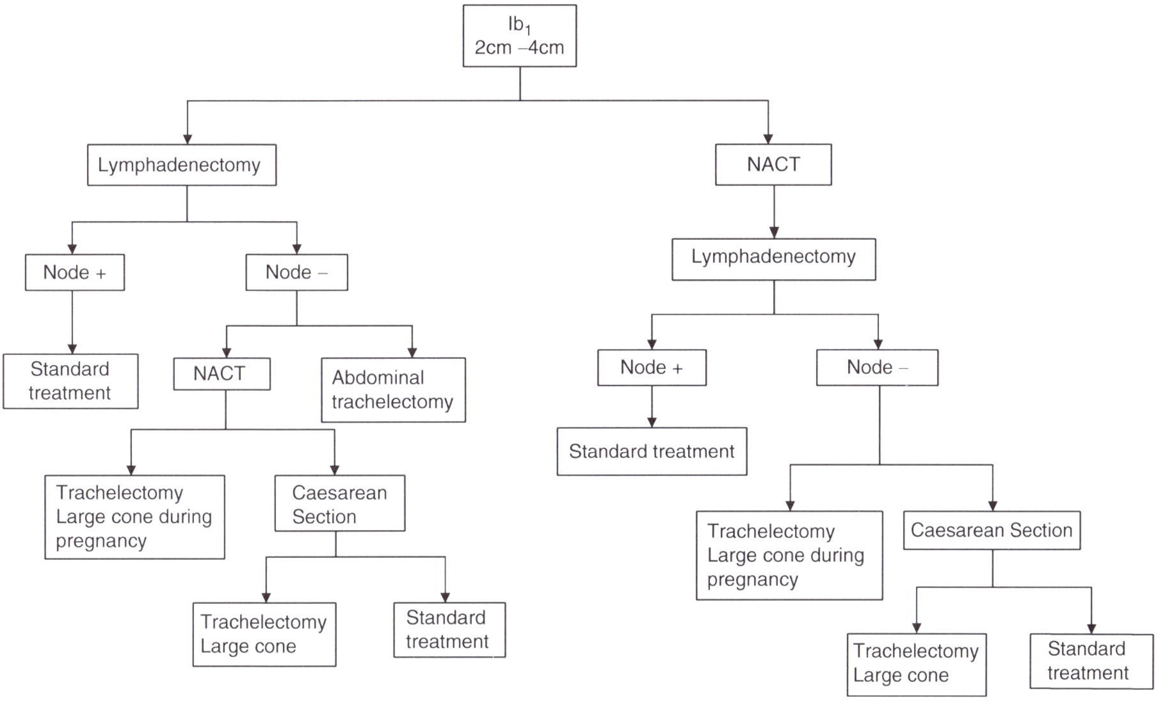

Fig. 21.2 Algorithm for treatment of cervical cancer stage Ib1, 2–4 cm treated during the second trimester of pregnancy in patients wishing to preservethe pr egnancya ndf ertility

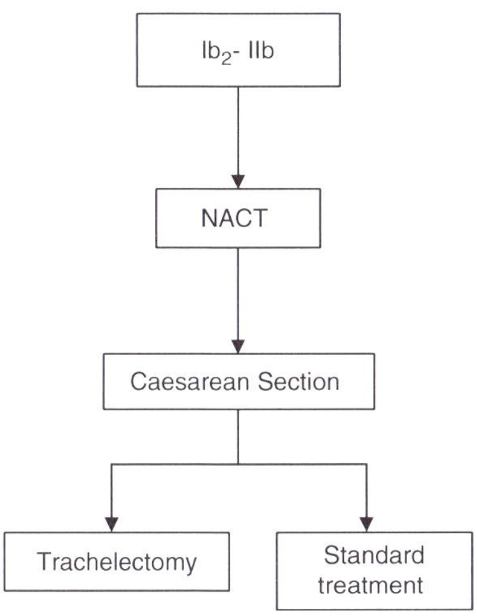

Fig. 21.3 Algorithm for treatment of cervical cancer stage IB2–IIB treated during the second trimester of pregnancy in patients wishingtopre serve thepr egnancya ndf ertility

is postponed until after delivery, when radical trachelectomy or standard treatment is opted for.

During the third trimester, fetal maturity is awaited and a cesarean section followed by standard treatment is proposed.

The route of delivery is determined by the presence or absence of tumor. When the cervix is cleared from tumor, a vaginal delivery is possible. In the presence of tumor, a cesarean section is the preferred route of delivery to prevent (fatal) recurrences in the episiotomy scar [17, 30, 62, 64, 71, 88, 120, 162, 165]. Since abdominal wall recurrences also (but less) have been described following a cesarean section,[109, 148] a wound protective system or a corporeal uterine incision might be useful when the tumor is large.

21.4.3 Vulvar Cancer

Epidemiological evidence to date suggests that vulva carcinogenesis originates from two etiologic pathways [97]. The first type is often seen in women over the age of 50 and is associated with non-neoplastic epithelial disorders. The second type is often seen in women under the age of 50, is frequently multifocal, and is associated with human papillomavirus infection [97]. Approximately 26% of vulvar intraepithelial neoplasia

(VIN) and 19% of invasive vulvar cancer occur in womenyo ungertha n40ye ars [151].

Although single cases of leiomyosarcoma, angiomyxoma, epithelioid sarcoma, and melanoma during pregnancy are reported,[5, 14, 42, 115] experience is mainly available with VIN and squamous vulvar cancer.

Diagnosis of VIN is made on a biopsy specimen. VIN can be treated with laser skinning or surgical excision, at every stage of pregnancy. Invasive (>1 mm) vulvar cancer with clinical negative nodes during pregnancy should be treated as in nonpregnant women with hemi- or total vulvectomy and uni- or bilateral inguinofemoral lymphadenectomy or sentinel procedure [34, 60]. Narrow margins should be avoided since recurrence during pregnancy has been described [125] and since postoperative radiotherapy during pregnancy is contraindicated. From a technical point of view, the increased vascularization of the pelvis during pregnancy increases the perioperative blood loss and meticulous hemostasis should be aimed for. After surgery for vulvar cancer, the route of delivery should be discussed with the gynecologic oncologist. Problematic wound healing, important scarring, or a periurethral or perianal scar are considered relative contraindications for a vaginal delivery.

The prognosis is poor if inguinal nodes are involved. Adequate treatment is needed without delay. Evidence for the benefit of chemotherapy is low. Termination of pregnancy with immediate treatment is advocated during the first and second trimester in patients with metastatic inguinofemoral lymph nodes. During the third trimester, delivery followed by standard treatment is suggested in these patients. Given the potential for spilling in the episiotomy wound and subsequent risk for an episiotomy scar recurrence, a cesarean section is preferred.

Vulvar melanoma deserves the same treatment as in nonpregnant patients. Patients harboring poor-prognosis disease should be informed about the high risk of relapse and death. Metastatic melanoma carries a risk for placental involvement with an approximate risk for fetal metastasis of 22% [5, 6].

21.4.4 Endometrial Cancer

Here, we define endometrial cancer related to pregnancy as any endometrial cancer diagnosed during pregnancy or during the puerperium (defined as the period 6 weeks after delivery). Using our definition, we found 28 published cases [11, 50, 77, 79, 144, 159]. Diagnosis was made during curettage ($n=17$, 61%), second to third trimester at birth ($n=8$, 28%) or during the puerperium ($n=3$, 11%). Distribution of pathological type and grading was as follows (n, %): grade I endometrioid (21, 75%), grade I–III endometrioid (6, 21%) or serous (1, 4%). In all but one case, the uterus was empty when the diagnosis was made [169]. In the absence of a fetus, standard treatment for endometrial cancer should be offered.

21.4.5 Ovarian Neoplasm

Surgical intervention is indicated for persistent adnexal masses with an unsure biological behavior. The clinician needs to make the balance between operating too early (risk for miscarriage and adnexectomy with loss of luteal function during the first trimester) and late surgery (torsion, rupture or bleeding of benign masses, higher stage ovarian cancer [50], premature labor). A midline laparotomy with minimal uterine manipulation during the second trimester is preferred. Perforation of a pregnant uterus by a Verres needle is a risk. An open laparoscopic procedure is only allowed in the absence of malignant signs and in experienced hands that minimize the risk for spilling, ideally between the 16th and 20th week of pregnancy [104, 175].

The incidence of ovarian cancer during gestation fluctuates around 1/10,000–100,000 [132]. Malignant tumors are more likely to present at early stage, due to frequent obstetrical examinations in asymptomatic patients [96, 154].

Non-epithelial neoplasms (germ cell, sex-cord stromal tumors) are usually stage I and can be treated with unilateral salpingo-oophorectomy, omentectomy, peritoneal cytology and blind biopsies during pregnancy. Uterine manipulations should be limited in order to prevent preterm contractions. Lymphadenectomy is not indicated, unless enlarged nodes were noticed during staging or intraoperatively. Adjuvant chemotherapy is not indicated for FIGO stage I grade I immature teratoma, or FIGO stage I dysgerminoma. Adjuvant chemotherapy for higher stages or non-dysgerminoma tumors is needed. Close surveillance instead of adjuvant chemotherapy has been propagated [131]; however, tumor markers during pregnancy are less reliable [61]. If continuation of pregnancy is desired, tumor markers are not useful to determine the number of cycles, and 6 cycles of paclitaxel-carboplatin are recommended (bleomycin-etoposide-cisplatin second choice) (see paragraph on chemotherapy). Restaging after delivery should be considered based on imaging findings and tumor markers.

Borderline epithelial cancers during pregnancy are likely to be stage I and can be treated during pregnancy. Staging laparotomy with unilateral salpingo-oophorectomy, omentectomy and peritoneal biopsies is needed. For higher stages removal of tumor during pregnancy is aimed for with completion of the surgery after delivery. A vaginal delivery is allowed. Chemotherapy or lymphadenectomy are not indicated for borderline ovarian malignancies.

For invasive epithelial ovarian carcinoma, the potential to preserve the pregnancy and the type of surgery and chemotherapy depend on the stage and grade. For stage IA, grade I surgical staging is similar to borderline tumors. Post-delivery re-staging may be considered since the pouch of Douglas is difficult to assess. For stage IA grade II–III, IB, IC and IIA, additionally a lymphadenectomy and adjuvant platin-based chemotherapy is mandatory. If the patient is upstaged, chemotherapy during pregnancy and final surgery after delivery are needed.

Advanced-stage ovarian cancer during pregnancy was treated with different treatment strategies, including primary debulking with termination of pregnancy [96, 155] or delivery, [78, 179] expectant management [18, 96], surgery during pregnancy followed by postpartum chemotherapy [18, 96], surgery (including cytoreductive surgery) followed by chemo during pregnancy with final surgery during/after delivery [18, 49, 70, 98, 101, 107, 114, 133, 143, 150, 153]. These case reports show that ovarian cancer treatment during pregnancy is an option. After considering the maternal prognosis and wish to preserve the pregnancy, stage of disease and the gestational age will determine the treatment plan. Advanced stage ovarian cancer before 20 weeks is mostly incompatible with maintenance of pregnancy. Debulking surgery with removal of the pregnancy and subsequent chemotherapy are recommended. For epithelial ovarian cancer stage ≥IIB, continuation of the pregnancy is experimental but may be an option if NACT renders continuation until delivery, followed by interval debulking thereafter. After 20 weeks, any debulking procedure would be incomplete since the pouch of Douglas is inaccessible. Therefore, surgery should be limited to establish the diagnosis and incomplete debulking during pregnancy should be avoided. In such a scenario, the fetus would be exposed unnecessarily to major surgery, not accomplishing the goal of complete resection of the tumor. Paclitaxel-carboplatin chemotherapy until fetal maturity is the regimen of choice for preoperative chemotherapy. Vaginal delivery is preferred since it allows final surgery in the postpartum period.

21.4.6 Psychosocial and Ethical Concerns of Cancer Diagnosis During Pregnancy

Most pregnant women diagnosed with cancer experience high emotional distress and even long-term emotional sequelae [145] Cancer diagnosis brings fear of death, worry about continuation of the pregnancy, anxiety about the impact of cancer treatment on the fetus, fear for not being able to raise the child into adulthood, and anxiety about future fertility. Emotional and psychological support is imperative. The partner runs a risk of raising the child on his own and should be involved. This child may be a remaining sign of their affection. It is advisable to engage the expertise of other members of the healthcare team such as psychologists, social workers, and, depending on patient's religion, a pastoral worker, especially during the time that treatment decisions are being made. Such a decision comprises a balance between the (dis)advantages for mother and child. The prognosis, treatment modalities, gestational age, and the patients' preference are pivotal in the decision-making process on treatment during pregnancy or termination of pregnancy. Although most studies report that the prognosis of cancer during pregnancy is similar to the nonpregnant state, these statements should be interpreted cautiously. The series are not large enough to control for all prognostic factors and to draw firm conclusions [76, 177]. Ethically, a delivery before 28 weeks is an undue risk for the fetus, but a suboptimal treatment is an undue risk for the mother. The parents should be informed about the different treatment options and the possible consequences for the patient and the fetus. A supportive patient–physician relationship is required, as is close collaboration and feedback of all disciplines involved in the patient's care, aiming to assist the patient and her partner toward achieving a valuable informed consent. Ongoing psychological support during treatment and delivery should be available for the parents.

21.5 Conclusion

Termination of pregnancy because of a concurrent malignancy does not always result in an improved prognosis. It is possible that the maternal prognosis is similar as in the nonpregnant state. Oncological surgery and chemotherapy can safely be performed after the first trimester, but individualization is crucial. In any case, oncological treatment close to standard should be offered and unnecessary delay in treatment should be avoided. Continuation of pregnancy until full term is advocated in order to prevent neonatal and long-term cognitive problems induced by preterm birth. When confronted with a cancer case during pregnancy, there is no reason to overreact and to take urgent decisions. The time needed for consulting an expert is notw orseningprognos is.

References

1. Ackermann S, Gehrsitz C, Mehlhorn G, et al. Management and course of histologically verified cervical carcinoma in situ during pregnancy. Acta Obstet Gynecol Scand. 2006; 85:1134–7.
2. Affleck DG, Handrahan DL, Egger MJ, et al. The laparoscopic management of appendicitis and cholelithiasis during pregnancy. Am J Surg. 1999;178:523–9.
3. Aghajafari F, Murphy K, Matthews S, et al. Repeated doses of antenatal corticosteroids in animals: a systematic review. Am J Obstet Gynecol. 2002;186:843–9.
4. Albo D, Wayne JD, Hunt KK, et al. Anaphylactic reactions to isosulfan blue dye during sentinel lymph node biopsy for breast cancer. Am J Surg. 2001;182:393–8.
5. Alexander A, Harris RM, Grossman D, et al. Vulvar melanoma: diffuse melanosis and metastasis to the placenta. J Am Acad Dermatol. 2004;50:293–8.
6. Alexander A, Samlowski WE, Grossman D, et al. Metastatic melanoma in pregnancy: risk of transplacental metastases in the infant. J Clin Oncol. 2003;21:2179–86.
7. Alouini S, Rida K, Mathevet P. Cervical cancer complicating pregnancy: implications of laparoscopic lymphadenectomy. Gynecol Oncol. 2008;108:472–7.
8. Ancel PY, Livinec F, Larroque B, et al. Cerebral palsy among very preterm children in relation to gestational age and neonatal ultrasound abnormalities: the EPIPAGE cohort study. Pediatrics. 2006;117:828–35.
9. Ashraf M, Boyd CB, Beresford WA. Ectopic decidual cell reaction in para-aortic and pelvic lymph nodes in the presence of cervical squamous cell carcinoma during pregnancy. J Surg Oncol. 1984;26:6–8.
10. Aviles A, Neri N, Nambo MJ. Long-term evaluation of cardiac function in children who received anthracyclines during pregnancy. Ann Oncol. 2006;17:286–8.
11. Ayhan A, Gunalp S, Karaer C, et al. Endometrial adenocarcinoma in pregnancy. Gynecol Oncol. 1999;75:298–9.
12. Bader AA, Petru E, Winter R. Long-term follow-up after neoadjuvant chemotherapy for high-risk cervical cancer during pregnancy. Gynecol Oncol. 2007;105:269–72.
13. Bader AA, Schlembach D, Tamussino KF, et al. Anhydramnios associated with administration of trastuzumab and paclitaxel for metastatic breast cancer during pregnancy. Lancet Oncol. 2007;8:79–81.
14. Bagga R, Keepanasseril A, Suri V, et al. Aggressive angiomyxoma of the vulva in pregnancy: a case report and review of management options. MedGenMed. 2007;9:16.
15. Bakri YN, Given Jr FT. Normal pregnancy and delivery following conservative surgery and chemotherapy for ovarian endodermal sinus tumor. Gynecol Oncol. 1984;19:222–5.
16. Baldauf JJ, Dreyfus M, Ritter J, et al. Colposcopy and directed biopsy reliability during pregnancy: a cohort study. Eur J Obstet Gynecol Reprod Biol. 1995;62:31–6.
17. Baloglu A, Uysal D, Aslan N, et al. Advanced stage of cervical carcinoma undiagnosed during antenatal period in term pregnancy and concomitant metastasis on episiotomy scar during delivery: a case report and review of the literature. Int J Gynecol Cancer. 2007;17:1155–9.
18. Behtash N, Karimi ZM, Modares GM, et al. Ovarian carcinoma associated with pregnancy: a clinicopathologic analysis of 23 cases and review of the literature. BMC Pregnancy Childbirth.2008; 8:3.
19. Benedetti PP, Bellati F, Pastore M, et al. An update in neoadjuvant chemotherapy in cervical cancer. Gynecol Oncol. 2007;107:S20–2.
20. Bernhard LM, Klebba PK, Gray DL, et al. Predictors of persistence of adnexal masses in pregnancy. Obstet Gynecol. 1999;93:585–9.
21. Blanford AT, Murphy BE. In vitro metabolism of prednisolone, dexamethasone, betamethasone, and cortisol by the human placenta. Am J Obstet Gynecol. 1977;127:264–7.
22. Brenner DJ, Hall EJ. Computed tomography – an increasing source of radiation exposure. N Engl J Med. 2007;357: 2277–84.
23. Burnett RA, Millan D. Decidual change in pelvic lymph nodes: a source of possible diagnostic error. Histopathology. 1986;10:1089–92.
24. Cailliez D, Moirot MH, Fessard C, et al. Placental localisation of cancer of the cervix. J Gynecol Obstet Biol Reprod (Paris).1980; 9:461–3.
25. Caluwaerts S, Van Calsteren K, Mertens L, et al. Neoadjuvant chemotherapy followed by radical hysterectomy for invasive cervical cancer diagnosed during pregnancy: report of a case and review of the literature. Int J Gynecol Cancer. 2006;16:905–8.
26. Cardonick E, Iacobucci A. Use of chemotherapy during human pregnancy. Lancet Oncol. 2004;5:283–91.

27. Caubel P, Giovangrandi Y, Lasry S, et al. Ovarian seminoma and pregnancy. Apropos of a new case. J Gynecol Obstet Biol Reprod (Paris). 1989;18:487–91.
28. Chelghoum Y, Vey N, Raffoux E, et al. Acute leukemia during pregnancy: a report on 37 patients and a review of the literature. Cancer. 2005;104:110–7.
29. Christman JE, Teng NN, Lebovic GS, et al. Delivery of a normal infant following cisplatin, vinblastine, and bleomycin (PVB) chemotherapy for malignant teratoma of the ovary during pregnancy. Gynecol Oncol. 1990;37:292–5.
30. Cliby WA, Dodson MK, Podratz KC. Cervical cancer complicated by pregnancy: episiotomy site recurrences following vaginal delivery. Obstet Gynecol. 1994;84:179–82.
31. Cobb CJ. Ectopic decidua and metastatic squamous carcinoma: presentation in a single pelvic lymph node. J Surg Oncol.1988;38:126–9.
32. Cohen-Kerem R, Railton C, Oren D, et al. Pregnancy outcome following non-obstetric surgical intervention. Am J Surg.2005;190:46 7–73.
33. Coppola A, Sorosky J, Casper R, et al. The clinical course of cervical carcinoma in situ diagnosed during pregnancy. Gynecol Oncol. 1997;67:162–5.
34. Couvreux-Dif D, Lhomme C, Querleu D, et al. Cancer of the vulva and pregnancy: two cases and review of the literature. J Gynecol Obstet Biol Reprod (Paris). 2003;32:46–50.
35. Covell LM, Disciullo AJ, Knapp RC. Decidual change in pelvic lymph nodes in the presence of cervical squamous cell carcinoma during pregnancy. Am J Obstet Gynecol. 1977;127:674–6.
36. Crivellaro M, Senna G, Dama A, et al. Anaphylaxis due to patent blue dye during lymphography, with negative skin prick test. J Investig Allergol Clin Immunol. 2003;13:71–2.
37. Crowley P, Chalmers I, Keirse MJ. The effects of corticosteroid administration before preterm delivery: an overview of the evidence from controlled trials. Br J Obstet Gynaecol. 1990;97:11–25.
38. Crowther CA, Doyle LW, Haslam RR, et al. Outcomes at 2 years of age after repeat doses of antenatal corticosteroids. N Engl J Med. 2007;357:1179–89.
39. Cuvier C, Espie M, Extra JM, et al. Vinorelbine in pregnancy. Eur J Cancer. 1997;33:168–9.
40. De Santis M, Lucchese A, De Carolis S, et al. Metastatic breast cancer in pregnancy: first case of chemotherapy with docetaxel. Eur J Cancer Care. 2000;9:235–7.
41. de Vries A, Holmes MC, Heijnis A, et al. Prenatal dexamethasone exposure induces changes in nonhuman primate offspring cardiometabolic and hypothalamic-pituitary-adrenal axis function. J Clin Invest. 2007;117:1058–67.
42. Di Gilio AR, Cormio G, Resta L, et al. Rapid growth of myxoid leiomyosarcoma of the vulva during pregnancy: a case report. Int J Gynecol Cancer. 2004;14:172–5.
43. Doll R, Wakeford R. Risk of childhood cancer from fetal irradiation. Br J Radiol. 1997;70:130–9.
44. Douvier S, Filipuzzi L, Sagot P. Management of cervical intra-epithelial neoplasm during pregnancy. Gynecol Obstet Fertil.2003;31:851–5.
45. Doyle LW. Neonatal intensive care at borderline viability – is it worth it? Early Hum Dev. 2004;80:103–13.
46. duBois A, Quinn M, Thigpen T, et al. 2004 consensus statements on the management of ovarian cancer: final document of the 3rd International Gynecologic Cancer Intergroup Ovarian Cancer Consensus Conference (GCIG OCCC 2004). Ann Oncol. 2005;16 Suppl 8:viii7–12.
47. Economos K, Perez VN, Delke I, et al. Abnormal cervical cytology in pregnancy: a 17-year experience. Obstet Gynecol.1993; 81:915–8.
48. Elit L, Bocking A, Kenyon C, et al. An endodermal sinus tumor diagnosed in pregnancy: case report and review of the literature. Gynecol Oncol. 1999;72:123–7.
49. Ferrandina G, Distefano M, Testa A, et al. Management of an advanced ovarian cancer at 15 weeks of gestation: case report and literature review. Gynecol Oncol. 2005;97: 693–6.
50. Foersterling DL, Blythe JG. Ovarian carcinoma, endometrial carcinoma, and pregnancy. Gynecol Oncol. 1999;72: 425–6.
51. Frith U. What framework should we use for understanding developmental disorders? Dev Neuropsychol. 2001;20: 555–63.
52. Gadducci A, Cosio S, Fanucchi A, et al. Chemotherapy with epirubicin and paclitaxel for breast cancer during pregnancy: case report and review of the literature. Anticancer Res. 2003;23:5225–9.
53. Gainford MC, Clemons M. Breast cancer in pregnancy: are taxanes safe? Clin Oncol. 2006;18:159.
54. Garcia-Manero M, Royo MP, Espinos J, et al. Pregnancy associated breast cancer. Eur J Surg Oncol. 2008;35:215–8.
55. Garrido M, Clavero J, Huete A, et al. Prolonged survival of a woman with lung cancer diagnosed and treated with chemotherapy during pregnancy. Review of cases reported. Lung Cancer. 2008;60:285–90.
56. Gentilini O, Cremonesi M, Trifiro G, et al. Safety of sentinel node biopsy in pregnant patients with breast cancer. Ann Oncol. 2004;15:1348–51.
57. Giacalone PL, Laffargue F, Benos P. Chemotherapy for breast carcinoma during pregnancy: a French national survey. Cancer. 1999;86:2266–72.
58. Giacalone PL, Laffargue F, Benos P, et al. Cis-platinum neoadjuvant chemotherapy in a pregnant woman with invasive carcinoma of the uterine cervix. Br J Obstet Gynaecol. 1996;103:932–4.
59. Giles W, Bisits A. Preterm labour. The present and future of tocolysis. Best Pract Res Clin Obstet Gynaecol. 2007;21: 857–68.
60. Gitsch G, van Eijkeren M, Hacker NF. Surgical therapy of vulvar cancer in pregnancy. Gynecol Oncol. 1995;56: 312–5.
61. Giuntoli RL, Vang RS, Bristow RE. Evaluation and management of adnexal masses during pregnancy. Clin Obstet Gynecol.2006; 49:492–505.
62. Goldman NA, Goldberg GL. Late recurrence of squamous cell cervical cancer in an episiotomy site after vaginal delivery. Obstet Gynecol. 2003;101:1127–9.
63. Gonzalez-Angulo AM, Walters RS, Carpenter Jr RJ, et al. Paclitaxel chemotherapy in a pregnant patient with bilateral breast cancer. Clin Breast Cancer. 2004;5:317–9.
64. Gordon AN, Jensen R, Jones III HW. Squamous carcinoma of the cervix complicating pregnancy: recurrence in episiotomy after vaginal delivery. Obstet Gynecol. 1989;73: 850–2.
65. Gralla RJ, Osoba D, Kris MG, et al. Recommendations for the use of antiemetics: evidence-based, clinical practice

guidelines. American Society of Clinical Oncology. J Clin Oncol.1999;17:2971–94.
66. Guariglia L, Conte M, Are P, et al. Ultrasound-guided fine needle aspiration of ovarian cysts during pregnancy. Eur J Obstet Gynecol Reprod Biol. 1999;82:5–9.
67. Gustafsson L, Ponten J, Zack M, et al. International incidence rates of invasive cervical cancer after introduction of cytological screening. Cancer Causes Control. 1997;8:755–63.
68. Hahn KM, Johnson PH, Gordon N, et al. Treatment of pregnant breast cancer patients and outcomes of children exposed to chemotherapy in utero. Cancer. 2006;107:1219–26.
69. Han JY, Nava-Ocampo AA, Kim TJ, et al. Pregnancy outcome after prenatal exposure to bleomycin, etoposide and cisplatin for malignant ovarian germ cell tumors: report of 2 cases. Reprod Toxicol. 2005;19:557–61.
70. Henderson CE, Elia G, Garfinkel D, et al. Platinum chemotherapy during pregnancy for serous cystadenocarcinoma of the ovary. Gynecol Oncol. 1993;49:92–4.
71. Heron DE, Axtel A, Gerszten K, et al. Villoglandular adenocarcinoma of the cervix recurrent in an episiotomy scar: a case report in a 32-year-old female. Int J Gynecol Cancer. 2005;15:366–71.
72. Hertel H, Possover M, Kuhne-Heid R, et al. Laparoscopic lymph node staging of cervical cancer in the 19th week of pregnancy. A case report. Surg Endosc. 2001;15:324.
73. Hogg R, Ungar L, Hazslinszky P. Radical hysterectomy for cervical carcinoma in pregnant women – a case of decidua mimicking metastatic carcinoma in pelvic lymph nodes. Eur J Gynaecol Oncol. 2005;26:499–500.
74. Horbelt D, Delmore J, Meisel R, et al. Mixed germ cell malignancy of the ovary concurrent with pregnancy. Obstet Gynecol.1994;84 :662–4.
75. Hubalek M, Smekal-Schindelwig C, Zeimet AG, et al. Chemotherapeutic treatment of a pregnant patient with ovarian dysgerminoma. Arch Gynecol Obstet. 2007;276:179–83.
76. Ibrahim EM, Ezzat AA, Baloush A, et al. Pregnancy-associated breast cancer: a case-control study in a young population with a high-fertility rate. Med Oncol. 2000;17: 293–300.
77. Ichikawa Y, Takano K, Higa S, et al. Endometrial carcinoma coexisting with pregnancy, presumed to derive from adenomyosis: a case report. Int J Gynecol Cancer. 2001;11: 488–90.
78. Ishioka S, Hayashi T, Endo T, et al. Advanced epithelial ovarian carcinoma during pregnancy. Int J Clin Oncol. 2007;12:375–8.
79. Itoh K, Shiozawa T, Shiohara S, et al. Endometrial carcinoma in septate uterus detected 6 months after full-term delivery: case report and review of the literature. Gynecol Oncol.2004;93:242–7.
80. Jackson H, Granger S, Price R, et al. Diagnosis and laparoscopic treatment of surgical diseases during pregnancy: an evidence-based review. Surg Endosc. 2008;22:1917–27.
81. Johnson S. Cognitive and behavioural outcomes following very preterm birth. Semin Fetal Neonatal Med. 2007;12: 363–73.
82. Jonker JW, Smit JW, Brinkhuis RF, et al. Role of breast cancer resistance protein in the bioavailability and fetal penetration of topotecan. J Natl Cancer Inst. 2000;92:1651–6.
83. Kal HB, Struikmans H. Radiotherapy during pregnancy: fact and fiction. Lancet Oncol. 2005;6:328–33.
84. Karam A, Feldman N, Holschneider CH. Neoadjuvant cisplatin and radical cesarean hysterectomy for cervical cancer in pregnancy. Nat Clin Pract Oncol. 2007;4:375–80.
85. Karimi ZM, Behtash N, Modares GM. Good pregnancy outcome after prenatal exposure to bleomycin, etoposide and cisplatin for ovarian immature teratoma: a case report and literature review. Arch Gynecol Obstet. 2008;277:75–8.
86. Karlan BY, Marrs R, Lagasse LD. Advanced-stage ovarian carcinoma presenting during infertility evaluation. Am J Obstet Gynecol. 1994;171:1377–8.
87. Keleher A, Wendt III R, Delpassand E, et al. The safety of lymphatic mapping in pregnant breast cancer patients using Tc-99m sulfur colloid. Breast J. 2004;10:492–5.
88. Khalil AM, Khatib RA, Mufarrij AA, et al. Squamous cell carcinoma of the cervix implanting in the episiotomy site. Gynecol Oncol. 1993;51:408–10.
89. Kim DS, Park MI. Maternal and fetal survival following surgery and chemotherapy of endodermal sinus tumor of the ovary during pregnancy: a case report. Obstet Gynecol. 1989;73:503–7.
90. Kim JH, Kim HS, Sung CW, et al. Docetaxel, gemcitabine, and cisplatin administered for non-small cell lung cancer during the first and second trimester of an unrecognized pregnancy. Lung Cancer. 2008;59:270–3.
91. Knopik VS, Sparrow EP, Madden PA, et al. Contributions of parental alcoholism, prenatal substance exposure, and genetic transmission to child ADHD risk: a female twin study. Psychol Med. 2005;35:625–35.
92. Krauer B, Krauer F, Hytten FE. Drug disposition and pharmacokinetics in the maternal-placental-fetal unit. Pharmacol Ther.1980; 10:301–28.
93. Langley K, Turic D, Rice F, et al. Testing for gene x environment interaction effects in attention deficit hyperactivity disorder and associated antisocial behavior. Am J Med Genet B Neuropsychiatr Genet. 2008;147B:49–53.
94. Lowe SA. Diagnostic radiography in pregnancy: risks and reality. Aust N Z J Obstet Gynaecol. 2004;44:191–6.
95. Lycette JL, Dul CL, Munar M, et al. Effect of pregnancy on the pharmacokinetics of paclitaxel: a case report. Clin Breast Cancer. 2006;7:342–4.
96. Machado F, Vegas C, Leon J, et al. Ovarian cancer during pregnancy: analysis of 15 cases. Gynecol Oncol. 2007;105: 446–50.
97. Madeleine MM, Daling JR, Carter JJ, et al. Cofactors with human papillomavirus in a population-based study of vulvar cancer. J Natl Cancer Inst. 1997;89:1516–23.
98. Malfetano JH, Goldkrand JW. Cis-platinum combination chemotherapy during pregnancy for advanced epithelial ovarian carcinoma. Obstet Gynecol. 1990;75:545–7.
99. Malhotra N, Sood M. Endodermal sinus tumor in pregnancy. Gynecol Oncol. 2000;78:265–6.
100. Malone JM, Gershenson DM, Creasy RK, et al. Endodermal sinus tumor of the ovary associated with pregnancy. Obstet Gynecol.1986; 68:86S–9.
101. Mantovani G, Gramignano G, Mais V, et al. Use of chemotherapy for ovarian cancer during human pregnancy: case report and literature review. Eur J Obstet Gynecol Reprod Biol.2007; 131:238–9.
102. Marana HR, de Andrade JM, Silva Mathes AC, et al. Chemotherapy in the treatment of locally advanced cervical cancer and pregnancy. Gynecol Oncol. 2001;80:272–4.

103. Martinez-Onsurbe P, Ruiz VA, Sanz Anquela JM, et al. Aspiration cytology of 147 adnexal cysts with histologic correlation. Acta Cytol. 2001;45:941–7.
104. Mathevet P, Nessah K, Dargent D, et al. Laparoscopic management of adnexal masses in pregnancy: a case series. Eur J Obstet Gynecol Reprod Biol. 2003;108:217–22.
105. McNeish IA, Kanfer EJ, Haynes R, et al. Paclitaxel-containing high-dose chemotherapy for relapsed or refractory testicular germ cell tumours. Br J Cancer. 2004;90: 1169–75.
106. Mead GM, Cullen MH, Huddart R, et al. A phase II trial of TIP (paclitaxel, ifosfamide and cisplatin) given as second-line (post-BEP) salvage chemotherapy for patients with metastatic germ cell cancer: a medical research council trial. Br J Cancer. 2005;93:178–84.
107. Mendez LE, Mueller A, Salom E, et al. Paclitaxel and carboplatin chemotherapy administered during pregnancy for advanced epithelial ovarian cancer. Obstet Gynecol. 2003; 102:1200–2.
108. Mennes M, Stiers P, Lagae L, et al. Long-term cognitive sequelae of antenatal maternal anxiety: involvement of the orbitofrontal cortex. Neurosci Biobehav Rev. 2006;30: 1078–86.
109. Method MW, Brost BC. Management of cervical cancer in pregnancy. Semin Surg Oncol. 1999;16:251–60.
110. Meyer-Wittkopf M, Barth H, Emons G, et al. Fetal cardiac effects of doxorubicin therapy for carcinoma of the breast during pregnancy: case report and review of the literature. Ultrasound Obstet Gynecol. 2001;18:62–6.
111. Michael CW, Esfahani FM. Pregnancy-related changes: a retrospective review of 278 cervical smears. Diagn Cytopathol.1997; 17:99–107.
112. Mikkola K, Ritari N, Tommiska V, et al. Neurodevelopmental outcome at 5 years of age of a national cohort of extremely low birth weight infants who were born in 1996–1997. Pediatrics.2005;1 16:1391–400.
113. Milad MP, Olson E. Factors that increase the risk of leakage during surgical removal of benign cystic teratomas. Hum Reprod. 1999;14:2264–7.
114. Modares GM, Karimi ZM, Behtash N, et al. Preservation of pregnancy in a patient with advanced ovarian cancer at 20 weeks of gestation: case report and literature review. Int J Gynecol Cancer. 2007;17:1140–3.
115. Moore RG, Steinhoff MM, Granai CO, et al. Vulvar epithelioid sarcoma in pregnancy. Gynecol Oncol. 2002;85: 218–22.
116. Motegi M, Takakura S, Takano H, et al. Adjuvant chemotherapy in a pregnant woman with endodermal sinus tumor of the ovary. Obstet Gynecol. 2007;109:537–40.
117. Murdoch WJ. Ovarian surface epithelium, ovulation and carcinogenesis. Biol Rev Camb Philos Soc. 1996;71:529–43.
118. Nagayama M, Watanabe Y, Okumura A, et al. Fast MR imaging in obstetrics. Radiographics. 2002;22:563–80.
119. National Institutes of Health Consensus Development Panel. Antenatal corticosteroids revisited: repeat courses – National Institutes of Health Consensus Development Conference Statement, August 17–18, 2000. Obstet Gynecol.2001;98 :144–50.
120. Neumann G, Rasmussen KL, Petersen LK. Cervical adenosquamous carcinoma: tumor implantation in an episiotomy scar. Obstet Gynecol. 2007;110:467–9.
121. Ni Mhuireachtaigh R, O'Gorman DA. Anesthesia in pregnant patients for nonobstetric surgery. J Clin Anesth. 2006;18:60–6.
122. Nieto Y, Santisteban M, Aramendia JM, et al. Docetaxel administered during pregnancy for inflammatory breast carcinoma. Clin Breast Cancer. 2006;6:533–4.
123. Obel C, Linnet KM, Henriksen TB, et al. Smoking during pregnancy and hyperactivity-inattention in the offspring – comparing results from three Nordic cohorts. Int J Epidemiol.2008.doi :10.1093/ije/dym290.
124. Oehler MK, Wain GV, Brand A. Gynaecological malignancies in pregnancy: a review. Aust N Z J Obstet Gynaecol. 2003;43:414–20.
125. Ogunleye D, Lewin SN, Huettner P, et al. Recurrent vulvar carcinoma in pregnancy. Gynecol Oncol. 2004;95:400–1.
126. Otton G, Higgins S, Phillips KA, et al. A case of early-stage epithelial ovarian cancer in pregnancy. Int J Gynecol Cancer.2 001;11:413–7.
127. Ozer H, Armitage JO, Bennett CL, et al. 2000 update of recommendations for the use of hematopoietic colony-stimulating factors: evidence-based, clinical practice guidelines. American Society of Clinical Oncology Growth Factors Expert Panel. J Clin Oncol. 2000;18:3558–85.
128. Palaia I, Pernice M, Graziano M, et al. Neoadjuvant chemotherapy plus radical surgery in locally advanced cervical cancer during pregnancy: a case report. Am J Obstet Gynecol.2007; 197:e5–6.
129. Palle C, Bangsboll S, Andreasson B. Cervical intraepithelial neoplasia in pregnancy. Acta Obstet Gynecol Scand. 2000;79:306–10.
130. Pandit-Taskar N, Dauer LT, Montgomery L, et al. Organ and fetal absorbed dose estimates from 99mTc-sulfur colloid lymphoscintigraphy and sentinel node localization in breast cancer patients. J Nucl Med. 2006;47:1202–8.
131. Patterson DM, Murugaesu N, Holden L, et al. A review of the close surveillance policy for stage I female germ cell tumors of the ovary and other sites. Int J Gynecol Cancer. 2008;18:43–50.
132. Pavlidis NA. Coexistence of pregnancy and malignancy. Oncologist.2002; 7:279–87.
133. Picone O, Lhomme C, Tournaire M, et al. Preservation of pregnancy in a patient with a stage IIIB ovarian epithelial carcinoma diagnosed at 22 weeks of gestation and treated with initial chemotherapy: case report and literature review. Gynecol Oncol. 2004;94:600–4.
134. Potluri V, Lewis D, Burton GV. Chemotherapy with taxanes in breast cancer during pregnancy: case report and review of the literature. Clin Breast Cancer. 2006;7:167–70.
135. Raffles A, Williams J, Costeloe K, et al. Transplacental effects of maternal cancer chemotherapy. Case report. Br J Obstet Gynaecol. 1989;96:1099–100.
136. Reddy UM, Filly RA, Copel JA. Prenatal imaging: ultrasonography and magnetic resonance imaging. Obstet Gynecol.2008; 112:145–57.
137. Ring AE, Smith IE, Jones A, et al. Chemotherapy for breast cancer during pregnancy: an 18-year experience from five London teaching hospitals. J Clin Oncol. 2005;23: 4192–7.
138. Rizzo AG. Laparoscopic surgery in pregnancy: long-term follow-up. J Laparoendosc Adv Surg Tech A. 2003; 13:11–5.

139. Robova H, Pluta M, Hrehorcak M, et al. High-dose density chemotherapy followed by simple trachelectomy: full-term pregnancy. Int J Gynecol Cancer. 2008;18:1367–71.
140. Robova H, Rob L, Hrehorcak M, et al. Endodermal sinus tumor diagnosed in pregnancy: a case report. Int J Gynecol Cancer.2007; 17:914–6.
141. Robova H, Rob L, Pluta M, et al. Squamous intraepithelial lesion-microinvasive carcinoma of the cervix during pregnancy. Eur J Gynaecol Oncol. 2005;26:611–4.
142. Rodriguez A, Miettunen J, Henriksen TB, et al. Maternal adiposity prior to pregnancy is associated with ADHD symptoms in offspring: evidence from three prospective pregnancy cohorts. Int J Obes. 2008;32:550–7.
143. Sankaranarayanan R, Ferlay J. Worldwide burden of gynaecological cancer: the size of the problem. Best Pract Res Clin Obstet Gynaecol. 2006;20:207–25.
144. Schammel DP, Mittal KR, Kaplan K, et al. Endometrial adenocarcinoma associated with intrauterine pregnancy. A report of five cases and a review of the literature. Int J Gynecol Pathol. 1998;17:327–35.
145. Schover LR. Psychosocial issues associated with cancer in pregnancy. Semin Oncol. 2000;27:699–703.
146. Sekar R, Stone PR. Trastuzumab use for metastatic breast cancer in pregnancy. Obstet Gynecol. 2007;110:507–10.
147. Sinclair KD, Lea RG, Rees WD, et al. The developmental origins of health and disease: current theories and epigenetic mechanisms. Soc Reprod Fertil Suppl. 2007;64:425–43.
148. Sivanesaratnam V, Jayalakshmi P, Loo C. Surgical management of early invasive cancer of the cervix associated with pregnancy. Gynecol Oncol. 1993;48:68–75.
149. Smit JW, Huisman MT, van Tellingen O, et al. Absence or pharmacological blocking of placental P-glycoprotein profoundly increases fetal drug exposure. J Clin Invest. 1999;104:1441–7.
150. Sood AK, Shahin MS, Sorosky JI. Paclitaxel and platinum chemotherapy for ovarian carcinoma during pregnancy. Gynecol Oncol. 2001;83:599–600.
151. Stroup AM, Harlan LC, Trimble EL. Demographic, clinical, and treatment trends among women diagnosed with vulvar cancer in the United States. Gynecol Oncol. 2008; 108:577–83.
152. Syme MR, Paxton JW, Keelan JA. Drug transfer and metabolism by the human placenta. Clin Pharmacokinet. 2004;43:487–514.
153. Tabata T, Nishiura K, Tanida K, et al. Carboplatin chemotherapy in a pregnant patient with undifferentiated ovarian carcinoma: case report and review of the literature. Int J Gynecol Cancer. 2008;18:181–4.
154. Takeuchi T, Suzuki S, Hayashi Z, et al. Primary ovarian tumor undergoing surgical management during pregnancy. J Nippon Med Sch. 2002;69:39–42.
155. Tewari K, Brewer C, Cappuccini F, et al. Advanced-stage small cell carcinoma of the ovary in pregnancy: long-term survival after surgical debulking and multiagent chemotherapy. Gynecol Oncol. 1997;66:531–4.
156. Tewari K, Cappuccini F, Gambino A, et al. Neoadjuvant chemotherapy in the treatment of locally advanced cervical carcinoma in pregnancy: a report of two cases and review of issues specific to the management of cervical carcinoma in pregnancy including planned delay of therapy. Cancer. 1998;82:1529–34.
157. Undevia SD, Gomez-Abuin G, Ratain MJ. Pharmacokinetic variability of anticancer agents. Nat Rev Cancer. 2005;5: 447–58.
158. Ungar L, Smith JR, Palfalvi L, et al. Abdominal radical trachelectomy during pregnancy to preserve pregnancy and fertility. Obstet Gynecol. 2006;108:811–4.
159. Vaccarello L, Apte SM, Copeland LJ, et al. Endometrial carcinoma associated with pregnancy: A report of three cases and review of the literature. Gynecol Oncol. 1999;74:118–22.
160. Van Calsteren K, Verbesselt R, Paridaens R, et al. Pregnancy induces decreased doxorubicin plasma levels and tissue toxicity. Oral presentation, 14th International Meeting of the European Society of Gynaecological Oncology (ESGO), Berlin.2007.
161. Van Calsteren K, Berteloot P, Hanssens M, et al. In utero exposure to chemotherapy: effect on cardiac and neurologic outcome. J Clin Oncol. 2006;24:e16–7.
162. Van Calsteren K, Vergote I, Amant F. Cervical neoplasia during pregnancy: diagnosis, management and prognosis. Best Pract Res Clin Obstet Gynaecol. 2005;19:611–30.
163. van de Nieuwenhof HP, van Ham MA, Lotgering FK, et al. First case of vaginal radical trachelectomy in a pregnant patient. Int J Gynecol Cancer. 2008;18:1381–5.
164. Van den Bergh BR, Van Calster B, Smits T, et al. Antenatal maternal anxiety is related to HPA-axis dysregulation and self-reported depressive symptoms in adolescence: a prospective study on the fetal origins of depressed mood. Neuropsychopharmacology.2008; 33:2301.
165. Van den Broek NR, Lopes AD, Ansink A, et al. "Microinvasive" adenocarcinoma of the cervix implanting in an episiotomy scar. Gynecol Oncol. 1995;59:297–9.
166. Van der Zee AG, Oonk MH, De Hullu JA, et al. Sentinel node dissection is safe in the treatment of early-stage vulvar cancer. J Clin Oncol. 2008;26:884–9.
167. Vergote I, De Brabanter J, Fyles A, et al. Prognostic importance of degree of differentiation and cyst rupture in stage I invasive epithelial ovarian carcinoma. Lancet. 2001;357: 176–82.
168. Vlahos G, Rodolakis A, Diakomanolis E, et al. Conservative management of cervical intraepithelial neoplasia (CIN(2–3)) in pregnant women. Gynecol Obstet Invest. 2002;54:78–81.
169. Wall JA, Lucci Jr JA. Adenocarcinoma of the corpus uteri and pelvic tuberculosis complicating pregnancy; report of case with delivery of live infant and successful recovery. Obstet Gynecol. 1953;2:629–35.
170. Wapner RJ, Sorokin Y, Mele L, et al. Long-term outcomes after repeat doses of antenatal corticosteroids. N Engl J Med.2007; 357:1190–8.
171. Webb JA, Thomsen HS, Morcos SK. The use of iodinated and gadolinium contrast media during pregnancy and lactation. Eur Radiol. 2005;15:1234–40.
172. Wood NS, Marlow N, Costeloe K, et al. Neurologic and developmental disability after extremely preterm birth. EPICure Study Group. N Engl J Med. 2000;343:378–84.
173. Yahata T, Numata M, Kashima K, et al. Conservative treatment of stage IA1 adenocarcinoma of the cervix during pregnancy. Gynecol Oncol. 2008;109:49–52.
174. Yost NP, Santoso JT, McIntire DD, et al. Postpartum regression rates of antepartum cervical intraepithelial neoplasia II and III lesions. Obstet Gynecol. 1999;93:359–62.

175. Yuen PM, Ng PS, Leung PL, et al. Outcome in laparoscopic management of persistent adnexal mass during the second trimester of pregnancy. Surg Endosc. 2004;18:1354–7.
176. Zanotti-Fregonara P, Champion C, Trebossen R, et al. Estimation of the beta+ dose to the embryo resulting from 18F-FDG administration during early pregnancy. J Nucl Med.2008;49:679–82.
177. Zemlickis D, Lishner M, Degendorfer P, et al. Maternal and fetal outcome after invasive cervical cancer in pregnancy. J Clin Oncol. 1991;9:1956–61.
178. Zemlickis D, Lishner M, Erlich R, et al. Teratogenicity and carcinogenicity in a twin exposed in utero to cyclophosphamide. Teratog Carcinog Mutagen. 1993;13: 139–43.
179. Zhao XY, Huang HF, Lian LJ, et al. Ovarian cancer in pregnancy: a clinicopathologic analysis of 22 cases and review of the literature. Int J Gynecol Cancer. 2006; 16:8–15.

Index

N. Reed et al. (eds.), *Rare and Uncommon Gynecological Cancers*,
DOI: 10.1007/978-3-642-13492-0, © Springer-Verlag Berlin Heidelberg 2011

Printed by Printforce, the Netherlands